Drug Guide

Eileen Trigoboff, RN, APRN/PMH-BC, DNS, DABFN, CIP
Clinical Nurse Specialist, Director of Nursing Research, Buffalo Psychiatric Center, Buffalo, New York

Billie Ann Wilson, RN, PhD
Professor and Director, Department of Nursing, Loyola University New Orleans, New Orleans, Louisiana

Margaret T. Shannon, RN, PhD
Professor and Dean, Division of Nursing, Our Lady of Holy Cross College, New Orleans, Louisiana

Carolyn L. Stang, PharmD
Vice President, Clinical Program Development, Caremark Inc., Northbrook, Illinois

PEARSON
Prentice Hall

Upper Saddle River, New Jersey 07458

CONTENTS

ABOUT THE AUTHORS

Eileen Trigoboff is a Clinical Nurse Specialist with a specialty in adult psychiatry–mental health in a private psychotherapy practice in western New York. An important part of her practice is the national and international interdisciplinary supervision of, and consultation with, other mental health and health care professionals. She has positions as the director of nursing research and as a Clinical Nurse Specialist in psychiatry at the Buffalo Psychiatric Center in Buffalo, New York. Dr. Trigoboff is active on the Institutional Review Board at the facility that reviews, modifies, and supervises all scientific research in health-related issues. She has taught associate degree, bachelor's degree, and graduate-level nursing students on all aspects of the nursing process, research methodologies, statistics, and pharmacology. Dr. Trigoboff earned her B.S.N., her M.S. as a clinical nurse specialist in psychiatric nursing, and her Doctorate in Nursing Science (D.N.S.) in psychiatric nursing from the State University of New York at Buffalo. She received a National Institutes of Mental Health Individual National Research Service Award Pre-Doctoral Research Fellowship for her research on medication teaching and psychopharmacology. She is a diplomate in the American College of Forensic Examiners, on the American Board of Forensic Nursing (DABFN), and is board certified as a Certified Institutional Review Board Professional (CIP).

Billie Ann Wilson is currently professor and director of the Department of Nursing at Loyola University in New Orleans, Louisiana. Prior to entering nursing, she taught natural and physical sciences at the secondary and collegiate levels. She holds a B.S. in biology from Boston College, an M.S. in biology from Purdue University, a B.S. in nursing from Northwestern State University of Louisiana, a master of nursing from Louisiana State University Health Sciences Center, and a Ph.D. in curriculum and instruction from the University of New Orleans.

Margaret T. Shannon is currently professor and dean of the Division of Nursing at Our Lady of Holy Cross College, New Orleans, Louisiana. Her educational preparation includes a B.S. in chemistry and an M.S. in chemistry, both from Saint Louis University; an M.A. in teaching biology from Saint Mary's College, a B.S. in nursing from Northwestern State University of Louisiana, a master of nursing from Louisiana State University Health Sciences Center, and a Ph.D. in curriculum and instruction from the University of New Orleans. Prior to entering nursing, she taught physical science, natural science, and mathematics at the secondary and collegiate levels.

Carolyn L. Stang is currently vice president for clinical program development at Caremark Inc. She has worked in hospital and community pharmacies, home health care, and the pharmaceutical industry. Dr. Stang has been a freelance medical writer and an assistant professor at Rutgers University College of Pharmacy. She holds a B.S. in pharmacy from The Ohio State University and a doctor of pharmacy from the University of Tennessee, Memphis, and completed a fellowship in family medicine at the Medical University of South Carolina, Charleston.

PREFACE

Medications still comprise the primary treatment mode of intervention in psychiatry. They do not form the *only* treatment necessary, but are used in many cases with various therapies to achieve the goal of promoting hope and recovery from a mental illness. Because psychopharmacology can become a part of someone's life for years, knowledge about these medications will help providers keep a holistic view of the individual. To work effectively with people who have mental illnesses, treatment providers must know as much about the many ways psychiatric medications affect people's lives as they do about the actual mental illnesses. *Prentice Hall's Psychiatric Drug Guide* looks at those impacts in a variety of ways.

How to Use *Prentice Hall's Psychiatric Drug Guide*

The psychiatric medications covered in this psychiatric drug book are listed according to the overall class or psychiatric use of the medication and alphabetically by generic name. Pronunciations are given in parentheses. The names following the generic name are the trade names, including those used in Canada and Europe. The index includes the generic and the brand names of these medications. When a medication treats a nonpsychiatric condition as well as psychiatric disorders (such as valproic acid for mania), the psychiatric dosing and information is accentuated.

Pregnancy Category

Drugs have their pregnancy category indicated as A, C, D, or X according to the risk–benefit ratio for the mother and the fetus. A is the lowest risk and X is the highest risk.

Controlled Substances

Controlled substances such as narcotics are categorized in the United States as belonging to one of the five schedules (indicated by Roman numerals I–V). Inclusion in a schedule class depends on the potential for abuse of the compound. Schedule I has the highest abuse potential, Schedule V the lowest.

Availability

Medications come in a variety of dosages and forms (such as liquid, tablet, capsule, extended release, etc.) for administration. The available options at the time of publication are listed in this section.

Action and Therapeutic Effects

This entry for each monograph describes the mechanism by which the specific drug produces physiologic and biochemical changes at the cellular, tissue, and organ levels. This information helps the user understand how the drug works in the body and makes it easier to learn its side effects, adverse reactions, and cautions. The therapeutic effects are the reasons why a drug is prescribed. Therapeutic effectiveness of the drug can be determined by monitoring improvement in the condition for which the drug is prescribed.

Uses and Unlabeled Uses

The therapeutic applications of each drug are described in terms of approved, or labeled, uses and unlabeled uses. An unlabeled use is literally one that does not appear on the drug label or in the manufacturer's literature on the use of the drug. The unlabeled use is, nevertheless, an accepted use for the drug supported by the medical literature.

Contradictions and Cautious Use

Many drugs have contraindications and therefore should not be used in specific conditions, such as during pregnancy, or with particular drugs or foods. In other cases, the drug should be used with great caution because of a greater than average risk of untoward effects.

Route and Dosages

Route of administration is specified as SC, IM, IV, PO, PR, nasal, ophthalmic, vaginal, topical, aural, intradermal, or intrathecal. Dosages are listed according to indication or use. One of the hallmarks of this drug guide is the comprehensive dosage information it provides. The guide includes adult, geriatric, and pediatric dosages, as well as dosages for neonates and infants. This section also indicates dosage adjustments for renal impairment (based on creatinine clearance) and for impaired hepatic function whenever applicable. In all monographs, the routes and dosages are highlighted in a gray box to facilitate quick reference.

Administration

Drug administration is an important primary role for the nurse. Organized by different routes, this section lists comprehensive instructions for administering, handling, and storing medications.

Intravenous Drug Administration

Within the Administration section of each monograph, the authors have added a section highlighting intravenous drugs. Indicated by a vertical bar, this section provides users with comprehensive instructions on how to Prepare and Administer direct, intermittent, and continuous intravenous medications. It also includes Solution/Additive and Y-Site incompatibility for every monograph where appropriate to indicate which drugs and solutions should not be mixed with the intravenous drug. This is crucial information for drug administration.

Adverse Effects

Virtually all drugs have adverse or side effects that may be bothersome to some individuals but not to others. In each monograph, adverse effects with an incidence of ≥1% are listed by body system or organs. The most common adverse effects appear in *italic type,* while those that are life threatening are underlined. Users of the drug guide will find a key at the bottom of every page as a quick reminder.

Diagnostic Test Interference

This section describes the effect of the drug on various diagnostic tests, and alerts the nurse to possible misinterpretations of test results when applicable. The specific altered element is highlighted in bold italic type.

Interactions

The authors have expanded this section to include herbal interactions. Whenever appropriate, this section lists individual drugs, drug classes, foods, and herbs that interact with the drug discussed in the monograph. Drugs may interact to inhibit or enhance one another. Thus, drug interactions may improve the therapeutic response, lead to therapeutic failure, or produce specific adverse reactions. Only drugs that have been shown to cause clinically significant interactions with the drug discussed in the monograph are listed in this section. Note that generic drugs appear in **bold type,** and drug classes appear in SMALL CAPS.

Pharmacokinetics

This section identifies how the drug moves throughout the body. It lists the mechanisms of absorption, distribution, metabolism, elimination, and half-life when known. It also provides information about onset, peak, and duration of the drug action.

Nursing Implications

The Nursing Implications section of each drug monograph is formatted in an easy-to-use manner so that all the pertinent information that nurses need is listed under two headings: Assessment & Drug Effects and Client & Family Education. Under these headings, the user can quickly and easily identify needed information and incorporate it into the appropriate steps of the nursing process. Before administering a drug, the nurse should read both sections to determine the assessments that should be made before and after administration of the drug, the indicators of drug effectiveness, laboratory tests recommended for individual drugs, and the essential client or family education related to the drug.

Client & Family Education

The Client & Family Education section is unique in that information for each medication focuses on what the client and/or family members would want to know. The practical features and considerations of a medication are highlighted and explained. This section provides specific information for the clinician. It will ease discussion with clients, remind you of the major points to bring up when prescribing, and help you conduct ongoing medication teaching.

Appendixes

This edition includes several helpful appendixes, including Appendix A, U.S. Schedules of Controlled Substances; Appendix B, FDA Pregnancy Categories; Appendix C, Oral Dosage Forms That Should Not Be Crushed; Appendix D, Glossary of Key

Terms, Clinical Conditions, and Associated Signs and Symptoms; and Appendix E, Abbreviations.

Index

The index in the ***Prentice Hall's Psychiatric Drug Guide*** is perhaps the most often used section in the entire book. All generic, trade, and combination drugs are listed in this index. Whenever a trade name is listed, the generic drug monograph is listed in parentheses. Additionally, classifications are listed and identified in SMALL CAPS, while all prototype drugs are highlighted in **bold type.**

ACKNOWLEDGMENTS

I could not have asked for better people to work with on a project like this than those at Prentice Hall. Everyone has been a source of encouragement and support. Sladjana Repic, assistant editor, provided, coordinated, suggested, and generally facilitated. Reviewers read and critiqued drafts—thank you for the generosity of your insightful comments. They are Harvey "Skip" Davis, RN. Ph.D. CARN, PHN, San Francisco State University; Nancy Kostin, B.S.N., M.S.N., Madonna University; and Virginia Lester, RN MSN, Angelo State University.

The co-authors of this Guide are to be especially acknowledged. Billie Ann Wilson, Margaret T. Shannon, and Carolyn L. Stang gave a great deal to the creation of this project. Their professionalism and knowledge made it all happen as it should. All the clinicians I have worked with over the years contributed to this text by thinking and talking about psychopharmacology with me and they deserve an acknowledgement as well. And, of course, I recognize my husband's contributions through his caring and his expertise. Thank you all.

Eileen Trigoboff

CLASSIFICATION SCHEME

Acetylcholinesterase Inhibitors 49
Donepezil Hydrochloride (Aricept) 49
Galantamine Hydrobromide (Reminyl) 51
Memantine (Axura, Ebixa, Namenda) 53
Rivastigmine Tartrate (Exelon) 55
Tacrine (Cognex) 57

Antianxiety Agents 60
Alprazolam (Xanax) 60
Buspirone Hydrochloride (BuSpar) 62
Chlordiazepoxide Hydrochloride (Librium, Lipoxide, Medilium, Novopoxide, Sereen, Solium) 64
Clonazepam (Klonopin, Rivotril) 68
Clonidine Hydrochloride (Catapres, Catapres-TTS, Dixaril, Duraclon) 71
Clorazepate Dipotassium (Novoclopate, Tranxene, Tranxene-SD) 74
Diazepam (Apo-Diazepam, Diastat, Diazemuls, E-Pam, Meval, Novodipam, Valium, Valrelease, Vivol) 77
Diazepam Emulsified (Dizac) 77
Droperidol (Inapsine) 80
Halazepam (Paxipam) 83
Hydroxyzine Hydrochloride (Atarax, Hyzine-50, Quiess, Vistacon, Vistaject-25 &, -50, Vistaril IM) 85
Hydroxyzine Pamoate (Hy-Pam, Vamate, Vistaril Oral) 85
Lorazepam (Ativan) 88
Meprobamate (Equanil, Meprospan, Miltown) 91
Oxazepam (Ox-Pam, Serax, Zapex) 93

Anticonvulsants/Mood Stabilizers and Antiaggression Agents 96
Carbamazepine (Apo-Carbamazepine, Carbatrol, Epitol, Mazepine, PMS-Carbarmazepine, Tegretol, Tegretol-XR) 96
Clorazepate Dipotassium (Novoclopate, Tranxene, Tranxene-SD) *See* Antianxiety Agents 100

Felbamate (Felbatol) 100
Gabapentin (Neurontin) 102
Lamotrigine (Lamictal) 105
Levetiracetam (Keppra) 107
Lithium Carbonate (Eskalith, Eskalith CR, Lithane, Lithobid, Lithonate, Lithotabs) 109
Lithium Citrate (Cibalith-S) 109
Olanzapine, Fluoxetine Hydrochloride (Symbyax) 113
Oxcarbazepine (Trileptal) 118
Tiagabine Hydrochloride (Gabitril Filmtabs) 121
Topiramate (Topamax) 123
Valproic Acid (Depacon, Depakene, Depakote, Depakote ER, Depakote Sprinkle, Epival) 125
Zonisamide (Zonegran) 129

Antidepressants 131
Bupropion Hydrochloride (Wellbutrin, Wellbutrin SR, Zyban) 131
Nefazodone (Serzone) 134
Trazodone Hydrochloride (Desyrel, Desyrel Dividose) 136

Antidepressants, Monoamine Oxidase Inhibitors 138
Isocarboxazid (Marplan) 138
Phenelzine Sulfate (Nardil) 141
Tranylcypromine Sulfate (Parnate) 145

Antidepressants, Selective Norepinephrine- and Serotonin-Reuptake Inhibitor 147
Venlafaxine (Effexor, Effexor XR) 147

Antidepressants, Selective Serotonin-Reuptake Inhibitors 149
Citalopram Hydrobromide (Celexa) 149
Escitalopram Oxalate (Lexapro) 152
Fluoxetine Hydrochloride (Prozac, ProzacWeekly, Sarafem) 154
Fluvoxamine (Luvox) 157
Paroxetine (Asimia, Paxil, Paxil CR) 159
Sertraline Hydrochloride (Zoloft) 162

Antidepressants, Tetracyclic 164
Maprotiline Hydrochloride (Maprotiline HCl) 164
Mirtazapine (Remeron, Remeron SolTab) 167

PART ONE

PSYCHOPHARMACOLOGY

Psychiatric medications form the primary treatment for many psychiatric diagnoses. The past six decades have shown us the beginning use, then enormous leaps of generations of compounds with major impacts, and even success, in treating many of the serious symptoms of mental illness. The impacts that psychopharmacology has had on serious mental illness indicates that the physiologic and behavioral responses are in answer to the physiologic impairment of the mental illness. Just like the symptoms of an endocrine disorder such as diabetes responds to treatment with insulin, mental illness is an imbalance of brain chemicals that can be addressed or corrected with medications.

Psychopharmacology is a primary treatment mode of psychiatric–mental health nursing care and requires nurses to monitor client response as well as identify problems or side effects. Ours is a holistic function, incorporating the client's life, likes, and activities along with symptomatology into a comprehensive focus of treatment. The aim of psychopharmacologic nursing interventions is to teach clients about their medications, including over-the-counter medications and supplements, and assist in problem solving (American Nurses Association [ANA], 2000).

Psychopharmacology and Nursing

The area of psychopharmacology has grown considerably in recent years. Psychiatric–mental health nursing has similarly grown, and our responsibilities to recipients of mental health care services involve, to a large degree, psychopharmacologic expertise. Our national professional organization, the American Nurses Association (ANA), examined this issue and the ANA's Task Force on Psychopharmacology set forth guidelines for this aspect of our nursing practice (ANA, 1994). The guidelines delineate three areas that unite the practice of psychiatric–mental health nursing with expertise in psychopharmacology. We must:

1. Integrate current data from the neurosciences.
2. Demonstrate knowledge of psychopharmacologic principles.
3. Provide safe and effective clinical management of clients taking these medications through assessment, diagnosis, and treatment.

Psychiatric–mental health nurses must understand current advances in psychobiology to maintain an updated knowledge base for clinical work. The goal of psychopharmacologic interventions is to promote clients' physiologic stability, so they can achieve psychologic, social, and spiritual growth.

The word *drugs* conjures up a variety of powerful positive and negative images. Media messages concerning the devastating effects of IV drug use, alcoholism, and crack cocaine exemplify the negative image. Another image leaps from the pages of nursing and medical journals; pharmaceutical advertisements show people leading productive lives or smiling nurses, allegedly grateful for a medication that controls psychiatric symptoms. Yet another drug-related image is that of schoolchildren being inoculated against diphtheria, polio, and pertussis. All these images are powerful, and each is backed by truth.

THE CLIENT'S CULTURAL PERSPECTIVE

A vital aspect to competent care is accounting for the client's cultural perspective or meaning behind the behavior (Lambert, Lambert, Davidson, Anders, O'Brien, Yunibhand, Wong, Lee, Kim, & Kawano, 2003). Refusing to take medication may be more than paranoia or misunderstanding; it may be intrinsically representative of a cultural standard—for example, the belief that illness is caused by a supreme being, and that prayer and good wishes from others are the only acceptable routes to healing. Nurses often act as liaisons between the health care system and the culture of clients, making a bridge between the health care system and the client's belief system. This can be accomplished by being open and nonjudgmental about the cultural practice while promoting healthy aspects of its use. Psychiatric–mental health nurses may be especially challenged by certain cultural differences, however (Leighton, 2003). A client's native language may provide a more detailed, or a more restricted, description of events than the English language. Nurses need to examine interventions and plans for care in light of the client's culture and commonly held views. For example, individualism is a dominant theme in the Western world; however, this focus may not fit with people of a minority ethnicity who may hold values defining caretaking as a collective, rather than an individual, responsibility (Gerrish, 2000; Carrese & Rhodes, 2000).

It has been argued that it is difficult to incorporate non-Western sensibilities into our present psychiatric classification system. Your recognition of the validity of cultural backgrounds other than Western will promote client rights and afford clients legitimate entry into health care delivery systems (Gaskin, O'Brien, & Hardy, 2003). An awareness of the issues relating to culture helps minimize the problem and is necessary for providing quality mental health care.

Biologic Impact on Ethnically Distinct Groups

In addition to assessing for cultural impacts on behavior, you must also assess for the biologic impacts of medications on ethnically distinct groups. Factors such as benefits received from drug treatment, drug toxicity levels, and addiction liabilities are not the same for all groups of individuals (Dimsdale, 2000).

One important factor is the variation in metabolic rates among ethnic groups (an important point in evaluating the effectiveness of a medication). A high metabolic rate may produce effects below the optimal level, resulting in ineffective treatment. A low metabolic rate increases side effects. Because Asians have low metabolic rates, almost all Asians (95%) experience extrapyramidal side effects (EPSEs), as compared to European- and African-Americans, two-thirds of whom experience EPSE (Morita et al., 2000). Also because of metabolic differences, the therapeutic range for lithium differs among Asian, African-American, and Caucasian groups. The determination of effective lithium levels must take ethnicity into account.

The relationships between a client with a mental illness and the family have been examined for their psychobiologic (the study of the basics of psychiatry through biologic, chemical, and genetic impacts on thinking, mood, and behavior) impact. Typically, Mexican-Americans exude warmth and regard, which can positively affect a client's course of recovery. If a family is warm and they respond readily to a family member with schizophrenia, it is not as likely that the client will relapse as quickly as someone with schizophrenia staying in the midst of a family with low warmth (Lopez & Guarnaccia, 2000). Interestingly, the relapse rates of Anglo-Americans were unrelated to warmth.

Recognizing how ethnicity and phenotype determine response to drugs promotes the provision of culturally competent care. How ethnicity affects the expression of abnormal biologic processes is a growing field of study. Exploring the related literature will help you to incorporate this expanding knowledge base into your psychiatric–mental health nursing practice and promote your cultural competence.

ASSESSMENT OF THE CLIENT TAKING PSYCHIATRIC MEDICATIONS

Our responsibilities as nurses to clients receiving psychotropic medications are very different from the responsibilities of nurses in other settings. A nurse working with clients having cardiac difficulties, for example, may have clear physiologic indicators for the administration of drugs such as isosorbide dinitrate or nitroglycerin, but psychiatric nurses rarely have comparable consistent complexes of symptoms on which to base clinical judgments. In psychiatric work, nurses must often observe client behaviors closely to be aware of the sometimes subtle nature of the presenting symptom. Pacing, mild diaphoresis, slight increases in blood pressure or pulse, heightened muscle tone, and hypervigilant posture may be indicative of escalating anxiety, but they may also point to other problems such as caffeine toxicity, excessive use of tobacco, or side effects of psychopharmacologic agents. Accurate nursing assessment of client behavior is crucial if medications are to be given effectively and appropriately. Psychiatric nurses must also be attuned to the circumstances of adjunct pharmacotherapy (taking different medications at the same time).

Assessment is not a static process. It takes shape over time and includes a wide range of nursing knowledge. Similar behaviors indicating a wide array of vastly different sources often exist with psychiatric clients. A sleepy, isolated client with schizophrenia may be experiencing paranoid ideation, may have negative symptoms of the illness, may be having sedating side effects of the antipsychotic medication, or may be depressed as well as schizophrenic. Your assessment of this client and your clinical judgment will direct the nursing care. Whether you decide to administer a PRN antipsychotic, hold the next dose of antipsychotic, develop a treatment plan that includes motivational aspects, or discuss the possibility of depression with the other treatment team members depends upon your ongoing assessment of this client.

DRUG ADMINISTRATION

Administering psychiatric medications demands more than the six rights: the right medication, the right dose, the right route, the right time, to the right client, and using the right technology. These aspects of medication administration in psychiatry are confounded by the psychiatric illness. Knowing the side effects of the medication, in addition to the interactive effects with other psychiatric and medical–surgical medications, is another facet to psychiatric–mental health nursing.

The right medication in a psychiatric setting depends on the nursing assessment skills of the nurse. The right medication may be one of a number of choices. A medication may be ordered by mouth (PO) for routine administration, but the client may refuse the medication. Assessment skills come into play here as well; you must determine whether the client needs a liquid or a pill, or whether a PRN injection is necessary. The right client, client identification regarding medication administration, is different than in medical–surgical settings because clients usually do not wear wristbands. They may be confused or have psychiatric symptoms that encourage them to spontaneously assume the identity of another client for any number of reasons including an effort to please the staff.

Documenting the rationale for the effect of medications is an important nursing responsibility. Follow-up documentation on a medication that was given as a PRN will simplify treatment decisions for the client. Did the PRN work? How did you determine the value of the PRN's effect? What behavioral indicators are you using in your evaluation of a medication's effectiveness?

CLIENT AND FAMILY EDUCATION

Nursing responsibilities include educating clients about their medication. Adherence to medication regimens is often an issue for psychiatric clients, and nurses have explored the efficacy of teaching as a way of improving client adherence to medication regimens after discharge from inpatient settings. Variables related to adherence include socioeconomic status, marital status, number of concurrent medications, diagnosis, side effects, health benefits, and health values. Clients' individual differences must be addressed in the course of the teaching-learning process.

An issue of great concern to many nurses is the planning of teaching-learning experiences for chronically mentally ill clients. Although this population has learning needs concerning care and treatment, teaching is often difficult, depending on the severity and chronicity of the illness.

Recidivism, the tendency to relapse into a previous mode of behavior requiring readmission to a treatment program, can be linked to a psychiatric client's psychoeducation. Helping a client change health-related behavior requires a thoughtful, comprehensive approach. Interventions designed to match the client's learning, and teaching in the most relevant manner, can reduce recidivism and promote healthier behavior.

Another concern for nurses working with psychiatric clients is the need to assess their learning capacity at different points in their disorders. For example, when clients are first admitted to an inpatient unit, they may be too disorganized and symptomatic to focus on specific learning tasks. Depressed clients may be so psychomotorally slowed, because of hormonal shifts and dysfunctional neurotransmission, that they may be unable to learn. Given appropriate treatment and care, however, a client's psychobiologic disequilibrium may be corrected, making learning possible.

Even when a nurse perceives that a client is ready to learn (cognitive abilities are intact), learning will not necessarily occur. Many nurses conduct medication groups on an acute psychiatric unit to not only address the importance of assessing cognitive abilities but also to explore affective and social issues that may contribute to effective learning experiences. After considering the client's readiness, knowledge, background, environment, beliefs, preferences, and lifestyle, involving the client and significant others in the design and implementation of the medication treatment plan will help ensure the client's active collaboration in his or her care.

In many ways, psychiatric clients are no different from other learners. When presented with material that is clearly beneficial to them, they are likely to be more interested in the learning process. An evaluation of teaching efforts is essential to completing the teaching–learning process. This part of the process can be as informal or formal as you choose or deem necessary to check the client's knowledge of information taught. You will not be able to evaluate a client's understanding of information unless, at minimum, the client verbally reiterates information or performs a return demonstration of the skill. A change in behavior over time is a powerful indication of learning. If you desire a more extensive evaluation you may consider using a "pretest/posttest" format.

You can develop a written test to cover the content of the teaching and have the client complete the test *before* you begin teaching (a pretest). This provides a written measure of the client's learning needs and level of knowledge. After you implement and complete the teaching plan, the client completes the same examination (a posttest). Comparison of the pretest and posttest results yields a documented measure of how much learning has occurred as a result of your teaching intervention.

NEUROLEPTICS AND PSYCHOTROPICS

Recently, there has been significant change in the use of classes of medications for psychiatric symptomatology. In previous years, there were clear delineations between what was an antipsychotic and what was not. Empirical data and clinical expertise have led us to a less rigid application of chemical compounds. The complexities of psychiatric disorders and the desire to address the difficulties facing people who have these symptoms have resulted in a number of innovative medication regimens. Research further expanded our knowledge and a clearer vision of the capabilities of these compounds emerged. Now many medications have multiple indications beyond their original ones, which have necessitated more global terms to describe the medication. We still use classification names like "antipsychotic" and "antidepressant"; however, this is changing and some medications are labeled as being a "neuroleptic" or a "psychotropic" with the understanding that this medication can be used across some diagnostic groups.

Examples of this phenomenon include fluoxetine (Prozac), an initial antidepressant, indicated as an antiobsessional drug and in premenstrual dysphoria disorder (PMDD); and risperidone (Risperdal), a newer antipsychotic, indicated for use in stabilizing the manic phase of bipolar disorder. There are also clinical applications of psychiatric medications to a different diagnostic group, or for a different set of psychiatric symptoms, than originally intended. There may not be a Food and Drug Administration (FDA) indication for the drug in those circumstances; however, clinical appropriateness has established the use pattern. This holds true for risperidone as treatment in dementia with agitation.

Clinical application of nonpsychiatric medications to treat a psychiatric diagnostic group or a set of psychiatric symptoms has also occurred. The most apparent example of a class of nonpsychiatric medications being used to treat psychiatric treatment is the anticonvulsant class. Valproic acid (Depakote), carbamazepine (Tegretol), and gabapentin (Neurontin) are all used as mood stabilizers as well as for their original indications.

Antipsychotic Medications

The discovery of the first **antipsychotic drug,** chlorpromazine (Thorazine), is a prime example of the role chance has played in the history of psychopharmacology. Chlorpromazine was initially synthesized as an antihistamine and was not tried as a tranquilizer for clients with schizophrenia until 1952. Its effects on the behavior, thinking, affect, and perception of schizophrenic clients were so profound that knowledge of its properties was rapidly disseminated, and it became widely used within 3 to 4 years. Chlorpromazine's effects on the hospital practice of psychiatry were staggering. Its use contributed to reversing a steadily increasing population in U.S. mental institutions, and that population has progressively decreased ever since. One might say that chlorpromazine gave birth to the modern notions of psychiatric treatment—unlocked wards, milieu treatment, occupational and recreational therapy, and supervised living environments. The entire field of community mental health is ultimately linked to its discovery because it enabled clients to return to their homes or otherwise live outside an inpatient facility.

PSYCHOBIOLOGIC CONSIDERATIONS

Understanding the psychobiology of antipsychotic medications requires a basic knowledge of the functions of the central nervous system. An extended discussion of how these drugs work to reduce symptoms is beyond the scope of this chapter, but here is a brief overview of the basic mechanisms of action.

Generally, neuroleptics work by blocking a variety of CNS receptors. Drugs such as antipsychotics do not work only on the neurotransmitter system. Therefore, it is likely that several types of neurotransmitters and neuromodulators are affected by the administration of a single medication. While most neuroleptics have an affinity for several types of neurotransmitters, others are more specific and work more selectively. These differences account for the effects of the various neuroleptic medications.

MAJOR EFFECTS

The beneficial effects of antipsychotic medications in all psychotic states have been demonstrated beyond question. Multiple and varied criteria have been used to measure improvement. These drugs have been used successfully in clients with delusional thinking, confusion, motor agitation, and motor retardation. Antipsychotic drug treatment also decreases formal thought disorder, blunted affect, bizarre behavior, social withdrawal, hallucinations, belligerence, and uncooperativeness.

The most common disintegrative condition treated with antipsychotic drugs is the group of symptoms traditionally labeled schizophrenia. The problem of assessment is complicated by the fact that many diseases can cause syndromes with features like those of schizophrenia. For example, delusions may indicate a variety of *DSM-IV-TR* conditions, including schizophrenia and dementia, Alzheimer's type, with delusions. The finer points of differentiation between these two conditions include cognitive functioning and the client's presenting history. All clients manifesting psychotic symptoms should give a thorough medical history and take a physical examination, to rule out treatable medical illnesses, many of which are accompanied by behaviors considered psychotic or psychobiologic.

THE CHOICE OF A SPECIFIC DRUG

There are many antipsychotic medications on the market, and you may have noticed the recent expansion of this class of drugs. Drugs will have varying success rates with clients as individual responses frequently dictate use. The choice of a particular medication, then, depends on knowledge of the pharmacologic properties and side effects, the client's or a family member's history of drug response, and the prescriber's experience with various compounds. Important client variables are past successes with specific drugs, a history of allergies, and a history of serious or intolerable side effects. Some medications may have side effects with certain clients (sedation), which while not necessarily desired by the prescriber, may nevertheless prove to be helpful in treatment. Expect a certain amount of trial and error with each clinical application.

Table 1–1 summarizes the characteristics of the major antipsychotic medications. The list is extensive and growing, and it makes sense for each member of the treatment team to become familiar with just a few representative drugs, their predictable effects, and their common side effects. The characteristics covered in the table are discussed in the sections that follow.

TABLE 1–1 Antipsychotic Medications

Class	Generic Name	Trade Name	Usual Dosage Range (mg/day)	Side Effects		
				Sedative	Extrapyramidal*	Anticholinergic*
Phenothiazines						
Aliphatic	Chlorpromazine	Thorazine	150–1500	Very strong	Moderate	Strong
Piperidine	Thioridazine	Mellaril	150–800	Moderate	Minimal	Moderate
Piperazine	Trifluoperazine	Stelazine	10–60	Weak	Strong	Weak
	Fluphenazine	Prolixin	3–45	Weak	Strong	Weak
	Perphenazine	Trilafon	12–60	Weak	Strong	Weak
Butyrophenones	Haloperidol	Haldol	2–40	Weak	Strong	Weak
Thioxanthenes	Thiothixene	Navane	10–60	Weak	Strong	Weak
	Chlorprothixene	Taractan	40–600	Strong	Moderate	Strong
Dihydroindolones	Molindone	Moban	15–225	Weak	Moderate	Weak
Dibenzoxazepines	Loxapine	Loxitane	10–100	Moderate	Strong	Moderate
Dibenzodiazepines	Clozapine	Clozaril	12.5–900	Moderate	Weak	Strong
Benzisoxazole derivative	Risperidone	Risperdal	4–6	Weak	Weak	Weak
Thienobenzodiazepine	Olanzapine	Zyprexa	10–20	Moderate	Weak	Weak
Dibenzothiazepine derivative	Quetiapine	Seroquel	300–400	Moderate	Weak	Weak
Benzisothiazolyl piperazine derivative	Ziprazidone	Geodon	40–200	Moderate	Weak	Moderate

**Extrapyramidal and anticholinergic side effects are discussed later in this chapter.*

There are now more than seven distinct chemical classes of antipsychotic medications commonly used in the United States. (One class, the phenothiazines, is subdivided into three different types of medications.) Thus, there is a broad choice in terms of side effects and potential client responsiveness. A client who is unresponsive to one class may well respond to another that circumvents a problem in absorption, accumulation at neurotransmitter receptor sites, or metabolism.

Table 1–1 also shows the wide range among these medications in milligram-per-milligram potency. This fact is most relevant when treating clients who require large doses. In such cases, a potent medication is best. Consumer issues and clinician concerns are addressed at www.FDA.gov, the Website for the Food and Drug Administration in the United States.

NEWER ANTIPSYCHOTICS

The newer antipsychotics (they were called atypicals when they were first marketed) are those medications with a drastically different physiologic action than the traditional or conventional antipsychotics. The conventional antipsychotics primarily affected the positive symptoms of psychotic disorders, with little or no effect on the negative or cognitive symptoms. Their mechanism of action is thought to occur through nonselectively blocking the neurotransmitter dopamine D_2 receptors in the brain. To be clinically effective, these medications occupy between 70% and 90% of the D_2 receptors while the advent of EPSEs occurs at above 80% occupancy. The newer antipsychotics have a much reduced affinity for D_2 receptors, plus they all have an affinity for the serotonin receptors, a profile that appears to mitigate against EPSEs and has an impact on the negative symptoms of psychotic disorders (Rummel, Hamann, Kissling, & Leucht, 2004).

These medications provide new options for the care and treatment of clients suffering from psychotic conditions. The search continues for psychopharmacologic treatments for psychoses. Medications are being researched and tested every day, and if they provide relief from symptoms without undue side effects, they will enhance our psychopharmacologic arsenal.

Clozapine (Clozaril)

The first on the market was clozapine (Clozaril). Clozapine is an antipsychotic drug with an unusual pharmacologic and clinical profile. It was used in Europe for several years and is now generally used in the U.S. with clients who cannot tolerate the EPSEs of other antipsychotics, or who have a treatment-resistant or treatment-refractory psychosis, as is the case with certain schizophrenic clients. Reviews of studies regarding the effectiveness of clozapine have demonstrated its decided impact on both negative and positive symptoms, with improvement evident on follow-up as well.

Serious Side Effects. Despite its capacity to ameliorate symptoms of some very recalcitrant clients, clozapine has some serious side effects. The most serious is agranulocytosis (a marked decrease in granulated white blood cells), which occurs in less than 1% of clients taking this medication. It is essential to monitor white blood cell (WBC) counts of clients taking clozapine. Immediately discontinuing the medication when agranulocytosis is detected and before signs of an infection develop will usually resolve the episode. If a client experiences agranulocytosis as a result of using clozapine, the drug cannot be reinstituted. There is a risk for agranulocytosis with a variety of other psychotropic medications (conventional antipsychotics, benzodiazepines); however, there is a higher risk with clozapine. This compound requires cautiously adjusting this rate to a lower level. There have been rates of agranulocytosis at significantly lower levels than the currently estimated 1% (i.e., 0.3%) (Wahlbeck, Cheine, & Essali, 2004; Kilian & Lawrence, 1999). One of the important questions for clozapine treatment remains, "Is there a specific risk period for agranulocytosis, and if there is, when does it occur?" The risk period establishes the frequency of blood monitoring that can be an impediment to clients' initial and continued use of the antipsychotic. Currently, it is estimated that agranulocytosis may occur up to a year following initial treatment with clozapine, although the vast majority of cases appear within 6 months. As a result of these data, blood monitoring for agranulocytosis is completed weekly for the first 6 months of therapy. If the WBC levels remain normal and regular use is not interrupted throughout those 6 months, then blood monitoring can be reduced to biweekly frequencies. Remember that blood monitoring must continue for 4 weeks following the discontinuation of clozapine.

Another serious side effect is the potential for seizure, which seems to be dose-related. Less acute but nonetheless important side effects include sedation, tachycardia, sialorrhea (drooling), weight gain, and hypotension.

Risperidone (Risperdal)

Risperidone was introduced in the United States in the spring of 1994. It is the first of a new class of antipsychotics, benzisoxazole derivatives, that does not clinically relate to any existing antipsychotic drug. Its unique feature is the relative absence of EPSE at the therapeutic dosing level. It addresses the positive, negative, and affective symptoms of schizophrenia and may also alleviate depression and anxiety. Risperidone has demonstrated an ability to suppress TD (discussed later in this chapter) without increasing parkinsonism (Rummel, Hamann, Kissling, & Leucht, 2004), somewhat like clozapine.

Dosage of this new medication has been described as "the 1-2-3" regimen, in which the client receives 1 mg BID, the next increase (slowly titrated according to client's tolerability and response) is to 2 mg BID, and the next increase after that is to 3 mg BID. This places the client at 6 mg/day, which is in the therapeutic window of 4 to 8 mg/day currently recommended. Doses less than 5 mg/day have been linked with a better outcome than those receiving higher doses (Conley, 2000). Risperidone can be administered up to 16 mg/day, but the absence of EPSEs fades over 10 mg/day. Response within 1 to 10 weeks gives the drug a fair trial. Dosage for older clients is lower, generally cutting the initial dosage in half (0.5 mg BID, 1 mg BID, and 1.5 mg BID) and taking at least a full week between dosage changes.

This medication has been very useful in the treatment of psychotic symptoms, and the clinical knowledge gained from using it regularly has been valuable. The opportunity to have risperidone available in a depot form is now being examined. Once the current trials have been completed, the additional administration mode for this medication will offer another choice in the array of treatments for psychotic symptoms.

DOSAGE

Dosage ranges of antipsychotic medications vary widely among clients. Medications must be titrated against the psychotic target symptoms and the appearance of side effects. Most clients are initially given a relatively low dose of an antipsychotic to test for adverse effects for 1 to 2 hours. Consider chlorpromazine, with an initial dose of 20 to 50 mg orally (PO) or 25 mg intramuscularly (IM). Then the medication is typically given in 300 to 400 mg (or IM equivalent) per day, and gradually increased by 25% to 50% each day until maximum improvement is noted or intolerable side effects are encountered. This type of progression is common with the various antipsychotic medications.

The treatment setting frequently influences the drug regimen. In a crowded hospital emergency room, for example, hourly doses of medication may be given until a client is sedated. In more completely staffed, private inpatient units, a client may be observed for several days before medication is given. However, in terms of long-term outcome and length of eventual remission, neither approach is superior to the other (Bagnall, Jones, Ginnelly, Lewis, Glanville, Gilbody, Davies, Torgerson, & Kleijnen, 2003).

Clients who are extremely agitated, violent, severely withdrawn, or catatonic require significant doses during the first few days of treatment, delivered by injection to ensure rapid relief. Chlorpromazine, 50 to 100 mg IM, may be used, particularly if sedation is required. The nurse must be aware that this is an irritating drug; injections must be deeply intramuscular in either the buttocks or upper arms, and sites must be rotated. Substantial IM doses of the more potent antipsychotics, such as haloperidol 10 mg or trifluoperazine 10 mg, may be given to agitated clients. This approach frequently avoids some of the more troublesome side effects while ameliorating behavioral and cognitive symptoms.

Because antipsychotic medications have a rather long biologic half-life and many have significant sedative effects, there is little reason to give divided doses of medication after the initial days of treatment. It is recommended that the drugs, particularly the sedative ones such as chlorpromazine, be given in substantial doses at bedtime. In addition to promoting sleep, decreasing the chances the client will forget to take a dose after discharge, and saving nursing time in the hospital, this method saves money because large-dose capsules or tablets cost less than an equivalent amount of medication prepared in smaller doses.

After maximum clinical improvement has been obtained, antipsychotic medications are generally reduced gradually. Continuing to give a client modest doses of an antipsychotic following a psychotic episode lowers the chances of relapse and rehospitalization. Psychotherapy with schizophrenic clients may not be particularly effective without maintenance medications in conventional treatment settings, but it does improve psychosocial functioning in clients who are also taking maintenance medications. It is generally believed that clients should be kept on doses of antipsychotics sufficient to suppress symptoms for 3 months to 1 year following an acute episode. After such an interval, the client's course and life situation must be considered and treatment individualized. Some clients recover from a psychotic episode completely within 6 months. These clients, with schizophreniform disorder, should not receive long-term maintenance drug treatment. For individuals who have already experienced recurrent episodes of psychosis and demonstrate a deteriorating course, it is clearly advantageous to prevent relapses with drugs if possible.

THE DECISION TO USE A DRUG

Today, these general principles govern antipsychotic drug use:

- Drugs are given to treat target symptoms of schizophrenia or other psychotic disorders.
- Initial treatment may require parenteral doses. These are changed to oral pill or concentrate forms as the behavior disturbance subsides.
- Total dosages are tailored to individual needs; wide variations exist among clients.
- As soon as practical with drugs having sedating side effects, divided doses are changed to a single dose given at bedtime to maximize the drug's sedative properties.
- Most clients with a chronic course require maintenance doses for sustained improvement and to minimize the number of relapses.

Other considerations for using a particular medication include the use of adjunctive therapies (Bowen, Garry, & Sajbel, 2000). Do the medications needed to treat one problem blend well with any or all of the other medications the client may need? See Table 1–2 for antipsychotic drug interactions with other medications and substances to which your client may be exposed.

SPECIAL CONSIDERATIONS

These following special considerations apply to the use of antipsychotic medication.

A Unique Route of Administration

The phenothiazines fluphenazine (Prolixin) and haloperidol (Haldol) are available in long-acting intramuscular injectable forms that behave like timed-release capsules. These medications are gradually released over a long period of time, 2 to 3 weeks. Long-acting

TABLE 1–2 Antipsychotic Drug Interactions

Combining One of These:	With One of These Antipsychotics:	Can Lead to These Problems:
Carbamazepine	Haloperidol	Decreased effect of either medication
Carbamazepine	Clozapine	Additive bone marrow suppression
Anticholinergics	Clozapine	Potentiate anticholinergic effect of clozapine
Benzodiazepines	Clozapine	Respiratory arrest, circulatory difficulties
Anticholinergic medication	Antipsychotic	Increased level of neuroleptic in the system with extrapyramidal side effects
Antacids	Phenothiazine antipsychotic	Decreased phenothiazine effect
Coffee, Tea, Milk, or Fruit juices	Phenothiazine antipsychotic	Decreased phenothiazine effect
CNS depressants such as: Narcotics, Anxiolytics, Alcohol, Barbiturates, or Antihistamines	Antipsychotic	Additive CNS depression

fluphenazine and haloperidol are available in decanoate (long-acting depot injection) preparations. The main advantage of decanoate forms is that they reduce clients' ambivalence about taking medication and eliminate the need for constant pill taking. The treatment team must also honor the clients' civil liberties; truly involuntary treatment can be performed only according to due process, as required by a particular state's mental hygiene laws.

The psychiatric–mental health nurse in a community setting may frequently have occasion to administer long-acting fluphenazine or haloperidol. With a client whose treatment will include a long-acting medication, a dose of regular fluphenazine or haloperidol is usually taken first to rule out the possibility of allergic reactions. Such reactions can be devastating if discovered after a 2- or 3-week supply of medicine has been given as a depot treatment. If no adverse reactions are noted within 1 hour, the long-acting form is injected, usually in the upper outer quadrant of the buttock or the vastus lateralis site.

The depot form of the newer antipsychotic risperidone, once available, will be useful for clients with positive symptomatology as well as problems with executive functioning, memory, or adherence. It is delivered IM via saline—as opposed to the sesame oil used in haloperidol and fluphenazine decanoate IM injections. A depot antipsychotic with considerably fewer side effects than haloperidol and fluphenazine has the potential to prolong antipsychotic medication use and minimize dissatisfaction with and discontinuation of treatment.

Better routes for medication administration have been explored by various drug companies for years. As a result, there is yet another way to give olanzapine (Zyprexa) in a newly approved orally disintegrating tablet formulation. Called Zyprexa Zydis, these tablets begin disintegrating in the mouth within seconds. This allows them to be swallowed with or without liquid, thus limiting difficulties in swallowing and cheeking (hiding) behaviors. The Zydis form of medication is also being used with a variety of compounds in medical–surgical settings.

Medication Requirements of Certain Age Groups

In elderly clients, the agitation often associated with delirium, dementia, and related disorders is markedly responsive to antipsychotics. Other sedatives, such as barbiturates and benzodiazepines, may further compromise cerebral functioning, further depressing the level of awareness and concentration and thereby worsening the disorder. Doses of medications are generally reduced for older adults. Risperidone 1 mg/day, trifluoperazine (Stelazine) 5 to 20 mg/day, or haloperidol 1 to 6 mg/day might constitute adequate treatment.

Antipsychotic medications are effective in treating childhood psychoses and in managing the behavior problems associated with mental retardation. The general principle of reduced dosage is again applicable. The upper limit of the usual daily dosage for children under 12 might be 200 mg/day of chlorpromazine or thioridazine (Mellaril) or 20 mg/day per day of trifluoperazine. Amounts of individual IM injections of chlorpromazine must also be kept at 0.25 mg per pound of body weight every 6 to 8 hr, or not over 40 mg/day for up to 50 lb and not over 75 mg/day for children weighing 50 to 100 lb.

POTENTIAL SIDE EFFECTS OF ANTIPSYCHOTIC MEDICATIONS

Continuous contact with clients gives nurses an advantage over physicians and other professionals who may see a client only every other day or, at best, once a day. Both the dangerous and the more uncomfortable side effects frequently have a rapid onset and need attention promptly.

The side effects of antipsychotic medications that nurses must recognize can be divided into these classes:

- Autonomic nervous system
- Extrapyramidal
- Other central nervous system (CNS)
- Allergic
- Blood
- Skin
- Eye
- Endocrine
- Weight gain

Autonomic Nervous System Effects

The antipsychotics all possess anticholinergic side effects and antiadrenergic side effects; that is, they interfere with the normal transmission of nerve impulses by acetylcholine and epinephrine, in both central and peripheral nerves. The most common side effects are the anticholinergic ones. These include dry mouth, blurred vision, constipation, urinary hesitance or retention, and, under rarer circumstances, paralytic ileus.

Orthostatic hypotension, also known as postural hypotension, is a common antiadrenergic effect. The primary danger here is injury from a fall. Clients receiving parenteral medications, such as chlorpromazine intramuscularly, must have their blood pressure monitored lying and standing before and a half hour after each dose. Clients should be advised to rise from a supine position gradually and to sit down if they feel faint. Support stockings and a large intake of fluids may be indicated. This problem is much less significant with oral administration of the drug. However, nurses working with clients receiving oral antipsychotic medications should take both baseline and routine vital sign readings at regular intervals. This practice establishes the client's tolerance for medications without the untoward side effects of orthostatic hypotension and subsequent falls.

Extrapyramidal Side Effects

Another common and sometimes frightening group of adverse reactions results from the effects of antipsychotics on the extrapyramidal tracts of the central nervous system, which are involved in the production and control of involuntary movements. These extrapyramidal side effects (EPSEs) can be broken down into four types, each with distinguishing clinical characteristics and times of onset after the initiation of drug therapy.

Types of EPSEs. The earliest and most dramatic reactions are the *acute dystonic reactions*, forms of dystonia. These occur in the first days of treatment, sometimes after a single dose of medication. They involve bizarre and severe muscle contractions. These reactions can be physically painful and are almost always frightening to the individual. They are readily reversible.

Parkinsonian syndrome so named because of its striking resemblance to true Parkinson's disease, commonly occurs after a week or two of the therapy. It is the result of dopamine blockade caused by the neuroleptic drugs. Treatment with oral medication is usually sufficient, since urgency is seldom a consideration in the management of this syndrome.

A third reversible extrapyramidal side effect is known as akathisia. This characteristically is a motor restlessness perceived subjectively by the client and experienced as an urge to pace, a need to shift weight from one foot to another, or an inability to sit or stand still. Akathisia is generally a later complication of drug treatment, occurring weeks to months into the course of therapy.

Accurate observation of the course of therapy by the psychiatric nurse can promote prompt recognition and proper interpretation of EPSEs. If care is not taken, the health care provider may misinterpret the increasing withdrawal, emotional blunting, apathy, and lack of spontaneity as increasing schizophrenic behavior. This error in interpretation may lead to a mistaken increase in dosage of antipsychotic medication, which will aggravate the condition. Akathisia can also be confused with psychotic agitation, and this error also prompts an increase in medication. Clients with akathisia require a reduction in the dosage of offending agents and/or treatment with an antiparkinsonian drug. You can save the client many uncomfortable and worrisome days by being aware of the frequency with which these syndromes complicate treatment and by reporting any suspicious sign or symptom while reassuring the client of the reversibility of the syndrome in almost all cases.

Prophylactic Treatment. Whether clients should be treated prophylactically with antiparkinsonian agents, in view of the relatively high incidence of EPSEs, is open to debate. Some argue that the use of antiparkinsonian agents eventually leads to relatively higher antipsychotic doses, thereby increasing the probability of serious side effects. Another argument is that antiparkinsonian agents also pose risks and thus should be used only to counteract EPSEs, not to guard against their possible emergence. Moreover, a great many clients never develop the syndromes. If the likelihood of an extrapyramidal reaction is high (if, for example, the client has a history of them) and the possible consequences significant (the client may discontinue medication or drop out of treatment altogether), antipsychotic and antiparkinsonian agents are frequently initiated simultaneously.

Assessment of EPSEs. Nursing assessment of EPSEs is important to the quality care of clients receiving psychotropic medications (Kralik & Koch, 2003). One difficulty is *consistency* of assessment among caregivers. For example, nurses usually assess for the presence of cogwheeling or muscle rigidity in clients receiving psychotropic drugs. However, the reliability among those assessments is sorely lacking; what one nurse may consider moderate to severe side effects may be assessed as mild to moderate by another nurse.

Two assessment tools are the Simpson Neurological Rating Scale for the assessment of extrapyramidal side effects and the Abnormal Involuntary Movement Scale (AIMS) for the assessment of iatrogenic movements resulting from particular psychotropic drugs. These assessment tools can be found on the Companion Website for this book (AIMS is discussed later in this chapter). They are helpful in quantifying EPSEs prior to administering a medication to counteract the side effect. Readministering the instruments after the medication is given helps you assess the amelioration of the side effect. These data chart the course of a client's side effects and the effectiveness of medications to decrease them. This information is critical to quality nursing care.

The last EPSE to emerge in the course of treatment is also the most severe because it can be largely irreversible. This is tardive dyskinesia (TD), which frequently appears after years of antipsychotic drug treatment, although it can occur earlier. It usually appears after a maintenance dose is discontinued or reduced, and it can be masked—but not treated—by reinstituting the medication or the dosage or by switching to another drug (Ballesteros, Gonzalez-Pinto, & Bulbena, 2000).

Current estimates put the incidence of TD at 4% to 5% per year for young adults and as high as 25% after 1 year in elderly clients (Boyd, 2002). Early detection through regular examinations (at least every 6 months) is recommended.

There is no known cure for TD. There is no research evidence to support the formerly held view that stopping the neuroleptic would serve as a treatment for TD. It is clear that there is an increased risk of relapse with dosage reduction even though it may offer some benefit as a treatment for TD compared to remaining with current dose. There is a need to evaluate the utility of clozapine and the other atypical antipsychotics as treatments for established TD (McGrath & Soares-Weiser, 2004).

To properly assess the impacts psychopharmacology is having on your client, regular assessments must be completed, especially for evidence of TD. One commonly utilized tool to assess to the presence and the severity of TD is the Abnormal Involuntary Movement Scale or AIMS. Directions on the assessment tool and the examination procedure guide you through a careful and complete TD screen. It is helpful to use a goose-neck lamp to enhance your abilities to see minute movements particularly in the oral/facial areas. Clinical practice dictates an AIMS be completed every 6 months during treatment. Use of a videocamera allows clinicians to record these observations and make multiple comparisons of the regular exams.

With the emergence of the newer antipsychotic medications such as clozapine and risperidone, which can have an effect on TD and are not likely to cause a significant number of TD cases, the choices in this area are expanding. As noted above, five of the newer antipsychotics have been known to reduce tardive dyskinesia. The sixth and most recent antipsychotic, aripiprazole, is currently being evaluated in this regard.

Table 1–3 lists the commonly used antiparkinsonian medications for addressing EPSEs.

Other Central Nervous System Effects

CNS side effects of antipsychotic medications are sedation and reduction of the seizure threshold. Because antipsychotic drugs vary in their sedative effects, this side effect is troublesome, but it can be managed by changing to a less sedating agent. Seizures are not a contraindication for use of these drugs. However, their use requires close observation.

TABLE 1–3 Antiparkinsonian Medications

Generic Name	Trade Name	Maximum Daily Dosage	Available in Injectable Form
Amantadine	Symmetrel	300 mg	No
Benztropine	Cogentin	8 mg	Yes
Biperiden	Akineton	8 mg	Yes
Diphenhydramine	Benadryl	100 mg	Yes
Procyclidine	Kemadrin	15 mg	No
Trihexyphenidyl	Artane	15 mg	No

Allergic Effects

The principal allergic manifestation of the antipsychotics is cholestatic jaundice. This occurs much less frequently than in the early days of psychopharmacology, and it is usually a benign and self-limiting condition. Chlorpromazine, tricyclic antidepressants, and phenothiazines can all cause cholestatic jaundice, which is not universally thought to always be an allergic reaction. It is suggested that chlorpromazine exerts a direct toxic effect on the bile secretory mechanisms of the liver.

Many times, clients may have a record of an "allergic" reaction to a psychotropic medication without cholestatic jaundice or other evidence of allergic reactions documented. When these circumstances are clearly assessed, it may turn out that the client either experienced neuroleptic malignant syndrome (NMS) or a dystonic reaction. The dangers associated with NMS may have prompted an explanation to the client along the lines of the dangers associated with an allergic reaction. This communication may have been misinterpreted and was not detected or corrected.

The other false-positive report of an allergic reaction to a psychiatric medication is *dystonia*. A painful side effect such as dystonia is a negative experience to be avoided and may be communicated to caregivers as an allergy to assure avoidance of the compound at fault. Careful scrutiny of reports of allergies must be conducted regularly to determine true allergies so the client is protected from contact, but also to make sure no medications are removed from the array of effective treatments for that client.

Blood, Skin, and Eye Effects

Among the other side effects, agranulocytosis is the most serious. It is both potentially fatal and, fortunately, extremely rare. Usually the person gets an infection and deteriorates rapidly or begins to bleed spontaneously, requiring emergency medical attention. Many medications cause agranulocytosis, including benzodiazepines and antibiotics.

Skin eruptions, photosensitivity leading to severe sunburn, blue-gray metallic discolorations over the face and hands, and pigmentation changes in the eyes are all potential side effects. Clients are generally advised to avoid prolonged exposure to sunlight or to use a sunscreen agent when outdoors. These conditions usually remit.

One serious and permanent eye change is retinitis pigmentosa. This condition may occur in clients on dosages of thioridazine exceeding 800 mg/day. The condition may lead to blindness. Therefore, doses exceeding 800 mg per day are contraindicated.

Endocrine Effects

Lactation in females and gynecomastia and impotence in males lead a list of endocrine changes that can occur with antipsychotic drug treatments. *Hyperprolactinemia* is a common side effect that will affect many aspects of the client's sex life. Difficulties with libido, arousal, excitation, orgasm, male ejaculatory volume, and overall performance can occur to a disturbing degree with hyperprolactinemia. You can imagine how these side effects would affect the regular or long-term use of the medication. Hyperprolactinemia is also responsible for oligomenorrhea or amenorrhea in women, galactorrhea in women and rarely in men, and, in cases of prolonged hyperprolactinemia, osteoporosis (Perese & Perese, 2003). Be alert to these endocrine changes, as a nurse will likely be the professional told about such problems.

Another endocrine problem surfacing recently is diabetes in people who have schizophrenia. The baseline occurrence of diabetes is elevated with schizophrenia (twice the rate of the general population), and seems to be further escalated by endocrine changes from psychotropics. While weight gain can certainly propel one into an increased diabetic risk, some studies show diabetes occurring in clients who have not gained significant weight. The particular medication used may be contributing. You should be alert to any changes in body functions reported by clients taking these medications.

Weight Gain

Weight gain is a significant side effect that affects self-esteem and poses health risks for the client. Antipsychotics, tricyclic antidepressants, lithium, anticonvulsants, and other classes of medications have individual compounds within the class that can cause an increase in weight. As mentioned above, an increase in weight can put an individual at risk for health problems such as diabetes, hypertension, and coronary artery disease. The impact of weight gain can be more disturbing than EPSEs to a client. Over time, this side effect can be a devastating force to long-term treatment and quality of life. Assiduous attention paid to the potential for weight gain issues from the inception of treatment can help minimize this particular side effect.

Neuroleptic Malignant Syndrome

Neuroleptic malignant syndrome (NMS) is a severe and potentially life-threatening side effect of all psychotropic medications. This extreme condition is believed to be the result of dopamine blockade in the striatum of the brain or dopaminergic antagonism in the CNS. There are some interesting efforts to examine the genetic etiology of NMS; the search is on to discover phenotypes and genetic markers to this syndrome (Gurrera, 2000; Qureshi & Al-Habeeb, 2000). NMS occurs in 0.5 to 1% of clients taking neuroleptic medications. Men are affected more than women, approximately twice as much, and younger clients appear to be more susceptible than older ones (Silva, Munoz, Alpert, Perlmutter, & Diaz, 2000). NMS typically occurs within the first 2 weeks of treatment with a different medication or a dosage increase, but cases have been reported months after a new medication regimen has begun. Nurses are in the best position to assess for this condition because its symptoms are muscle rigidity, hyperpyrexia, altered consciousness, and diaphoresis. Because NMS often occurs in clients whose presentations are already complex, the nursing assessment can be difficult.

Treatment for NMS includes discontinuing all psychotropic medication immediately and supporting the client medically through the crisis. If cooling and rehydration are not achieved quickly, along with holding all psychotropics, the client may die. Caution in follow-up care is, of course, important. The pathology of NMS is complex and not completely understood at this time beyond the knowledge that the major symptoms of NMS are caused by the neuroleptic blockade of the dopamine receptors.

CLINICAL IMPLICATIONS

Nurses have many responsibilities to clients receiving neuroleptic drugs. To ensure the bioavailability and effectiveness of neuroleptic medications, it is important to understand the relationships between the medication and the liquid (or substance) you administer it with, as well as the relationships between medications. Some medications are not compatible with all substances.

In addition to the liquid and drug compatibilities you need to be aware of other problematic combinations. Recent practice has shown a specific problem with the combination of grapefruit juice with several psychiatric medications. For example, two anxiolytic medications, triazolam (Halcion) and buspirone (BuSpar) are specifically called to your attention. Triazolam will not be metabolized efficiently and therefore remains at higher levels in the body, and buspirone can have a blood level nine times normal when taken with grapefruit juice. The explanation for this resides in grapefruit juice's furanocoumarins, compounds within grapefruit juice, and their ability to inhibit a liver enzyme (cytochrome P_{450}3A4 or CYP3A4) from metabolizing the medication out of the system. This inhibition of the enzyme allows the medication and its metabolites to remain in the system longer than usual, accumulating and causing higher blood levels, enhanced effects of the medication, and greater side effects (Koth & Cassavaugh, 2000).

The entire field of study on the cytochrome P_{450}s (or CYPs) is an extensive one, covering the intricacies of drug interactions, metabolism, and co-administration cautions. Although it may be difficult to envision a liver enzyme having a tremendous influence on psychiatric symptomatology, you will be able to see the impacts of these effects with your clients. The above paragraph talks about the impacts of inhibiting these enzymes, which determines whether the metabolism of a medication will be delayed. There is another cytochrome P_{450} action important to clinical practice called activating the enzyme. Activating the CYP enzyme, which means the compound will be moving through the system at an accelerated pace, has an entirely different clinical presentation. When a medication does not have enough time to exert its power, it will appear to not be addressing symptoms competently or it will appear to be considerably less effective than if it had the time to be fully utilized by the client's body.

Ultimately, either of these mechanisms of cytochrome P_{450} activation or inhibition can be accomplished through a variety of interactions among drugs, foods, liquids, or substances (e.g., nicotine). Being aware of the total picture of your clients and their medications in a holistic manner will alert you to drug–drug interactions as well as the dynamism of drug metabolism.

Antidepressant Medications

Like antipsychotic drugs, the original antidepressant medications were discovered accidentally. Four classes of antidepressants currently exist: tricyclic antidepressants (TCAs), monoamine oxidase inhibitors (MAOIs), selective serotonin reuptake inhibitors (SSRIs), and phenethylamine antidepressants. There are also atypical antidepressants, called so because of their variety of formulation and actions. In the case of imipramine (Tofranil), the first of the tricyclic antidepressants, investigators were actually searching for effective antipsychotics similar to chlorpromazine. Iproniazid, a MAOI, was discovered when tuberculous clients regularly treated with a similar drug, isoniazid, became less depressed. The antidepressants have shed considerable light on the biochemical mechanisms of the brain in both normal and abnormal emotional expression.

PSYCHOBIOLOGIC CONSIDERATIONS

Knowledge about the pharmacology of antidepressant medications has led to a theory of the biochemistry of depression. Basically, all the true antidepressants make the neurotransmitters norepinephrine (NE) and serotonin (5-HT) more available to the synaptic receptors in the central nervous system. Tricyclics block the reuptake of these substances into the neuron after their release, thereby postponing their degradation. MAOIs interfere with the enzymes responsible for the actual breakdown of the neurotransmitter molecules. Since both are antidepressants, these observations have led to the theory that NE and 5-HT shortages in the brain cause depression, at least the type of depression that responds to drug therapy.

The initial distinction to be understood in the psychopharmacology of depression is between true antidepressants and stimulants or euphoriants. TCAs and MAOIs are not stimulants and will not induce euphoria in healthy people. In a single dose, they have a sedative effect. Amphetamines and methylphenidate (Ritalin), on the other hand, are stimulants but not antidepressants in the pharmacologic sense. They can induce an increased sense of well-being in certain individuals, but do nothing to combat depression on a lasting basis.

Tricyclic antidepressants are the "first generation" of antidepressant medications. This means they were among the first medications identified as effective in the treatment of depression.

Since that time, a number of medications have been developed to treat the symptoms of major depression and the depressive features of schizoaffective disorder. Among these medications are the MAOIs, the SSRIs, and a number of atypical antidepressants with a variety of neurotransmitter actions.

Bupropion (Wellbutrin) is an oral antidepressant drug that is not a TCA and is unrelated to other known antidepressants. Bupropion has been well tolerated in people experiencing orthostatic hypotension with TCAs. This medication has a dose-related potential for causing seizures to a greater extent than other antidepressants. It has few anticholinergic side effects and essentially no important cardiovascular effects. Bupropion is also indicated for use as an aid to smoking cessation and supports the client through the process of quitting the habit of smoking. There are sustained-release formulations of this medication under two trade names (Wellbutrin SR and Zyban). For smoking cessation, the medication is used for up to 12 weeks.

Of note is the cross-diagnostic use of medications initially indicated for other conditions. Fluoxetine (Prozac) is an antidepressant and was the first SSRI developed. This compound recently received an indication for yet another treatment regimen. Fluoxetine is formulated under the trade name Sarafem to treat the mood and physical symptoms of premenstrual dysphoric disorder (PMDD), which is differentiated from depression and other mental disorders. The dosing is flexible, with 10- or 20-mg pulvules available; 20 mg/day is the recommended dose.

As each new group of medications became available, practitioners initially used the new drugs to the partial exclusion of the old. When a client is not responding to a medication, it is helpful to have an array of choices from which to select further treatment. The side effect profiles of antidepressants remain one of the linchpins of successful care. If sedation is a side effect and the client is sleeping at a higher-than-preferred level, then a class of medications with less sedating side effects may be a better choice. Experience reinforces the truth that a number of treatment and medication options are necessary to effectively treat psychiatric disorders; therefore, all categories of antidepressants remain useful.

NURSING RESPONSIBILITIES WHEN CLIENTS RECEIVE UNCOMMON DRUG COMBINATIONS

As drug combinations and innovative psychobiologic therapies become more commonplace in the practice of psychiatry, psychiatric nurses must be observant for idiosyncratic responses among clients. Knowing the interactive effects of medications is an important feature of effective psychopharmacologic nursing. Planning and implementing care for this specialized client subpopulation are likely to be challenging, and you need to be aware of the underlying psychobiology to recognize potential drug-related behaviors among clients who are on multiple-drug regimens.

CLINICAL CONSIDERATIONS

The most important clinical consideration in the use of medications to treat depression is that antidepressant drugs are not effective in all cases of depressed mood. Evidence from research and clinical practice indicates that only a portion of depressive disorders respond to this category of drugs. For example, TCAs, MAOIs, and amphetamines are generally contraindicated in depression resulting from what commonly has been referred to as grief reaction or pathologic grief. Other types of depression, described in the DSM-IV-TR, may be more amenable to psychopharmacologic intervention. Thus, accurate diagnosis is necessary to ensure maximum effectiveness.

Clients for whom antidepressants are indicated usually suffer from characteristic symptoms: a severely depressed mood, loss of interest, an inability to respond to normally pleasurable events or situations, a depression that is worse in the morning and lessens slightly as the day goes on, early morning awakening (and an inability to fall asleep again), marked psychomotor retardation or agitation, appetite and weight changes, and excessive or inappropriate guilt. A significant, and commonly overlooked, clinical consideration is that antidepressants have a delayed-reaction onset. A client will not show lessening of depressed mood until 2 to 3 weeks after the institution of an adequate dose of TCAs, for example.

TRICYCLIC ANTIDEPRESSANTS (TCAs)

One of the most commonly used class of antidepressant drugs is TCAs. These compounds are close in chemical structure to phenothiazines and have many similar side effects, but they have profoundly different effects on mood, behavior, and cognition. TCAs are not antipsychotic agents when given to schizophrenic clients and may in fact aggravate a disintegrative pattern or precipitate overt symptoms in a client with latent disintegrative behavior. Imipramine (Tofranil) and amitriptyline (Elavil) are the two prime representative TCAs. Desipramine (Norpramin, Pertofrane), nortriptyline (Pamelor), and protriptyline (Vivactil) are compounds prepared in simpler forms (similar to the conversions made in normal metabolism) that are reported to reduce the incidence of side effects.

Dosage

What constitutes an adequate dose of tricyclics is a matter of debate. Using imipramine (considered the prototype TCA) as an example, most clinicians agree that most of the responsive clients with a major depression need doses of 50 to 300 mg/day. Dosages of other tricyclics, such as nortriptyline are not recommended above 150 mg/day.

After remission of the symptoms, clients who are put on a reduced maintenance dosage (perhaps 50% of the acute dosage) show less likelihood of relapse. Therefore, most clients are continued on treatment for 6 months to 1 year following a major depressive episode. Clients who have had repeated episodes may require longer drug maintenance or should be considered for treatment with a mood stabilizer because of the prophylactic effects on recurrent major depression and the depressive episodes of bipolar disorder.

Side Effects

Many of the common side effects of the tricyclic drugs are autonomic due to the anticholinergic characteristics of the medications. These side effects include dry mouth, blurred vision, constipation, palpitations, and urinary retention. Clients with glaucoma must be treated with caution. Some allergic skin reactions have been observed. TCAs also cause changes in the normal electrical conduction of the heart and are cardiotoxic, which is particularly significant in treating clients with a history of cardiovascular disease, especially heart block. Sudden death has occurred during tricyclic treatment. Clients with known heart disease and most elderly clients require electrocardiograms (ECGs) before, and periodically during, the course of tricyclic therapy. Several CNS effects may occur, including tremor, twitching, paresthesias, ataxia, and convulsions.

Overdose Effects

One aspect of TCA treatment that deserves attention is the consequences of an overdose. Significant overdoses may cause delirium; hyperthermia; convulsions; and even coma, shock, and respiratory failure. A lethal dose of an antidepressant such as amitriptyline is estimated at between ten and thirty times the usual daily therapeutic dose. Drug intake deserves close attention, because many clients treated with these drugs are severely suicidal. Serious overdosing is a medical emergency and may require resuscitative measures.

MONOAMINE OXIDASE INHIBITORS (MAOIs)

Clients who do not respond to tricyclic antidepressants may respond to another major class, MAOIs. These drugs generally are not as effective as tricyclics and are somewhat slower to act, sometimes requiring a month of treatment before improvement shows. Isocarboxazid (Marplan) is considered the most effective, with phenelzine (Nardil) and tranylcypromine (Parnate) slightly behind. Complicating the decision to use MAOIs is their association with several very severe side effects. Hepatic necrosis, commonly fatal, and hypertensive crisis leading to intracranial bleeding are among the most threatening. The latter reaction, heralded by severe headache, stiff neck, nausea, vomiting, and sharply increased blood pressure, follows the ingestion of foods that contain the amino acid tyramine and the ingestion of sympathomimetic medications.

Client and Family Education

The MAOI antidepressants require an especially strong, concerted teaching effort from nurses. These medications have many drawbacks that directly affect nursing intervention. For example, clients on MAOIs *must* avoid foods that contain even moderate amounts of tyramine; failure to do so will result in hypertensive crisis. Box 1–1 outlines the low-tyramine diet for clients taking MAOIs.

Box 1–1: Low-Tyramine Diet

The MAO inhibitors combine with certain foods and medications to produce a significant increase in blood pressure, which can be a health hazard. In general, foods that can cause this reaction are ones that have been *pickled, fermented, smoked,* or *aged*. The list below includes the main foods, fluids, and medications to avoid while taking an MAOI and for the 2 weeks after the MAOI is discontinued.

Foods and Beverages to Avoid Completely

Meats and fish	Pickled herring, dried fish, unrefrigerated fermented fish, liver, caviar, fermented sausage (bologna, salami, pepperoni, summer sausage), hoisin sauce (fermented oyster sauce used in Oriental dishes)
Vegetables	English broad peas, Chinese pea pods, Fava beans
Dairy products	Most cheeses (exceptions are listed under Allowed Foods), yogurt
Beverages	Chianti, aged wines, imported beers, aged beers
Combination foods	Pizza, lasagna, souffles, macaroni and cheese, quiche, liver pate, caesar salads, eggplant parmesan

All yeast products (such as Brewer's yeast) and yeast extracts (such as Marmite)

Foods and Beverages to Avoid Taking in Large Amounts

Dairy products	Processed American cheese
Fruits	Raisins, prunes, bananas, avocados, plums, canned figs
Caffeine sources	Coffee, chocolate, colas
Beverages	Domestic jug red wines; domestic beers, ales, and stouts; sherry

Medications to avoid	Cold medications, nasal decongestants (tablets, drops, sprays, etc.), hay fever and allergy medications, weight reduction preparations, "pep" pills, antiappetite medications, asthma inhalants

continued

Box 1–1: (continued)

Foods and Beverages That May Be Taken Without Problems

Beverages	White wines
Any baked goods raised with yeast	
Dairy products	Cottage cheese, cream cheese, milk, cream, ice cream

Note: Although white wines are listed as having no tyramine, alcohol is a depressant and should not be ingested by individuals in treatment for depression.

Tyramine Content of Some Cheeses

English Stilton	17.3 mg/serving
Mozzarella	2.4 mg/serving
Grated Parmesan	0.2 mg/serving
Cream cheese	0

The principles guiding the use of MAOI and TCA medications are as follows:

- Drug treatment does not preclude psychotherapy, electroconvulsive therapy, or behavioral treatments if they are also indicated.
- Other antidepressant treatment should be given first unless there are contraindications, clinical indications for MAOI, or a past history of unresponsiveness to other antidepressants.
- Dosage may vary and may be limited by significant side effects.
- A response is seen 2 to 3 weeks after the therapeutic dose is reached.
- Clients with recurrent major depressive episodes with melancholia may require long-term maintenance treatment, although doses are usually lower than those needed in acute episodes.

SELECTIVE SEROTONIN REUPTAKE INHIBITORS (SSRIs)

Further development of antidepressants has been the result of a scientific search for drugs with fewer toxic side effects and greater biologic predictability in the treatment of depression. They are believed to be more neurotransmitter–specific and better able to treat conditions related to dopamine, serotonin, or norepinephrine dysfunctions.

There are disadvantages with the early antidepressants. Uncomfortable and sometimes intolerable side effects, and a number of use restrictions with certain populations, combined with the dietary restrictions of the MAOIs, make these drugs for depression inappropriate for many people.

The next class of antidepressant medications developed was the SSRIs. A profound difference with this group of drugs is their side effects. While all chemically different, SSRIs inhibit the reuptake (and thus the deactivation) of the neurotransmitter serotonin, allowing for the increased availability of serotonin at synapses. The first SSRI developed was fluoxetine. There are now a number of medications with this action. They are potent and highly specific reuptake blockers of serotonin.

Side Effects

Although the side effects of SSRIs are less severe than those of other antidepressants, some may be intolerable for certain clients. Activation, a more energized state including decreased sleep and akathisia, is common. Special care must be taken with clients who have hypomania or mania in their histories. SSRIs may precipitate an emergence or a relapse.

An important consideration with clients taking SSRIs is the proximity of the administration of MAOIs. Fluoxetine and a MAOI together may cause serious and fatal interactions. The half-life of fluoxetine is such that there must be a 5-week gap between taking fluoxetine and taking a MAOI, and vice versa. Sertraline (Zoloft), paroxetine (Paxil), citalopram (Celexa), escitalopram (Lexapro) have shorter half-lives, and there must be a 1- or 2-week gap (both directions) with these medications and MAOIs.

NEW GENERATION ANTIDEPRESSANTS

Venlafaxine (Effexor) is the first in a class of medications called phenethylamine antidepressants. It has two mechanisms of action: inhibiting the reuptake of both serotonin and norepinephrine.

Anticholinergic-like side effects may occur with venlafaxine. There are also reports of sustained increases in blood pressure with some clients. This last side effect seems to be dose-related, so nursing management of clients taking venlafaxine should include regular blood pressure monitoring. There is also a need for a time buffer regarding MAOIs: a 14-day gap after discontinuing an MAOI before starting venlafaxine, and at least a 7-day gap after discontinuing venlafaxine before starting an MAOI.

The side effects of this medication include nervousness and anorexia. Medications such as this one that have an activation component can cause nervous feelings. Anorexia may be a difficult side effect for underweight individuals. Other reported side effects include:

- Nausea
- Somnolence
- Dry mouth
- Dizziness
- Constipation
- Nervousness
- Sweating
- Asthenia
- Abnormal ejaculation/orgasm
- Anorexia

The recommended starting dosage for venlafaxine is 75 mg/day, administered in divided doses and taken with food. The dose may be increased to 225 mg/day according to clinical needs, and even further increased to 375 mg/day. It is recommended that clients who have been taking venlafaxine for more than 1 week taper the dose when discontinuing the medication. Clients taking it for 6 weeks or more should time this taper over a 2-week period to minimize the risk of symptoms caused by discontinuing the medication.

Reboxetine (Vestra) is an antidepressant with a unique mechanism of action; the drug is the first in a new class of medications known as selective norepinephrine reuptake inhibitors (SNRIs). Reboxetine does not inhibit the reuptake of serotonin or dopamine nor does it inhibit monoamine oxidase. It has not been marketed as of this printing; however, it has received an FDA approval letter. Reboxetine is effective for moderate to severe depression and dysthymia. In addition, the medication is significantly more effective than placebo for relapse prevention, indicating long-term efficacy and tolerability. It is as effective as TCAs for major depression, and more effective than fluoxetine for depressive symptoms related to social functioning such as amotivation and negative self-perception. Onset of action may occur as early as 10 to 14 days after treatment initiation. Unlike the majority of SSRIs, reboxetine does not appreciably inhibit hepatic cytochrome isoenzymes, thereby lowering the potential for drug interactions. Reboxetine is currently available in the United Kingdom as Edronax but will be marketed in the United States under the trade name Vestra.

Issues of major concern to clinicians and recipients of psychopharmacologic treatments are drug interactions. With the wide range of medications available to treat each facet of psychiatric symptomatology comes the inevitable blending of incompatible agents.

OTHER DRUGS USED FOR DEPRESSION

Stimulants, such as amphetamines and methylphenidate (Ritalin), and the phenothiazines are less commonly used antidepressants. Stimulants are not a proven treatment. Phenothiazines may be particularly useful in the presence of agitation. Some clinicians and researchers believe that major depressive episodes with psychotic features (delusional depressions) respond better to a combination of an antidepressant and an antipsychotic agent or to electroconvulsive therapy (ECT) than to antidepressants alone. Others simply recommend higher-than-usual doses of antidepressants.

Mood Stabilizers

The earliest medication discovery was made in 1949 by Australian physician John Cade. Cade found that lithium worked to subdue wild behavior in animals. To the astonishment of his colleagues, he went one step further and gave lithium to humans. Lithium was the drug of choice for the treatment of bipolar mood disorder for many years.

The psychopharmacologic treatment of conditions collectively labeled mania used to be virtually synonymous with lithium carbonate therapy in the United States. Many well-controlled clinical studies indicate unequivocally that lithium was initially the most effective agent for treating the vast majority of acute manic and hypomanic episodes. In addition, because of the absence of sedative side effects, the client felt much more related to the environment and able to function normally while under the influence of lithium.

In the last few years, several drugs have been added to the list of pharmacologic treatments for bipolar disorder. It started with the use of carbamazepine as a treatment to control bipolar symptoms in people who either could not take lithium or did not respond therapeutically to it.

Recognizing the potential effectiveness of carbamazepine in certain mood disorders, another seizure medication was prescribed, divalproex (Depakote), to treat clients with diagnoses of bipolar mood disorder or schizoaffective disorder.

The development of pharmacologic treatments for bipolar disorder has grown and is substantially improved from the clinically efficacious choices available even a decade ago. New guidelines for bipolar treatment have been created and have thus expanded our abilities to care for clients with bipolar disorders. The four main treatment guidelines for bipolar disorders (Expert Consensus Guideline Series, 2000) highlight these key recommendations:

1. A mood stabilizer is used in all phases of treatment.
2. Atypical, or newer, antipsychotics are preferable to conventionals (first-line use only when mania is accompanied by psychosis).

3. Mild depression is treated initially with a mood stabilizer. Severe depression is treated from the beginning with an antidepressant plus a mood stabilizer.
4. Rapid cycling (mania or depression) is treated from the beginning with a mood stabilizer alone, preferably divalproex.

Treatment for mania consists of divalproex or lithium as the foundation of treatment for acute-phase and preventive treatment; alone or as adjunctive therapy with each other has been found to be desirable (McCabe, 2003). If the mania is accompanied by psychosis, the addition of an atypical antipsychotic is most effective. The medications that were effective during the acute manic phase are also used for long-term prevention of mania. Bipolar depression usually necessitates lithium to stabilize clients in monotherapy for depression. If, for some reason, lithium is not used, divalproex or even lamotrigine (Lamictal) can be used.

DOSAGE

The management of an acute manic episode involves rapid initiation of the selected mood stabilizer, increased to substantial doses during the first week of treatment. Lithium is available only in oral form in capsules and time-release tablets or as a liquid known as lithium citrate. Because lithium is an ion, its concentration can be measured in the blood. In the acute phase the blood level must usually attain a concentration of 1.0 to 1.5 mEq/L. After 1 week to 10 days, as the bipolar symptoms subside, the dosage of lithium can be decreased to 900 to 1,200 mg/day, with the blood level maintained in the range of 0.6 to 1.2 mEq/L for continuing control of symptoms.

The basic principles for lithium drug therapy are as follows:

- Blood levels must be monitored after each dosage increase.
- Blood levels are checked every 2 to 3 months or when there is a behavioral reason to suspect a change.

For symptoms of breakthrough depression seen with bipolar depression, the dosing of divalproex or lithium must be maximized before other stabilizing or antidepressant agents are added to the regimen. After that episode resolves, the doses of the antidepressant medication are tapered slowly over the following 2 to 6 months. Special assessment skills are called into service during the tapering process to detect any resurgence of depressive symptomatology.

Length of treatment with medication for bipolar disorder is a debated issue. Clinical practice suggests prophylactic use of a mood stabilizer, preferably the compound effective during the acute phase of treatment, for at least 2 years. If the client has no intention of taking the medication that long, there may be a premature recurrence of the mania.

The use of anticonvulsants as mood stabilizers has its own unique set of effects and termination of treatment issues. Divalproex, carbamazepine, gabapentin, and lamotrigine all have sedation, gastrointestinal (GI) disturbances, and dizziness as side effects, along with others more specific to each compound. The body needs time to adapt to the medication; therefore, some side effects are temporary. However, dosage adjustments can minimize the impact of these side effects so that the quality of life is not shifted downward. An important client teaching aspect when using anticonvulsants as mood stabilizers is the inability for the body to handle abrupt discontinuation of these medications. Frank discussions must highlight the increased chance of having a seizure, even if the client has never had one, if the dose is not tapered slowly to discontinuation.

SIDE EFFECTS

Lithium has a significant number of side effects that can be troublesome and, in some cases, quite dangerous. Significant side effects are usually correlated with blood levels of lithium above 1.2 mEq/L. Common side effects include tremor, nausea, thirst, and polyuria. Thyroid goiter has also been seen as a side effect. Severe lithium poisoning is a potential medical emergency. Early signs include vomiting and diarrhea, lethargy, and muscle twitching. These may progress to ataxia and slurred speech. The client may become semiconscious or comatose; seizures may occur; and electrolyte imbalances may lead to cardiac arrest. This syndrome of severe toxicity ordinarily occurs only when the client has a blood lithium level of 2 to 3 mEq/L. The client may have overdosed or severely restricted food or salt intake (or taken diuretics) to induce this state.

Occasionally, very violent, agitated, or paranoid individuals with mania require adjunctive antipsychotic medications at the beginning of their treatment. These can be started simultaneously with the mood stabilizer, raised to whatever level is required to control the disintegrative behavior, then gradually reduced, and eliminated after therapeutic mood stabilizer levels have been effective for about 1 week.

PSYCHOBIOLOGY OF LITHIUM

Although the specifics of bipolar disorder are difficult to delineate, much can be said about the psychobiology of lithium. Lithium, not unlike the antidepressants, affects neurotransmitters, especially norepinephrine and serotonin. In short, lithium aids in the reduction of neurotransmitter release into the synapse and enhances its return, yielding a lower overall amount of the neurotransmitter in the synapse. Behaviorally, these biologic changes can be observed as an absence of mania or depression. What is unclear is why lithium takes up to a few weeks to be fully effective, when the drug's effects can be observed on synaptic activity almost immediately. Also, why do some people with bipolar disorder *not* respond at all to lithium therapy? Many psychobiologists believe that lithium's effects are likely to be based on neurocellular changes that occur over weeks or months after a client begins lithium therapy. A similar explanation may hold true concerning the effectiveness of other mood stabilizers.

Anxiolytic Medications

Medications in this class are used to treat a variety of problems from high levels of anxiety and panic to insomnia.

EFFECTS

The anxiolytic medications or antianxiety agents—sedatives and hypnotics—have very similar pharmacologic attributes. All can be used in small or moderate doses to relieve anxiety and in larger doses to induce sleep. Although they share the major clinical effect of tranquilization or disinhibition (loss or reduction of an inhibition) of fear-induced behavior, their side effects, including their addictive potentials and overdose sequelae, make certain representations of this category of medications more suitable for routine use and others better to reserve for limited, special circumstances.

Antianxiety medications are sometimes called *minor tranquilizers,* but this is a misleading term. Their effects on anxiety are qualitatively, not quantitatively, different from those of the "major tranquilizers" or antipsychotic medications.

DRUG CLASSIFICATION

The major categories of drug classification separate medications into groups according to their chemical composition and properties.

Meprobamate

Meprobamate (Miltown, Equanil) was the first antianxiety agent to gain popularity in the 1960s. The result of controlled studies of the effects of meprobamate compared to placebos are generally favorable but not overwhelmingly convincing. This, and the addictive and fatal overdose potentials of the drug, prompted investigators to develop more effective and safer medications that have all but made meprobamate obsolete.

Benzodiazepines and Nonbenzodiazepines

The major class of drugs today in the management of anxiety is the benzodiazepines and nonbenzodiazepines. This group, represented by alprazolam (Xanax), lorazepam (Ativan), and others, accounts for a very high percentage of all the psychoactive medications prescribed in the United States. This fact usually evokes a mixed response in professional circles. The easy distribution of drugs for such a ubiquitous human phenomenon as anxiety fosters the development of a pill-oriented and pill-dependent society, say critics. Sympathizers focus on the proven effectiveness of the drugs, which help people achieve higher levels of functioning, more pleasurable experiences, and even more productive psychotherapies in some instances.

The dosing and the timing of an antianxiety medication can be the difference between effective treatment of anxiety and interfering with a client's ability to learn and cope. Anxiety is a normal human response to threats of varying intensities and is not necessarily an experience to be avoided at all costs. At low to moderate levels, anxiety can be motivating and instructive and provide cues to the environment. But when anxiety passes these stages and proceeds to excess, panic can occur. Extreme feelings of anxiety such as panic are not motivating—in fact, they are immobilizing and learning is not possible. The clinical application and purpose of antianxiety medications is primarily to support clients through episodes of stress and anxiety at moderate to high levels. Medicating such that higher levels of anxiety are prevented allows the individual to have enough anxiety in a given situation to manage that anxiety with the coping skills taught by nurses, and to gauge their effectiveness. If antianxiety medications are given without regard to the actual anxiety level and the learning of the individual, it is possible to obliterate the need to learn to cope with stress. The client learns instead to rely on the medication to cope. An opportunity to promote stress management through psychopharmacology includes attention to these important issues.

NEW DRUGS

In the last decade, anxiety-related research has expanded tremendously, and several new anxiolytic drugs have been introduced. The newer benzodiazepines give prescribers a wider range of therapies to target the often idiosyncratic manifestations of anxiety. Some of the new drugs have more rapid onsets and shorter half-lives (triazolam, quazepam [Doral]), while others have a usual benzodiazepine onset time and an extended half-life (clonazepam [Klonopin]).

With the psychobiologic knowledge explosion, a great variety of benzodiazepine drugs have been used in the treatment of a number of disorders. According to List, Axelsson, & Leijon (2003), benzodiazepines are used for many reasons:

- Anxiety disorders.
- Sleep disorders.
- Mood disorders.
- Anxiety associated with medical illness.
- Psychotic symptoms and disorders.
- Convulsive disorders.
- Involuntary movement disorders.
- Spastic disorders and acute muscle spasms.
- Intoxication and withdrawal from alcohol and other substances.
- Preanesthesia.
- Nausea and vomiting associated with chemotherapy.
- Anxiolytic, sedative, and amnestic effects in a wide range of stressful diagnostic procedures.

New drugs and new uses for existing drugs are accompanied by new side effects and the need for new teaching plans developed by nurses for use in client education. The assessment skills of nurses must be finely tuned to detect unusual behaviors in relation to benzodiazepine therapy.

USES FOR ANXIOLYTICS

There is no question that benzodiazepines offer a rapid, effective, and safe treatment for the emotional state commonly known as anxiety. Caffeine interferes with the effectiveness of these drugs, both pharmacologically and as an irritant to client's mood and systems.

These medications are absorbed much more rapidly and completely from the gastrointestinal tract than from intramuscular injection and are almost always administered orally. Exceptions are the intramuscular injections of lorazepam (Ativan) for extreme agitation and the use of intravenous diazepam (Valium) to induce sleep before anesthesia or to manage status epilepticus. Peak levels of chlordiazepoxide (Librium) are reached in the bloodstream 2 to 4 hours after oral ingestion, and peak levels of diazepam are reached in 1 to 2 hours.

The major side effects of benzodiazepines are related to their sedative qualities. Clients may complain of excessive drowsiness and must be cautioned against driving a car or operating other machinery.

Other drugs used to treat anxiety but generally less effective include the antihistamines diphenhydramine (Benadryl) and hydroxyzine (Vistaril, Atarax), the beta-blocker propranolol (Inderal), and methaqualone (Quaalude), a synthetic nonbarbiturate sedative. Methaqualone has been a much-abused drug, probably because of the intense euphoria associated with peak blood levels.

Another common use of benzodiazepines, especially diazepam and chlordiazepoxide, is in the detoxification of individuals addicted to alcohol. Given adequate doses of benzodiazepines to induce sedation (usually starting at 30 to 40 mg/day of diazepam or 150 to 350 mg/day of chlordiazepoxide), alcoholic clients can be smoothly withdrawn by stepwise reductions in chlordiazepoxide dose over a 1- to 2-week period, without encountering alcohol withdrawal delirium or grand mal seizures.

CLIENT/FAMILY EDUCATION AND NURSING CONSIDERATIONS

Client teaching is an especially important element in the care of clients taking antianxiety medications. As most people know, anxiety is a generally uncomfortable experience. Self-medication often becomes the relief-seeking behavior used by many with severe anxiety. Such a psychopharmacologic approach is *temporarily* helpful in the restoration of a person's capacities and internal comfort. When the client is able and ready to learn, however, other means of anxiety control *must* be taught. Many of the anxiolytic drugs (especially benzodiazepines) carry a potential for dependence and tolerance. Therefore, nurses have a responsibility to help clients control anxiety in the most effective and safest way possible.

PSYCHOBIOLOGY OF ANXIOLYTIC MEDICATIONS

Antianxiety drugs probably work through a process of synaptic activity involving the neurotransmitter gamma-aminobutyric acid (GABA) in the brain and spinal cord. Benzodiazepines most likely potentiate GABA, producing muscle relaxation. This mechanism involves a complex process of presynaptic and postsynaptic receptor activity. Recent research has yielded information about the presence of a postsynaptic receptor called the *benzodiazepine receptor*. As the term implies, benzodiazepines bind perfectly and with great specificity to these receptors, allowing for the sensation of relaxation. Two types of benzodiazepine receptors have been identified in the CNS. Type 1 receptors are located in parts of the brain responsible for sedation and nonbenzodiazepines bind exclusively to the Type 1 receptors. This makes the nonbenzodiazepines excellent choices for the treatment of sleep disturbances. Type 2 receptors are positioned in parts of the brain responsible for cognition, memory, and psychomotor functioning. Benzodiazepines bind with either Type 1 or Type 2 receptors.

Treatment for Insomnia

The pharmacologic management of insomnia presents an interesting and challenging clinical problem. Many of the truly hypnotic drugs tend to have undesirable effects, including physiologic addiction, fatal overdose potential, and dangerous interactions with other medications because of liver enzyme induction. The first principle of treatment is to assess whether the insomnia is related to one of the major mental disorders, such as schizophrenia or major depression. If so, the insomnia can and should be treated as part of the larger problem, and sedative antipsychotics or antidepressants may be given at bedtime for this purpose.

In the management of simple insomnia without an associated major mental disorder, sedative–hypnotics are indicated for short-term treatment. Overall, the available sedative–hypnotics include certain antidepressants, benzodiazepines, nonbenzodiazepines, over-the-counter (OTC) medications, barbiturates, and some miscellaneous substances such as chloral hydrate and alcohol (Bain, Weschules, Knowlton, & Gallagher, 2003). Prescription medications have better effectiveness than the OTCs, while barbiturates are rarely, if ever, prescribed due to safety and addiction problems. The benzodiazepine compound flurazepam (Dalmane), 15 to 30 mg at bedtime, is an example of a commonly used historical insomnia treatment. This drug can be used on consecutive nights for about 1 month. Other benzodiazepine compounds that are used for their hypnotic qualities include triazolam and lorazepam. The rapid absorption, within 30 minutes, along with efficient elimination and the minimal hangover effects of sedation the following day with nonbenzodiazepines, make them the treatment of choice for insomnia (Skaer, 2000).

Zolpidem (Ambien) and zaleplon (Sonata) are two nonbenzodiazepines that are structurally very different from each other while being equally effective in the treatment of insomnia. Fast-acting, competent sleep-inducing, and quickly eliminated medications such as these can be used to our advantage without the difficulties associated with the other commonly used compounds. Clients using zolpidem may find it a little more difficult to fall asleep the first night without the medication, but zaleplon is not associated with any withdrawal or rebound effects.

CLIENT/FAMILY EDUCATION AND NURSING CONSIDERATIONS

As with anxiolytics, insomnia preparations are generally intended for either occasional or short-term use. These medications are appropriate for clients newly admitted to a psychiatric inpatient unit or for clients in outpatient therapy who develop sleep disorders. As other medications (antidepressants, lithium, antipsychotics) start to yield a therapeutic effect, however, the need for sedative-hypnotic medication should almost, if not completely, abate.

Nurses working with clients in these situations need to help them regulate their sleep patterns. Here are some strategies to reinstitute regular sleep patterns:

- Avoid caffeine and nicotine.
- Exercise several hours before bedtime.
- Use relaxation techniques, including white noise.
- Avoid alcoholic beverages before bed.

- Eat tryptophan-rich foods.
- Follow a regular routine of retiring and rising.
- Avoid bright light before sleep.

It is essential that the nurse teaching relaxation techniques assess the client's sleep patterns and presleep routines, to prescribe the correct technique to meet the client's needs. Ongoing evaluation of the effectiveness of the relaxation intervention allows for a change in approach if necessary.

Acetylcholinesterase Inhibitors

A new class of medications with specific abilities has entered the dementia treatment realm: acetylcholinesterase inhibitors. The title of this class describes the work done by these compounds in the CNS. The enzyme responsible for the breakdown of a particular neurotransmitter is inhibited from acting by the medication. The enzyme is acetylcholinesterase, and the neurotransmitter it specifically works on is acetylcholine. The cholinergic system is involved in memory, abilities to logically progress from one step to the next in problem solving, and identification of objects and people in the environment, among other skills. Clients with dementia of the Alzheimer's type (DAT) have acetylcholine neurotransmitter deficits at the root of some of their problems. When the breakdown of acetylcholine is slowed, it allows more of the neurotransmitter to remain in the synapse, thus promoting acetylcholine's purpose—to transmit information from one cell to another. In mild to moderately affected individuals, when there is more acetylcholine in the CNS, cognitive functioning and memory improve (Erkinjuntti, Skoog, Lane, & Andrews, 2003). This is essentially how these medications slow the progression of dementia in clients with early-stage DAT.

These medications are best utilized early in the dementing process when deficits are still only mild to moderate in scope. But the best time to institute treatment and the most effective use of the compounds are frequently thwarted by the realities of human nature. There are difficulties instituting treatment at early stages in that many people are not aware they are in the early stages of dementia. Frequently, there is an inability to grasp their own level of symptomatology combined with a general lack of information on the early signs, symptoms, or issues of dementia. Confabulation or denial prevent a client or loved ones from noting deficits or recognizing the implications of low-level difficulties. For example, a woman who is not able to tie her shoes may ask her husband to do that for her, while both of them attribute this situation to arthritis, musculoskeletal problems, or side effects from medications. Another example would be someone not balancing his checkbook anymore, stating the bank has always been correct, when in reality the simple math required to do so is a lost skill.

Think of this medication class as you would a similar psychopharmacologic class used to treat other psychiatric illnesses. It is a treatment for specific symptoms, not a cure. Acetylcholinesterase inhibitors do not alter the course of the underlying disease process or have an impact on the progressive nature of the disease. They are a way to temporarily improve neurotransmission and thus ameliorate memory deficits. The first of the acetylcholinesterase inhibitors was tacrine (Cognex). While not able to help all clients with DAT, it was the first step in the direction of active treatment for a major portion of people with dementing processes. There were problems with this medication in that it caused some liver toxicity, which could be controlled, and had several common side effects including GI disturbances and headache. From this beginning, subsequent compounds were developed. Donepezil (Aricept) and rivastigmine (Exelon) are newer acetylcholinesterase inhibitors with improved impacts on DAT and fewer difficulties from side effects. GI disturbances occur at a much lower level than the original compound, and headaches are reported at only a slightly higher level than clients taking placebo. There is even hope that these medications can somehow play a role in preventing individuals with cognitive deficits from converting to DAT.

Herbal Medicines

Herbal medicines are widely used as an alternative or complementary therapy. One quarter of prescription drugs and hundreds of OTC drugs are derived from plants. Many herbal agents have powerful medicine-like actions and side effects. Herbs and plants generally take longer to act than pharmaceuticals, and few have the potency of a prescription.

One of the critical features of safe and effective nursing care is communication about alternative and complementary treatments. Keep in mind the variety of phrases used to describe alternative and complementary practices (complementary medicine, botanical, nutriceutical, herbal medicine, home remedy, natural remedy, health food, vitamin therapy, hemeopathic remedy, dietary supplement, phytomedicine, herbal tea).

The concomitant use of herbal medicines with psychiatric pharmaceuticals can be accomplished safely only when health providers know that their clients use them and their safety and effectiveness for the client's specific condition has been thoroughly appraised. Be sure to assess your clients for the use of herbal medicines.

There are many benefits to using alternative substances. For example:

- Self-treatment can be empowering.
- The very low concentrations of these substances could be helpful and might not be harmful.
- People feel safer using these "natural" products when distrust and fear is associated with chemical formulations.
- Standard labeling and dosing is possible.

However, there are potential problems with the use of alternative substances in psychiatry even though these alternative substances have lower potencies. Psychiatric indications for alternative substances currently exist only for St. John's wort for depression and ginkgo biloba for dementia, although alternative substances are frequently used for several other psychiatric symptoms and disorders. You may encounter clients using ma huang (ephedra) for general malaise, kava for anxiety and stress, and ginseng and SAMe for depression. Competent assessment and evaluation requires our awareness of the potential for difficulties with alternative substances. Problems with using herbs may include:

- Contaminated product.
- Dosing inconsistencies.
- Delayed absorption of other coadministered medications.
- Worsening of high blood pressure, potassium imbalance, and coagulation problems.
- Side effects such as nerve damage, kidney damage, and liver damage.
- Advertising that makes unproven claims.
- Aggravation of allergic reactions.
- Interference with breast-feeding.
- Thinking that one is treating the problem, when in reality the symptoms could continue to worsen, making effective treatment much more difficult.

ASSESSING HERB TAKING

Many clients do not tell health care providers about their herbal use for fear of being ridiculed or criticized. How do you find out what alternative therapies your clients are taking? Good interviewing skills will bring much of your client's life into the light for you. Use of these skills requires tolerance, a nonjudgmental stance, and some expressive questions. Questions such as "Do you do anything to improve your health?" or "What do you buy at the grocery store or health food store besides food?" can open the subject.

Be aware of the client's need to talk to a knowledgeable professional. The client may tell you about someone else who is taking alternatives while watching for your reaction. A nonjudgmental response to this information would include questions about what the client thinks about it, whether it has helped the individual, or whether the client would consider using this particular treatment. Not knowing about your client's use of botanicals risks dangerous drug interactions or costly/painful tests or treatments when a herb causes an unrecognized side effect.

PART TWO

PSYCHIATRIC MEDICATIONS

ACETYLCHOLINESTERASE INHIBITORS

DONEPEZIL HYDROCHLORIDE

(don-e′pe-zil)

Aricept

Classifications: AUTONOMIC NERVOUS SYSTEM AGENT; CHOLINERGIC (PARASYMPATHOMIMETIC); ACETYLCHOLINESTERASE INHIBITOR

Pregnancy Category: C

AVAILABILITY 5 mg, 10 mg tablets

ACTIONS In early stages of Alzheimer's disease, pathologic changes in neurons result in deficiency of acetylcholine.

THERAPEUTIC EFFECTS Aricept, a cholinesterase inhibitor (also called an acetylcholinesterase inhibitor), presumably elevates acetylcholine concentrations in the cerebral cortex by slowing degradation of acetylcholine released by remaining intact neurons.

USES Mild to moderate dementia of Alzheimer's type.

CONTRAINDICATIONS Hypersensitivity to donepezil or piperidine derivatives.

CAUTIOUS USE Anesthesia, sick sinus rhythm, bradycardia, hypotension; hyperthyroidism; history of ulcers, GI bleeding, abnormal liver function; clients with asthma or obstructive pulmonary disease, history of seizures, urinary tract obstruction, intestinal obstruction; pregnancy (category C). Safety and efficacy during lactation or in children are not established.

ROUTE & DOSAGE

Alzheimer's Disease
Adult: **PO** 5–10 mg h.s.

ADMINISTRATION

Oral
- Give at h.s. just prior to going to bed.
- Increase dosage to 10 mg ONLY after 4–6 wk of therapy with the 5-mg dose.
- Store at 15°–30° C (59°–86° F).

ADVERSE EFFECTS (≥1%) **Body as a Whole:** *Headache,* fatigue. **CNS:** *Insomnia,* dizziness, depression, tremor, irritability, vertigo, ataxia. **CV:** Syncope, hypertension, atrial fibrillation, hot flashes, hypotension. **GI:** *Nausea, diarrhea, vomiting, muscle cramps, anorexia,* GI bleeding, bloating, fecal incontinence, epigastric pain. **Respiratory:** Dyspnea. **Skin:** Pruritus, sweating, urticaria. **Other:** Ecchymoses, muscle cramps, dehydration, blurred vision, urinary incontinence, nocturia.

INTERACTIONS Drug: Ketoconazole, quinidine may inhibit donepezil metabolism; **carbamazepine, dexamethasone, phenobarbital, phenytoin, rifampin** may increase donepezil elimination; donepezil may interfere with the action of ANTICHOLINERGIC AGENTS.

PHARMACOKINETICS Absorption: Rapidly absorbed from GI tract. **Peak plasma concentration:** 3–4 h. **Distribution:** 96% protein bound. **Metabolism:** Metabolized in the liver by CYP2D6 and CYP3A4 to at least 2 active metabolites. **Elimination:** Primarily excreted in urine. **Half-Life:** 70 h.

NURSING IMPLICATIONS

Assessment & Drug Effects
- Monitor therapeutic effectiveness; check for improvement as noted on the Alzheimer's Disease Assessment Scale.
- Monitor closely for S&S of GI ulceration and bleeding, especially with concurrent use of NSAIDs.
- Monitor carefully clients with a history of asthma or obstructive pulmonary disease.

- Monitor cardiovascular status; drug may have vagotonic effect on the heart, causing bradycardia, especially in presence of conduction abnormalities.

Client & Family Education

- Exercise caution. Fainting episodes related to slowing of the heart rate may occur.
- Report immediately to prescriber any S&S of GI ulceration or bleeding (e.g., "coffee-grounds" emesis, tarry stools, epigastric pain).
- This medication only slows the progression of the disease. At some point, the medication will have minimal impact.

GALANTAMINE HYDROBROMIDE

(ga-lan′ta-meen)

Reminyl

Classifications: AUTONOMIC NERVOUS SYSTEM AGENT; CHOLINERGIC (PARASYMPATHOMIMETIC); ACETYLCHOLINESTERASE INHIBITOR

Pregnancy Category: B

AVAILABILITY 4 mg, 8 mg, 12 mg tablets

ACTIONS Competitive and reversible inhibitor of acetylcholinesterase, which is the enzyme responsible for the hydrolysis (breakdown) of the neurotransmitter acetylcholine.

THERAPEUTIC EFFECTS Believed to increase concentration of the neurotransmitter acetylcholine in the CNS. If this mechanism is correct, the effect of drug will lessen as disease progresses and because fewer neurons stimulated by acetylcholine remain functionally intact.

USES Treatment of mild to moderate dementia of Alzheimer's type.

CONTRAINDICATIONS Hypersensitivity to galantamine. Not recommended with severe renal or hepatic impairment; pregnancy (category B), lactation, or in children.

CAUTIOUS USE Bradycardia, heart block or other cardiac conduction disorders; asthma, COPD; potential bladder outflow obstruction; a history of seizures or GI bleeding; concurrent use of drugs that slow the heart rate, drugs that may cause syncope, NSAIDs, or neuromuscular blocking agents during anesthesia.

ROUTE & DOSAGE

Alzheimer's Disease

Adult: **PO** Initiate with 4 mg b.i.d. times at least 4 wk; if tolerated may increase by 4 mg b.i.d. q4wk to target dose of 12 mg b.i.d. (8–16 mg b.i.d.)

Hepatic Impairment Not recommended with severe hepatic impairment

Renal Impairment Cl_{cr} <9 mL/min: Not recommended

ADMINISTRATION

Oral

- Give with meals (breakfast and dinner) to reduce the risk of nausea.
- Make increases in dosage increments at 4-wk intervals.
- If drug is interrupted for several days or more, restart at the lowest dose and gradually increase to the current dose.
- Store at 15°–30° C (59°–86° F).

ADVERSE EFFECTS (≥1%) **Body as a Whole:** Weight loss, fatigue, rhinitis, syncope. **CNS:** Dizziness, headache, depression, insomnia, somnolence, tremor. **CV:** Bradycardia, chest pain. **GI:** *Nausea, vomiting,* diarrhea, anorexia, abdominal pain, dyspepsia, flatulence. **Hematologic:** Anemia. **Urogenital:** UTI, hematuria, incontinence.

INTERACTIONS Drug: Additive effects with other ACETYLCHOLINESTERASE INHIBITORS (e.g., **succinylcholine, bethanecol**); **cimetidine, erythromycin, ketoconazole, paroxetine** may increase levels and toxicity.

PHARMACOKINETICS Absorption: Rapidly and completely absorbed. **Peak:** 1 h. **Distribution:** Mainly distributes to red blood cells. **Metabolism:** Metabolized in liver primarily by CYP2D6 and CYP3A4. **Elimination:** 95% excreted in urine. **Half-Life:** 7 h (4.4–10 h).

NURSING IMPLICATIONS

Assessment & Drug Effects

- Monitor cardiovascular status including baseline and periodic EKG and BP readings. Assess for postural hypotension.

- Monitor respiratory status; report worsening of preexisting asthma or COPD.
- Monitor I&O rates and pattern for urinary incontinence or urinary retention.
- Monitor appetite and food intake; weigh weekly and report significant weight loss.
- Lab tests: Baseline ALT/AST, BUN, and creatinine; periodic blood glucose, alkaline phosphatase, urinalysis, stool for occult blood.

Client & Family Education

- Report any of the following to a health care provider immediately: Loss of weight, urinary retention, chest pain, palpitations, difficulty breathing, fainting, dark stools, blood in the urine.
- This medication only slows the progression of the disease. At some point, the medication will have minimal impact.

MEMANTINE

(me-man′teen)

Axura, Ebixa, Namenda

Classifications: CENTRAL NERVOUS SYSTEM AGENT; *N*-METHYL-D-ASPARTATE (NMDA) RECEPTOR ANTAGONIST (not an ACETYLCHOLINESTERASE INHIBITOR but included here as treatment for dementia of Alzheimer's type)

Pregnancy Category: B

AVAILABILITY 5 mg, 10 mg tablets

ACTIONS Glutamate activation at the NMDA receptor is needed for memory and learning processes in the brain. Excess glutamate may play a role in Alzheimer's disease by overstimulating NMDA receptors, thus causing increased Ca^{2+} movement into neurons, leading to neuronal damage. Memantine is a low-affinity, uncompetitive antagonist at NMDA receptors in the brain. Blockade of NMDA receptors by memantine may slow intracellular calcium accumulation and help to prevent further nerve damage without interfering with the physiological actions of glutamate that are required for memory and learning.

THERAPEUTIC EFFECTS Improves cognitive functioning in moderate to severe dementia of Alzheimer's type and in mild to moderate vascular dementia.

USES Treatment of symptoms of moderate to severe dementia of the Alzheimer's type.

UNLABELED USES Treatment of moderate to severe vascular dementia.

CONTRAINDICATIONS Safety and efficacy in children are unknown.

CAUTIOUS USE Moderate to severe renal impairment; concurrent use with carbonic anhydrase inhibitors or sodium bicarbonate, pregnancy (category B), lactation.

ROUTE & DOSAGE

Alzheimer's Disease

Adult: **PO** Initiate with 5 mg once daily; increase dose by 5 mg/wk over a 3-wk period to target dose of 10 mg b.i.d.

ADMINISTRATION

Oral

- The recommended interval between dose increases is 1 wk.
- Dose reductions should be considered with moderate renal impairment.
- Store between 15°–30° C (59°–86° F).

ADVERSE EFFECTS (≥1%) **Body as a Whole:** Fatigue, pain, flu-like symptoms, peripheral edema. **CNS:** Dizziness, headache, confusion, somnolence, hallucinations, agitation, insomnia, abnormal gait, depression, anxiety, syncope, TIA, vertigo, ataxia, hypokinesia, aggressive reaction. **CV:** Hypertension, cardiac failure. **GI:** Constipation, vomiting, diarrhea, nausea, anorexia. **Hematologic:** Anemia. **Metabolic:** Weight loss, increased alkaline phosphatase. **Musculoskeletal:** Back pain, arthralgia. **Respiratory:** Coughing, dyspnea, bronchitis, upper respiratory infections, pneumonia. **Skin:** Rash. **Special Senses:** Conjunctivitis. **Urogenital:** Urinary incontinence, UTI, frequent micturition.

INTERACTIONS Drug: Drugs that increase the pH of the urine (CARBONIC ANHYDRASE INHIBITORS, **sodium bicarbonate**) may increase levels of memantine; may enhance the effects of **amantadine, dextromethorphan, ketamine, bromocriptine, pergolide, pramipexole**, and **ropinirole**; may enhance the adverse effects of **levodopa**-containing drugs.

NURSING IMPLICATIONS

Assessment & Drug Effects

- Monitor respiratory and CV status, especially with preexisting heart disease.

- Assess for and report S&S of focal neurologic deficits (e.g., TIA, ataxia, vertigo).
- Lab tests: Periodic Hct & Hgb, serum sodium, alkaline phosphatase, and blood glucose.
- Monitor diabetics for loss of glycemic control.

Client & Family Education

- Report any of the following to the physician: Problems with vision, skin rash, shortness of breath, swelling in throat or tongue, agitation or restlessness, confusion, dizziness, or incontinence.
- Do not drive or engage in other hazardous activities until reaction to drug is known.

RIVASTIGMINE TARTRATE

(ri-va-stig′-meen)

Exelon

Classifications: AUTONOMIC NERVOUS SYSTEM AGENT; CHOLINERGIC (PARASYMPATHOMIMETIC); ACETYLCHOLINESTERASE INHIBITOR

Pregnancy Category: B

AVAILABILITY 2 mg/mL solution

ACTIONS Inhibits acetylcholinesterase G1 form of this enzyme.
THERAPEUTIC EFFECTS The G1 form of acetylcholinesterase is found in higher levels in the brains of clients with Alzheimer's disease. Rivastigmine inhibits acetylcholinesterase more specifically in the brain (hippocampus and cortex) than the heart or skeletal muscle.

USES Treatment of mild to moderate dementia of Alzheimer's type.

CONTRAINDICATIONS Hypersensitivity to rivastigmine or carbamate derivatives; lactation.
CAUTIOUS USE History of toxicity to cholinesterase inhibitors (e.g., tacrine); diabetes mellitus, cardiovascular/pulmonary disease; GI disorders including intestinal obstruction and peptic ulcer disease; concurrent use of other cholinergic or anticholinergic agents; urogenital tract obstruction; Parkinson's disease; pregnancy (category B); hepatic or renal insufficiency; concurrent use of NSAIDs.

ROUTE & DOSAGE

Alzheimer's Disease

Adult/Geriatric: **PO** Start with 1.5 mg b.i.d with food, may increase by 1.5 mg b.i.d. q4wk if tolerated; target dose 3–6 mg b.i.d. (max 12 mg b.i.d.) [if discontinued for a few doses, restart at ≤ last dose; if treatment is interrupted for several days, reinitiate with 1.5 mg b.i.d. and titrate q4wk as above]

ADMINISTRATION

Oral

- Give both capsules and liquid with food.
- Give liquid form undiluted or mixed with water, juice, or soda (do not mix with other liquids). Stir completely to dissolve. Ensure that entire mixture is swallowed.
- Discontinue drug for several days if significant anorexia, nausea, or vomiting occurs. When adverse effects subside, restart at same or lower dose level (see ROUTE & DOSAGE).
- Store capsules and oral solution below 25° C (77° F). Ensure that bottle of liquid is in an UPRIGHT position.

ADVERSE EFFECTS (≥1%) **Body as a Whole:** Asthenia, increased sweating, syncope, fatigue, malaise, flu-like syndrome. **CV:** Hypertension. **GI:** *Nausea, vomiting, anorexia,* dyspepsia, *diarrhea, abdominal pain,* constipation, flatulence, eructation. **Metabolic:** Weight loss. **CNS:** *Dizziness, headache,* somnolence, tremor, insomnia, confusion, depression, anxiety, hallucination, aggressive reaction. **Respiratory:** Rhinitis.

INTERACTIONS Drug: May exaggerate muscle relations with **succinylcholine** and other NEUROMUSCULAR BLOCKING AGENTS; may attenuate effects of ANTICHOLINERGIC AGENTS.

PHARMACOKINETICS Absorption: Well absorbed; 40% reaches systemic circulation. **Peak:** 1 h. **Duration:** 10 h. **Distribution:** Crosses blood–brain barrier with CSF peak concentrations in 1.4–2.6 h; 40% protein bound. **Metabolism:** Metabolized by cholinesterase-mediated hydrolysis. **Elimination:** Excreted in urine. **Half-Life:** 1.5 h.

NURSING IMPLICATIONS

Assessment & Drug Effects

- Monitor cognitive function and ability to perform ADLs.
- Monitor for and report S&S of GI distress: Anorexia, weight loss, nausea, and vomiting.
- Lab tests: Periodic ECG, serum electrolytes, Hgb & Hct, urinalysis, blood glucose HbA_{1C}, especially with long-term therapy.

- Monitor ambulation because dizziness is a common adverse effect.
- Monitor diabetics for loss of glycemic control.

Client & Family Education

- Review instruction sheet provided with liquid form of the drug.
- Monitor weight at least weekly.
- Report any of the following to the prescriber: Loss of appetite, weight loss, significant nausea, and/or vomiting.
- Supervise activity because there is a high potential for dizziness.
- This medication only slows the progression of the disease. At some point, the medication will have minimal impact.

TACRINE

(tac′rine)

Cognex

Classifications: AUTONOMIC NERVOUS SYSTEM AGENT; CHOLINERGIC (PARASYMPATHOMIMETIC); ACETYLCHOLINESTERASE INHIBITOR

Pregnancy Category: C

AVAILABILITY 10 mg, 20 mg, 30 mg, 40 mg capsules

ACTIONS Cholinesterase inhibitor, presumably elevates acetylcholine in the cerebral cortex by slowing degradation of acetylcholine release by the remaining intact neurons. Balance pathologic changes in neurons that result in deficiency of acetylcholine in early stages of dementia of Alzheimer's type.

THERAPEUTIC EFFECTS Slows manifestations of dementia of Alzheimer's type.

USE Improvement of memory in mild to moderate Alzheimer's dementia.

UNLABELED USES HIV infection (severe dementia), tardive dyskinesia, acute anticholinergic syndrome with possible advantage over physostigmine.

CONTRAINDICATIONS Hypersensitivity to tacrine; clients who develop jaundice while taking tacrine.

CAUTIOUS USE Anesthesia, sick sinus rhythm, bradycardia; history of ulcers, GI bleeding, abnormal liver function; clients with asthma, hypotension, hyperthyroidism, urinary tract obstruction, intestinal obstruction; pregnancy (category C), lactation. Safety and efficacy in children are not established.

ROUTE & DOSAGE

Alzheimer's Disease

Adult: **PO** 10 mg q.i.d. (taken between meals if tolerated); increase in 40 mg/d increments not sooner than q6wk (max 160 mg/d)

Hepatic Impairment Dose-related hepatotoxic effects have been observed; use with caution or not at all in clients with history of past or current liver disease

ADMINISTRATION

Oral

- Give at least 1 h before meals; bioavailability reduced 30–40% when taken with food. Effectiveness depends on administration at regular intervals.
- Titrate dose upward as long as serum transaminase (ALT) levels remain less than or equal to 3 times upper limit of normal (ULN).
- Reduce daily dose by 40 mg/d when ALT exceeds 3 times but is less than or equal to 5 times ULN. Resume titration when ALT returns to normal.
- Stop treatment if ALT exceeds 5 times ULN.
- Store at room temperature, 15°–30° C (59°–86° F), away from moisture.

ADVERSE EFFECTS (≥1%) **CNS:** Agitation, dizziness and confusion, ataxia, insomnia, somnolence, hallucinations. **GI:** Nausea, *vomiting,* belching, *diarrhea,* abdominal discomfort, anorexia, *hepatotoxicity.* **Skin:** Purpura. **Urogenital:** Excessive micturition and incontinence with UTI infections. **Body as a Whole:** Diaphoresis.

INTERACTIONS Drug: Prolongs action of **succinylcholine** and possibly other NEUROMUSCULAR BLOCKING AGENTS due to inhibition of plasma pseudocholinesterase. Increases **theophylline** concentrations twofold. **Cimetidine** increases concentration of tacrine by 64%. **Herbal: Echinacea** may increase risk of hepatotoxicity.

PHARMACOKINETICS Absorption: Approximately 17% absorbed from GI tract. Food decreases rate and extent of absorption by 30–40%. **Onset:** 30–90 min. **Peak:** 2 h. Steady state in 24–36 h. **Distribution:** Penetrates blood–brain barrier. Protein binding is

55%. **Metabolism:** Metabolized in the liver by cytochrome P-450 system. At least three hydroxylated metabolites have been identified that may be biologically active. Females have lower activity in cytochrome P-450 isoenzymes so plasma levels are approximately 50% higher than men with same dose. **Elimination:** Less than 3% of dose recovered in urine in 24 h. **Half-Life:** 3.5 h.

NURSING IMPLICATIONS

Assessment & Drug Effects

- Monitor for clinical improvement (defined as a 4-point improvement in Alzheimer's Disease Assessment Scale/Cognitive Subscale). Improvement has been observed after 1–4 wk; may take 6 mo for maximum benefit.
- Lab tests: Monitor serum transaminase (ALT) levels according to following schedule: Every 2 wk for first 16 wk, then monthly for 2 mo, then every 3 mo thereafter; resume weekly monitoring for 6 wk with each dose increase; continue weekly monitoring if ALT remains more than 2 times normal; if therapy is interrupted more than 4 wk and then restarted, resume full ALT monitoring schedule.
- Monitor I&O because tacrine may cause bladder outflow obstruction.
- Monitor for seizure activity and take appropriate precautions.
- Monitor clients with history of angle-closure glaucoma for a worsening of this condition.
- Monitor for GI distress and bleeding, especially in clients with a history of peptic ulcer disease or clients on concurrent NSAID therapy.
- Supervise ambulation because dizziness occurs in more than 10% of clients.
- Monitor cardiovascular status, including periodic ECG monitoring. Assess for fluid retention and worsening of CHF.
- Monitor periodically for development of drug-induced diabetes.

Client & Family Education

- Be aware of adverse effects related to initiation of therapy or dosage increases (e.g., nausea, vomiting, diarrhea) as well as delayed effects (e.g., rash, GI bleeding, jaundice). Report adverse effects to the prescriber.
- Do not abruptly discontinue or reduce dosage of 80 mg/d or more because such action may precipitate acute deterioration of cognitive function.

- Make sure to have regular follow-up and liver function tests.
- Tacrine may induce seizures, vertigo, and syncope. Use appropriate precautions.
- Understand that tacrine therapy is not a cure and will become ineffective at some point as the disease progresses.

ANTIANXIETY AGENTS

ALPRAZOLAM

(al-pra′zoe-lam)

Xanax, Xanax XR

Classifications: CNS AGENT; BENZODIAZEPINE ANXIOLYTIC; SEDATIVE-HYPNOTIC

Pregnancy Category: D

Controlled Substance: Schedule IV

AVAILABILITY 0.25 mg, 0.5 mg, 1 mg, 2 mg tablets; 0.5 mg/5 mL, 1 mg/mL oral solution

ACTIONS CNS depressant. Mode of action not known but appears to act at the limbic, thalamic, and hypothalamic levels of the CNS. It is associated with significantly less drowsiness. Has antidepressant as well as anxiolytic actions.
THERAPEUTIC EFFECTS Drug has antidepressant as well as antianxiety actions.

USES Management of anxiety disorders or for short-term relief of anxiety symptoms. Also used as adjunct in management of anxiety associated with depression and agitation and for panic disorders, such as agoraphobia.

CONTRAINDICATIONS Sensitivity to benzodiazepines; acute narrow-angle glaucoma; pulmonary disease; use alone in primary depression or psychotic disorders; during pregnancy (category D), in nursing mothers and children <18 y.
CAUTIOUS USE Impaired renal or hepatic function; history of alcoholism; geriatric and debilitated clients. Effectiveness for long-term treatment (>4 mo) not established.

ROUTE & DOSAGE

Anxiety Disorders

Adult: **PO** 0.25–0.5 mg t.i.d. (max 4 mg/d).
Geriatric: **PO** 0.125–0.25 mg b.i.d.

Panic Attacks

Adult: **PO** 1–2 mg t.i.d. (max 8 mg/d)

ADMINISTRATION

- Alprazolam may be administered without regard to meals.
- Store in light-resistant containers at 15°–30° C (59°–86° F), unless otherwise directed.

ADVERSE EFFECTS CNS: *Drowsiness, sedation,* light-headedness, dizziness, syncope, depression, headache, confusion, insomnia, nervousness, fatigue, clumsiness, unsteadiness, rigidity, tremor, restlessness, paradoxical excitement, hallucinations. **CV:** Tachycardia, hypotension, ECG changes. **Other:** Blurred vision, dyspnea.

INTERACTIONS Drug: Alcohol and other CNS DEPRESSANTS, ANTICONVULSANTS, ANTIHISTAMINES, BARBITURATES, NARCOTIC ANALGESICS, BENZODIAZEPINES compound CNS depressant effects; **cimetidine, disulfiram** increase alprazolam effects (decreased metabolism); oral contraceptives may increase or decrease alprazolam effects. **Herbal: Kava-kava, valerian** may enhance sedation effects.

PHARMACOKINETICS Absorption: Rapidly absorbed. **Peak:** 1–2 h. **Distribution:** Crosses placenta. **Metabolism:** Oxidized in liver to inactive metabolites. **Elimination:** Renal elimination. **Half-Life:** 12–15 h.

NURSING IMPLICATIONS

Assessment & Intervention

- Clients receiving continuing therapy should have periodic blood counts, urinalyses, and blood chemistry studies.
- Drowsiness and sedation are the most common side effects. Monitor especially the elderly or debilitated, who may require supervised ambulation or side rails.
- Long-term use may lead to physical dependence.

Client & Family Education

- Adverse reactions, which may occur during early high-dose therapy, usually disappear with continuing therapy. Advise client to keep prescriber informed; dosage adjustments may be indicated. Instruct client to make position changes slowly and in stages.

- Only use this medication for the length of time prescribed, because prolonged use could lead to dependence on the drug.
- Alprazolam potentiates effects of ETOH and other CNS depressants; caution client not to use them or OTC medications containing antihistamines (sleep aids, cold, hay fever, or allergy remedies) without consulting prescriber.
- Advise client to avoid driving and other potentially hazardous activities until reaction to drug is determined.
- Following continuous use, dosage should be tapered off before drug is stopped. Abrupt discontinuation of drug may cause withdrawal symptoms: Nausea, vomiting, abdominal and muscle cramps, sweating, confusion, tremors, convulsions.

BUSPIRONE HYDROCHLORIDE

(byoo-spye′rone)

BuSpar

Classifications: CNS AGENT; ANXIOLYTIC

Pregnancy Category: B

AVAILABILITY 5 mg, 10 mg, 15 mg tablets

ACTIONS Nonbenzodiazepine unrelated to other psychotherapeutic agents. Does not have muscle relaxant or anticonvulsant effects. Abuse potential is minimal. Unlike other anxiolytics, it seems to cause less clinically significant impairment of cognitive and motor performance and produces minimal if any interaction with other brain depressants, including alcohol.

THERAPEUTIC EFFECTS Antianxiety effect is due to its serotonin reuptake inhibition and agonist effects on dopamine receptors of the brain.

USE Management of anxiety disorders and for short-term treatment of generalized anxiety.

CONTRAINDICATIONS Safe use in pregnancy (category B), lactation, or in children <18 y not established.

CAUTIOUS USE Renal or hepatic impairment.

ROUTE & DOSAGE

Anxiety

Adult: **PO** 7.5–15 mg in divided doses; may increase by 5 mg/d q2–3d as needed (max 60 mg/d).
Geriatric: **PO** 5 mg/d; may increase to max 60 mg/d

ADMINISTRATION

- Administer with food to decrease first-pass metabolism. Rate of absorption may be delayed, but administration with food increases bioavailability of drug.
- Do not give in conjunction with grapefruit juice.

ADVERSE EFFECTS CNS: Numbness, paresthesia, tremors, *dizziness, headache,* nervousness, *drowsiness,* light-headedness, dream disturbances, decreased concentration, excitement, mood changes. **CV:** Tachycardia, palpitation. **Special Senses:** Blurred vision. **GI:** *Nausea*, vomiting, dry mouth, abdominal/gastric distress, diarrhea, constipation. **GU:** urinary frequency, hesitancy. **Musculoskeletal:** arthralgias. **Respiratory:** hyperventilation, shortness of breath. **Skin:** rash, edema, pruritus, flushing, easy bruising, hair loss, dry skin. **Other:** fatigue, weakness.

DIAGNOSTIC TEST INTERFERENCE Buspirone may increase serum concentrates of ***hepatic aminotransferases*** (ALT, AST).

INTERACTIONS Drug: MAO INHIBITORS, hypertension; **trazodone,** possible increase in liver transaminases; increased **haloperidol** serum levels.

PHARMACOKINETICS Absorption: Readily absorbed from GI tract but undergoes first pass metabolism. **Onset:** 5–7 d. **Peak:** 1 h. **Duration:** 6–8 h. **Metabolism:** Metabolized in the liver. **Elimination:** 30–63% excreted in urine as metabolites within 24 h. **Half-Life:** 2–4 h.

NURSING IMPLICATIONS

Assessment & Intervention

- Buspirone may displace digoxin from its serum binding. This could increase the potential for toxic serum levels of digoxin.
- Benzodiazepines or sedative-hypnotic drugs are withdrawn gradually before buspirone therapy is started. Observe for rebound symptoms that may occur at varying times.

- Involuntary movements may manifest in a small number of clients early in therapy. This includes dystonia, motor restlessness, and involuntary repetitious movement of facial and cervical muscles.
- Observe for swollen ankles, decreased urinary output, changes in voiding pattern along with symptoms of hepatic impairment (jaundice, itching, nausea, vomiting).

Client & Family Education

- Buspirone should be taken exactly as prescribed without dose omissions, skipping, increasing, or decreasing.
- Advice of prescriber should be sought prior to concomitant use of OTC medications.
- Therapeutic response may initiate in 7–10 d; optimal results are usually achieved in 3–4 wk.
- Adverse effects occur early in therapy and subside without dosage changes.
- Advise prescriber if involuntary movements of face or neck or restlessness occurs.
- Cautious use of medication is required when client consumes alcohol.
- Rebound symptoms can occur at a low rate.

CHLORDIAZEPOXIDE HYDROCHLORIDE

(klor-dye-az-e-pox′-ide)

Librium, Lipoxide, Medilium, Novopoxide, Sereen, Solium

Classifications: CENTRAL NERVOUS SYSTEM AGENT; ANXIOLYTIC; SEDATIVE-HYPNOTIC; BENZODIAZEPINE

Pregnancy Category: D

Controlled Substance: Schedule IV

AVAILABILITY 5 mg, 10 mg, 25 mg capsules; 10 mg, 25 mg tablets; 100 mg/amp injection

ACTIONS Benzodiazepine derivative. Acts on the limbic, thalamic, and hypothalamic areas of the CNS. Has long-acting hypnotic properties. Causes mild suppression of REM sleep and of deeper phases, particularly stage 4, while increasing total sleep time.
THERAPEUTIC EFFECTS Produces mild anxiolytic (reduces anxiety), sedative, anticonvulsant, and skeletal muscle relaxant effects.

USES Relief of various anxiety and tension states, preoperative apprehension and anxiety, and for management of alcohol withdrawal.

UNLABELED USE Essential, familial and senile action tremors.

CONTRAINDICATIONS Hypersensitivity to chlordiazepoxide and other benzodiazepines; narrow-angle glaucoma, prostatic hypertrophy, shock, comatose states, primary depressive disorder or psychoses, pregnancy (category D), lactation, oral use in children <6 y, parenteral use in children <12 y, acute alcohol intoxication.
CAUTIOUS USE Anxiety states associated with depression, history of impaired hepatic or renal function; addiction-prone individuals, blood dyscrasias; in the older adult, debilitated clients, children; hyperkinesis, COPD.

ROUTE & DOSAGE

Mild Anxiety, Preoperative Anxiety

Adult: **PO** 5–10 mg t.i.d. or q.i.d. **IM/IV** 50–100 mg 1 h before surgery
Geriatric: **PO** 5 mg b.i.d. to q.i.d.
Child: **PO** 5 mg b.i.d. to q.i.d.; may be increased to 10 mg t.i.d.

Severe Anxiety and Tension

Adult: **PO** 20–25 mg t.i.d. or q.i.d. **IM/IV** 50–100 mg; then 25–50 mg t.i.d. or q.i.d.

Alcohol Withdrawal Syndrome

Adult: **PO** 50–100 mg prn up to 300 mg/d **IM/IV** 50–100 mg; may repeat in 2–3 h if necessary

ADMINISTRATION

Oral

- Give with or immediately after meals or with milk to reduce GI distress. If an antacid is prescribed, it should be taken at least 1 h before or after chlordiazepoxide to prevent delay in drug absorption.
- Supervise drug ingestion to prevent "cheeking" pills, a maneuver that leads to hoarding or omission of drug.

Intramuscular

- Prepare parenteral solution immediately before use; discard unused portion. Drug is unstable in light and when in solution.
- Use special diluent provided by manufacturer to make the IM solution. Add diluent carefully to avoid bubble formation; gently agitate until solution is clear. Resulting solution: 50 mg/mL. Discard diluent if it is not clear.

Intravenous

PREPARE **Direct:** Dilute each 100 mg ampule of dry powder with 5 mL sterile water for injection or NS. Agitate gently until dissolved. DO NOT use supplied diluent, which is for IM injection only.

ADMINISTER **Direct:** Give a rate of 100 mg or a fraction thereof over at least 1 min. The special diluent supplied by manufacturer for IM preparation should be kept refrigerated, preferably at 2°–8° C (36°–46° F) until ready for use.

ADVERSE EFFECTS **Body as a Whole:** Edema, pain in injection site, jaundice, hiccups, <u>respiratory depression</u>. **CV:** Orthostatic hypotension, tachycardia, changes in ECG patterns seen with rapid IV administration. **GI:** Nausea, dry mouth, vomiting, constipation, increased appetite. **CNS:**: *Drowsiness,* dizziness, *lethargy,* changes in EEG pattern; vivid dreams, nightmares, headache, vertigo, syncope, tinnitus, confusion, hallucinations, paradoxic rage, depression, delirium, ataxia. **Skin:** Photosensitivity, skin rash. **Urogenital:** Urinary frequency.

INCOMPATIBILITIES **Y-site: Cefepime.** Store in tight, light-resistant containers at room temperature unless otherwise specified by manufacturer.

DIAGNOSTIC TEST INTERFERENCE Chlordiazepoxide increases ***serum bilirubin, AST,*** and ***ALT;*** decreases ***radioactive iodine uptake;*** and may falsely increase readings for ***urinary 17-OHCS*** (modified ***Glenn-Nelson*** technique).

INTERACTIONS **Drug: Alcohol,** CNS DEPRESSANTS, ANTICONVULSANTS potentiate CNS depression; **cimetidine** increases **chlordiazepoxide** plasma levels, thus increasing toxicity; may decrease antiparkinsonian effects of **levodopa;** may increase **phenytoin** levels; smoking decreases sedative and antianxiety effects. **Herbal: Kava-kava, valerian** may potentiate sedation.

PHARMACOKINETICS **Absorption:** Well absorbed from GI tract; slow, erratic absorption from IM. **Peak:** 1–4 h PO; 15–30 min IM; 3–30 min IV. **Distribution:** Widely distributed throughout body; crosses placenta. **Metabolism:** Metabolized in liver to long-acting active metabolite. **Elimination:** Slowly excreted in urine (may last several days); excreted in breast milk. **Half-Life:** 5–30 h.

NURSING IMPLICATIONS

Assessment & Drug Effects

- Monitor for S&S of orthostatic hypotension and tachycardia, which occur more frequently with parenteral administration. Client should stay recumbent 2–3 h after IM or IV injection; observe closely and monitor vital signs.
- Check BP and pulse before giving benzodiazepine in early part of therapy. If blood pressure falls 20 mm Hg or more or if pulse rate is above 120 bpm, delay medication and consult prescriber.
- Lab tests: Periodic blood cell counts and liver function tests are recommended during prolonged therapy.
- Monitor for S&S of agranulocytosis: Sore throat or mouth, upper respiratory infection, fever, and malaise. Total and differential WBC counts should be ordered immediately, and protective isolation instituted.
- Monitor I&O until drug dosage is stabilized. Report changes in I&O ratio and dysuria to prescriber. Cumulative (overdosage) effects can result in renal dysfunction. Older adults are especially vulnerable.
- Monitor for S&S of paradoxic reactions—excitement, stimulation, disturbed sleep patterns, acute rage—which may occur during first few weeks of therapy in psychiatric clients and in hyperactive and aggressive children receiving chlordiazepoxide. Withhold drug and report to prescriber.
- Assess client's sleep pattern. If dreams or nightmares interfere with rest, notify prescriber. A change in the dosing schedule, dose, or an alternate drug may be prescribed.
- Supervise ambulation, especially with older adults and debilitated clients.
- Observe for signs of developing physical or psychologic dependency such as requests for change in drug regimen (dose and dose interval), diminishing favorable response (e.g., disturbed sleep pattern, increase in psychomotor activity), withdrawal symptoms.
- Investigate the symptoms of ataxia, vertigo, slurred speech; the client may be taking more than the prescribed dose.
- Abrupt discontinuation of drug in clients receiving high doses for long periods (≥4 mo) has precipitated withdrawal symptoms, but not for at least 5–7 d because of slow elimination.

Client & Family Education

- Take drug specifically as prescribed: Do not skip, increase, or decrease doses, change intervals, or terminate therapy without

prescriber's advice and do not lend or offer any of drug to another person.
- Can take medication with food or milk to ease stomach or bowel difficulties.
- Do not take OTC drugs unless prescribed or discussed with prescriber.
- Antacids can delay absorption of this medication. Wait 1 h between antacids and this medication.
- Long-term use of this drug may cause xerostomia. Good oral hygiene can alleviate the discomfort.
- Avoid activities requiring mental alertness until reaction to the drug has been evaluated.
- Avoid drinking alcoholic beverages. When combined with chlordiazepoxide, effects of both are potentiated.
- If pregnant during therapy or intending to become pregnant, communicate with prescriber about continuing therapy.
- Avoid excessive sunlight. Photosensitivity has been reported. Use sunscreen lotion (SPF 15 or above).
- Do not breast feed while taking this drug.

CLONAZEPAM

(kloe-na′zi-pam)

Klonopin, Klonopin Wafers, Rivotril

Classifications: CENTRAL NERVOUS SYSTEM AGENT; ANTICONVULSANT; BENZODIAZEPINE

Pregnancy Category: C

Controlled Substance: Schedule IV

AVAILABILITY 0.5 mg, 1 mg, 2 mg tablets

ACTIONS BENZODIAZEPINE derivative with strong anticonvulsant activity and several other pharmacologic properties characteristic of the drug class.

THERAPEUTIC EFFECTS Suppresses spike and wave discharge in absence seizures (petit mal) and decreases amplitude, frequency, duration, and spread of discharge in minor motor seizures.

USES Alone or with other drugs in absence, myoclonic, and akinetic seizures, Lennox-Gastaut syndrome, absence seizures refractory to succinimides or valproic acid, and for infantile spasms and restless legs.

UNLABELED USES Panic disorder, complex partial seizure pattern, and generalized tonic-clonic convulsions.

CONTRAINDICATIONS Hypersensitivity to benzodiazepines; liver disease; acute narrow-angle glaucoma; pregnancy (category C), lactation.

CAUTIOUS USE Renal disease; COPD; drug-controlled open-angle glaucoma; addiction-prone individuals; children (because of unknown consequences of long-term use on growth and development); client with mixed seizure disorders.

ROUTE & DOSAGE

Seizures

Adult: **PO** 1.5 mg/d in 3 divided doses, increased by 0.5–1 mg q3d until seizures are controlled or until intolerable adverse effects result (max recommended dose: 20 mg/d)
Child: **PO** *<10 y*, 0.01–0.03 mg/kg/d (not to exceed 0.05 mg/kg/d) in 3 divided doses; may increase by 0.25–0.5 mg q3d until seizures are controlled or until intolerable adverse effects result (max recommended dose: 0.2 mg/kg/d)

Panic Disorders

Adult: **PO** 1–2 mg/d in divided doses (max 4 mg/d)

ADMINISTRATION

Oral Give largest dose at bedtime if daily dose cannot be equally divided. If clonazepam is to replace a different anticonvulsant, verify whether or not the prior drug should be gradually tapered. Store in tightly closed container protected from light at 15°–30° C (59°–86° F) unless otherwise specified.

ADVERSE EFFECTS (≥1%) **CV:** Palpitations. **GI:** Dry mouth, sore gums, anorexia, coated tongue, increased salivation, increased appetite, nausea, constipation, diarrhea. **Hematologic:** Anemia, leukopenia, thrombocytopenia, eosinophilia. **CNS:** *Drowsiness, sedation, ataxia,* insomnia, aphonia, choreiform movements, coma, dysarthria, "glassy-eyed" appearance, headache, hemiparesis, hypotonia, slurred speech, tremor, vertigo, confusion, depression, hallucinations, aggressive behavior problems, hysteria, suicide attempt. **Respiratory:** Chest congestion, respiratory depression, rhinorrhea, dyspnea, hypersecretion in upper respiratory passages. **Skin:** Hirsutism, hair loss, skin rash, ankle and facial edema. **Special Senses:** Diplopia, nystagmus, abnormal eye movements. **Urogenital:** Increased libido, dysuria, enuresis, nocturia, urinary retention.

DIAGNOSTIC TEST INTERFERENCE Clonazepam causes transient elevations of ***serum transaminase*** and ***alkaline phosphatase.***

INTERACTIONS Drug: Alcohol, and other CNS DEPRESSANTS increase sedation and CNS DEPRESSION; may increase **phenytoin** levels. **Herbal: Kava-kava,** valerian may potentiate sedation.

PHARMACOKINETICS Absorption: Readily absorbed from GI tract. **Onset:** 60 min. **Peak:** 1–2 h. **Duration:** Up to 12 h in adults; 6–8 h in children. **Distribution:** Crosses placenta; distributed into breast milk. **Metabolism:** Metabolized in liver. **Elimination:** Excreted in urine primarily as metabolites. **Half-Life:** 18–40 h.

NURSING IMPLICATIONS

Assessment & Drug Effects

- Monitor I&O ratio and patterns: Excess accumulation of metabolites because of impaired excretion leads to toxicity.
- Assess carefully for signs of overdosage or drug interaction, i.e., increased depressant adverse effects, if multiple anticonvulsants are being given.
- Lab tests: Periodic liver function tests, platelet counts, blood counts, and renal function tests.
- Watch client to see that he or she does not cheek the tablet. Both psychological and physical dependence may occur in the client on long-term, high-dose therapy.
- Limit availability of large amounts of drug in the addiction-prone individual and the panic attack client who has depressive features to the illness.
- Monitor for S&S of overdose, including somnolence, confusion, irritability, sweating, muscle and abdominal cramps, diminished reflexes, coma.

Client & Family Education

- Do not abruptly discontinue this drug. Abrupt withdrawal can precipitate seizures even if the client did not have seizures prior to treatment. Other withdrawal symptoms include tremor, abdominal and muscle cramps, vomiting, sweating.
- Take drug as prescribed and do not alter dosing regimen without consulting prescriber.
- Do not self-medicate with OTC drugs before consulting the prescriber.
- Do not drive a car or engage in other activities requiring mental alertness and physical coordination until reaction to the drug is known. Drowsiness occurs in approximately 50% of clients.
- Do not breast feed while taking this drug.

CLONIDINE HYDROCHLORIDE

(kloe-ni-deen)

Catapres, Catapres-TTS, Dixaril ♣, Duraclon

Classifications: CARDIOVASCULAR AGENT; CENTRAL-ACTING ANTIHYPERTENSIVE; ANALGESIC

Pregnancy Category: C

AVAILABILITY 0.1 mg, 0.2 mg, 0.3 mg tablets; 0.1 mg/24 h, 0.2 mg/24 h; 0.3 mg/24 h transdermal patch; 100 mcg/mL, 500 mcg/mL injection

ACTIONS Centrally acting antiadrenergic derivative. Stimulates $alpha_2$-adrenergic receptors in CNS to inhibit sympathetic vasomotor centers. Central actions reduce plasma concentrations of norepinephrine. It decreases systolic and diastolic BP and heart rate. Orthostatic effects tend to be mild and occur infrequently. Also inhibits renin release from kidneys.

THERAPEUTIC EFFECTS Decreases systolic and diastolic BP and heart rate. Orthostatic effects tend to be mild and occur infrequently. Reportedly minimizes or eliminates many of the common clinical S&S associated with withdrawal of heroin, methadone, or other opiates.

USES Step 2 drug in stepped-care approach to treatment of hypertension, either alone or with diuretic or other antihypertensive agents. Epidural administration as adjunct therapy for severe pain.

UNLABELED USES Prophylaxis for migraine; treatment of dysmenorrhea, menopausal flushing, diarrhea, paroxysmal localized hyperhidroses; alcohol, smoking, opiate, and benzodiazepine withdrawal; in the clonidine suppression test for diagnosis of pheochromocytoma; Gilles de la Tourette syndrome; attention deficit hyperactivity disorder in children.

CONTRAINDICATIONS Pregnancy (category C), lactation. Use of clonidine patch in polyarteritis nodosa, scleroderma, SLE.

CAUTIOUS USE Severe coronary insufficiency, recent MI, sinus node dysfunction, cerebrovascular disease; chronic renal failure; Raynaud's disease, thromboangiitis obliterans; history of mental depression.

ROUTE & DOSAGE

Hypertension

Adult: **PO** 0.1 mg b.i.d. or t.i.d.; may increase by 0.1–0.2 mg/d until desired response is achieved (max 2.4 mg/d)
Transdermal 0.1 mg patch once q7d; may increase by 0.1 mg q1–2wk
Geriatric: **PO** Start with 0.1 mg once daily
Child: **PO** 5–10 mcg/kg/d divided q8–12h; may increase to 5–25 mcg/kg/d divided q6h (max 0.9 mg/d)

Severe Pain

Adult: **Epidural;** start infusion at 30 mcg/h and titrate to response. Use rates >40 mcg/h with caution
Child: **Epidural;** start infusion at 0.5 mcg/kg/h and titrate to response

ADHD

Child: **PO** 5 mcg/kg/d in 4 divided doses (average dose: 0.15–0.2 mg/d). **Transdermal** 0.2–0.3 mg/d q5–7d

ADMINISTRATION

- Give last PO dose immediately before client retires to ensure overnight BP control and to minimize daytime drowsiness.
- Oral dosage is increased gradually over a period of weeks so as not to lower BP abruptly (especially important in the older adult). Follow-up visits should be scheduled every 2–4 wk until BP stabilizes, then every 2–4 mo.
- Apply transdermal patch to dry skin, free of hair and rash. Avoid irritated, abraded, or scarred skin. Recommended areas for applying transdermal patch are upper outer arm and anterior chest. Less drug is absorbed from thighs. Rotate application sites and keep a record.
- During change from PO clonidine to transdermal system, PO clonidine should be maintained for at least 24 h after patch is applied. Consult prescriber.
- Do not abruptly discontinue drug. It should be withdrawn over a period of 2–4 d.
- Abrupt withdrawal resembles sympathetic stimulation and may result in restlessness and headache 2–3 h after a missed dose and a hypertensive crisis within 8–18 h.
- Store in tightly closed container at 15°–30° C (59°–86° F) unless otherwise directed.

ADVERSE EFFECTS (≥1%) **CV:** *Hypotension (epidural),* postural hypotension (mild), peripheral edema, ECG changes, tachycardia, bradycardia, flushing, rapid increase in BP with abrupt withdrawal. **GI:** *Dry mouth, constipation,* abdominal pain, pseudo-obstruction of large bowel, altered taste, nausea, vomiting, hepatitis, hyperbilirubinemia, weight gain (sodium retention). **CNS:** *Drowsiness, sedation,* dizziness, headache, fatigue, weakness, sluggishness, dyspnea, vivid dreams, nightmares, insomnia, behavior changes, agitation, hallucination, nervousness, restlessness, anxiety, mental depression. **Skin:** Rash, pruritus, thinning of hair, exacerbation of psoriasis; with transdermal patch: hyperpigmentation, recurrent herpes simplex, skin irritation, contact dermatitis, mild erythema. **Special Senses:** Dry eyes. **Urogenital:** Impotence, loss of libido.

DIAGNOSTIC TEST INTERFERENCE Possibility of decreased urinary excretion of ***aldosterone, catecholamines,*** and ***VMA*** (however, sudden withdrawal of clonidine may cause increases in these values); transient increases in ***blood glucose;*** weakly positive ***direct antiglobulin (Coombs') tests.***

INTERACTIONS Drug: Alcohol and other CNS DEPRESSANTS add to CNS depression; TRICYCLIC ANTIDEPRESSANTS may reduce antihypertensive effects. OPIATE ANALGESICS increase hypotension with epidural clonidine. Increased risk of bradycardia or AV block when epidural clonidine is used with DIGOXIN, ***CALCIUM CHANNEL BLOCKERS,*** or ***BETA-BLOCKERS.***

PHARMACOKINETICS Absorption: Readily absorbed from GI tract. **Onset:** 30–60 min PO; 1–3 d transdermal. **Peak:** 2–4 h PO; 2–3 d transdermal. **Duration:** 8 h PO; 7 d transdermal. **Distribution:** Widely distributed; crosses blood–brain barrier; not known if crosses placenta or distributed into breast milk. **Metabolism:** Metabolized in liver. **Elimination:** 80% excreted in urine, 20% in feces. **Half-Life:** 6–20 h.

NURSING IMPLICATIONS

Assessment & Drug Effects

- Monitor BP closely. Determine positional changes (supine, sitting, standing).
- With epidural administration, frequently monitor BP and HR. Hypotension is a common side effect that may require intervention.

- Monitor BP closely whenever a drug is added to or withdrawn from therapeutic regimen.
- Monitor I&O during period of dosage adjustment. Report change in I&O ratio or change in voiding pattern.
- Determine weight daily. Clients not receiving a concomitant diuretic agent may gain weight, particularly during first 3 or 4 d of therapy, because of marked sodium and water retention.
- Supervise closely clients with history of mental depression, because they may be subject to further depressive episodes.

Client & Family Education

- Although postural hypotension occurs infrequently, make position changes slowly, and in stages, particularly from recumbent to upright position, and dangle and move legs a few minutes before standing. Lie down immediately if faintness or dizziness occurs.
- Avoid potentially hazardous activities until reaction to drug has been determined due to possible sedative effects.
- Do not omit doses or stop the drug without consulting the prescriber.
- Do not take OTC medications, alcohol, or other CNS depressants without prior discussion with prescriber.
- Examine site when transdermal patch is removed and report to prescriber if erythema, rash, irritation, or hyperpigmentation occurs.
- If transdermal patch loosens, tape it in place. The patch should never be cut or trimmed.
- Do not breast feed while taking this drug.

CLORAZEPATE DIPOTASSIUM

(klor-az′e-pate)

Novoclopate ♣, Tranxene, Tranxene-SD

Classifications: CENTRAL NERVOUS SYSTEM AGENT; ANXIOLYTIC; SEDATIVE-HYPNOTIC; ANTICONVULSANT; BENZODIAZEPINE

Pregnancy Category: D

Controlled Substance: Schedule IV

AVAILABILITY 3.75 mg, 7.5 mg, 15 mg capsules and tablets; 11.25 mg, 22.5 mg long-acting tablets

ACTIONS Anxiolytic qualitatively similar to lorazepam. It has depressant effects on the CNS, thus controlling anxiety associated with stress.

THERAPEUTIC EFFECTS Effective in controlling anxiety and withdrawal symptoms of alcohol.

USES Management of anxiety disorders, short-term relief of anxiety symptoms, as adjunct in management of partial seizures, and symptomatic relief of acute alcohol withdrawal. Can be useful in treatment of agitation and aggression.

CONTRAINDICATIONS Hypersensitivity to clorazepate and other benzodiazepines; acute narrow-angle glaucoma; depressive neuroses, psychotic reactions, drug abusers. Safe use during pregnancy (category D), lactation, and in children <9 y not established.

CAUTIOUS USE Older adults; debilitated clients; hepatic disease; kidney disease.

ROUTE & DOSAGE

Anxiety

Adult: **PO** 15 mg/d h.s.; may increase to 15–60 mg/d in divided doses (max 60 mg/d)

Acute Alcohol Withdrawal

Adult: **PO** 30 mg followed by 30–60 mg in divided doses (max 90 mg/d); taper by 15 mg/d over 4 d to 7.5–15 mg/d until client is stable

Partial Seizures

Adult: **PO** 7.5 mg t.i.d.
Child: 9–12 y: **PO** 3.75–7.5 mg b.i.d.; may increase by no more than 3.75 mg/wk (max 60 mg/d)

ADMINISTRATION

Oral

- Give with food to minimize gastric distress. Give antacid no less than 1 h before or 1 h after drug ingestion.
- Ensure that sustained-release form of drug is not chewed or crushed. It must be swallowed whole.
- Taper drug dose gradually over several days when drug is to be discontinued. Abrupt termination may lead to memory impairment, severe GI symptoms, muscle pain, restlessness, irritability, fatigue, insomnia.
- Store in light-resistant container at 15°–30° C (59°–86° F) unless otherwise specified.

ADVERSE EFFECTS (≥1%) **Body as a Whole:** Allergic reactions. **CV:** Hypotension. **GI:** GI disturbances, abnormal liver function tests, xerostomia. **Hematologic:** Decreased Hct, blood dyscrasias. **CNS:**: *Drowsiness,* ataxia, dizziness, headache, paradoxical excitement, mental confusion, insomnia. **Special Senses:** Diplopia, blurred vision.

INTERACTIONS Drug: Alcohol and other CNS DEPRESSANTS compound CNS depression; clorazepate increases effects of **cimetidine, disulfiram,** causing excessive sedation. **Herbal: Ginkgo** may decrease anticonvulsant effectiveness.

PHARMACOKINETICS Absorption: Decarboxylated in stomach; absorbed as active metabolite, desmethyldiazepam. **Peak:** 1 h. **Duration:** 24 h. **Distribution:** Crosses placenta; distributed into breast milk. **Metabolism:** Metabolized in liver to oxazepam. **Elimination:** Excreted primarily in urine. **Half-Life:** 30–200 h.

NURSING IMPLICATIONS

Assessment & Drug Effects

- Drowsiness, a common side effect, is more likely to occur at initiation of therapy and with dose increments on successive days.
- Lab tests: Periodic blood counts and tests of liver and kidney function should be performed throughout therapy.
- Monitor client with history of cardiovascular disease in early therapy for drug-induced responses. If systolic BP drops more than 20 mm Hg or if there is a sudden increase in pulse rate, withhold drug and notify prescriber.

Client & Family Education

- Take drug as prescribed and do not change dose or abruptly stop taking the drug without prescriber's approval.
- Expectations of medication's effectiveness should be aligned with therapeutic goals. Discuss with prescriber and therapist.
- Do not self-dose with OTC drugs (cold remedies, sleep medications, antacids) without consulting prescriber.
- Avoid driving and other potentially hazardous activities until reaction to drug is known.
- Do not use alcohol and other CNS depressants while on clorazepate therapy.
- If a woman becomes pregnant during therapy or intends to become pregnant, communicate with prescriber about the desirability of discontinuing the drug.
- Do not breast feed while taking this drug.

DIAZEPAM

(dye-az′e-pam)

Apo-Diazepam ♣, Diastat, Diazemuls ♣, E-Pam ♣, Meval ♣, Novodipam ♣, Valium, Valrelease, Vivol ♣

DIAZEPAM EMULSIFIED

Dizac

Classifications: CENTRAL NERVOUS SYSTEM AGENT; BENZODIAZEPINE ANTICONVULSANT; ANXIOLYTIC

Pregnancy Category: D

AVAILABILITY 2 mg, 5 mg, 10 mg tablets; 1 mg/mL, 5 mg/mL, 5 mg/5 mL oral solution; 5 mg/mL injection; 2.5 mg, 5 mg, 10 mg, 15 mg, 20 mg rectal gel.

ACTIONS Psychotherapeutic agent related to chlordiazepoxide; reportedly superior in antianxiety and anticonvulsant activity, with somewhat shorter duration of action. Like chlordiazepoxide, it appears to act at both limbic and subcortical levels of CNS.

THERAPEUTIC EFFECTS Shortens REM and stage 4 sleep but increases total sleep time. Antianxiety and anticonvulsant agent.

USES Drug of choice for status epilepticus. Management of anxiety disorders, for short-term relief of anxiety symptoms, to allay anxiety and tension prior to surgery, cardioversion and endoscopic procedures, as an amnesic, and as treatment for restless legs. Also used to alleviate acute withdrawal symptoms of alcoholism, voiding problems in older adults, and adjunctively for relief of skeletal muscle spasm associated with cerebral palsy, paraplegia, athetosis, stiff man syndrome, tetanus.

CONTRAINDICATIONS Injectable Form: Shock, coma, acute alcohol intoxication, depressed vital signs, obstetrical clients, infants <30 d of age. **Tablet form:** Infants <6 mo of age, acute narrow-angle glaucoma, untreated open-angle glaucoma; during or within 14 d of MAO inhibitor therapy. Safe use during pregnancy (category D) and lactation is not established.

CAUTIOUS USE Epilepsy, psychoses, mental depression; myasthenia gravis; impaired hepatic or renal function; drug abuse, addiction-prone individuals. Injectable diazepam used with extreme caution in older adults, very ill clients, and clients with COPD.

ROUTE & DOSAGE

Status Epilepticus

Adult: **IV/IM** 5–10 mg; repeat if needed at 10–15 min intervals up to 30 mg; then repeat if needed q2–4h
Child: **IV/IM** *<5 y,* 0.2–0.5 mg slowly q2–5 min up to 5 mg; *>5y,* 1 mg slowly q2–5 min up to 10 mg; repeat if needed q2–4h

Anxiety, Muscle Spasm, Convulsions, Alcohol Withdrawal

Adult: **PO** 2–10 mg b.i.d. to q.i.d. or 15–30 mg/d sustained release **IV/IM** 2–10 mg; repeat if needed in 3–4 h
Geriatric: **PO** 1–2 mg 1–2 times/d (max 10 mg/d)
Child: **PO** *>6 mo,* 1–2.5 mg b.i.d. or t.i.d.

ADMINISTRATION

Note: Dizac emulsion is administered by IV only.

Oral

- Ensure that sustained-release form is not cut, chewed, or crushed. It MUST be swallowed whole. Give other tablets crushed with fluid or mixed with food if necessary.
- Supervise oral ingestion to ensure drug is swallowed.
- Avoid abrupt discontinuation of diazepam. Taper doses to termination.

Intramuscular

- Give deep into large muscle mass. Inject slowly. Rotate injection sites.
- Do NOT give emulsion form (Dizac) as IM or SC. It is for IV use only.

Intravenous

PREPARE **Direct:** Do not dilute or mix with any other drug.
ADMINISTER **Direct:** Give direct IV by injecting drug slowly, taking at least 1 min for each 5 mg (1 mL) given to adults and taking at least 3 min to inject 0.25 mg/kg body weight of children. ▪ If injection cannot be made directly into vein, inject slowly through infusion tubing as close as possible to vein insertion. ▪ The emulsion form is incompatible with polyvinyl chloride (PVC) infusion sets. ▪ Avoid small veins and take extreme care to avoid intra-arterial administration or extravasation.
INCOMPATIBILITIES **Solution/Additive: Bleomycin, benzquinamide, dobutamine, doxapram, doxorubicin, fluorouracil, glycopyrrolate, heparin, nalbuphone,**

sufentanil. Emulsion also incompatible with **morphine. Y-site: Furosemide, heparin, potassium chloride, vitamin B complex with C.** Emulsion also incompatible with **morphine.** Do not mix emulsion with any other drugs. Do not administer through **PVC** infusion sets.

- Store in tight, light-resistant containers at 15°–30° C (59°–86° F), unless otherwise specified by manufacturer. Store Dizac emulsion at 2°–8° C (36°–46° F). Do not freeze.

ADVERSE EFFECTS (≥1%) **Body as a Whole:** Throat and chest pain. **CNS:**: *Drowsiness*, fatigue, ataxia, confusion, paradoxic rage, dizziness, vertigo, amnesia, vivid dreams, headache, slurred speech, tremor; EEG changes, tardive dyskinesia. **CV:** Hypotension, tachycardia, edema, cardiovascular collapse. **Special Senses:** Blurred vision, diplopia, nystagmus. **GI:** Xerostomia, nausea, constipation, hepatic dysfunction. **Urogenital:** Incontinence, urinary retention, gynecomastia (prolonged use), menstrual irregularities, ovulation failure. **Respiratory:** Hiccups, coughing, laryngospasm. **Other:** Pain, venous thrombosis, phlebitis at injection site.

INTERACTIONS Drug: Alcohol, CNS DEPRESSANTS, ANTICONVULSANTS potentiate CNS depression; **cimetidine** increases diazepam plasma levels, increases toxicity; may decrease antiparkinsonian effects of **levodopa;** may increase **phenytoin** levels; smoking decreases sedative and antianxiety effects. **Herbal: Kava-kava, valerian** may potentiate sedation.

PHARMACOKINETICS Absorption: Readily absorbed from GI tract; erratic IM absorption. **Onset:** 30–60 min PO; 15–30 min IM; 1–5 min IV. **Peak:** 1–2 h PO. **Duration:** 15 min–1 h IV; up to 3 h PO. **Distribution:** Crosses blood–brain barrier and placenta; distributed into breast milk. **Metabolism:** Metabolized in liver to active metabolites. **Elimination:** Excreted primarily in urine. **Half-Life:** 20–50 h.

NURSING IMPLICATIONS

Assessment & Drug Effects

- Monitor for adverse reactions. Most are dose related. Prescriber will rely on accurate observation and reports of client response to the drug to determine lowest effective maintenance dose.
- Monitor for therapeutic effectiveness. Maximum effect may require 1–2 wk; client tolerance to therapeutic effects may develop after 4 wk of treatment.

- Observe necessary preventive precautions for suicidal tendencies that may be present in anxiety states accompanied by depression.
- Observe client closely and monitor vital signs when diazepam is given parenterally; hypotension, muscular weakness, tachycardia, and respiratory depression may occur.
- Lab tests: Periodic CBC and liver function tests during prolonged therapy.
- Supervise ambulation. Adverse reactions such as drowsiness and ataxia are more likely to occur in older adults and debilitated clients or in those receiving larger doses. Dosage adjustment may be necessary.
- Monitor I&O ratio, including urinary and bowel elimination.
- Note: Smoking increases metabolism of diazepam, lowering clinical effectiveness. Heavy smokers may need a higher dose than nonsmokers.
- Note: Psychological and physical dependence may occur in clients on long-term high-dosage therapy, in those with histories of alcohol or drug addiction, or in those who self-medicate.

Client & Family Education

- Avoid alcohol and other CNS depressants during therapy unless otherwise advised by prescriber. Concomitant use of these agents can cause severe drowsiness, respiratory depression, and apnea.
- Do not drive or engage in other potentially hazardous activities or those requiring mental precision until reaction to drug is known.
- Expectations of medication's effectiveness should be aligned with therapeutic goals. Discuss with prescriber and therapist.
- Tell prescriber if you become or intend to become pregnant during therapy; drug may need to be discontinued.
- Take drug as prescribed; do not change dose or dose intervals.
- Check with prescriber before taking any OTC drugs.
- Do not breast feed while taking this drug without consulting prescriber.

DROPERIDOL

(droe-per'i-dole)

Inapsine

Classifications: CENTRAL NERVOUS SYSTEM AGENT; BUTYROPHENONE; ANTIEMETIC

Pregnancy Category: C

AVAILABILITY 2.5 mg/mL injection

ACTIONS Butyrophenone derivative structurally and pharmacologically related to haloperidol. Antagonizes emetic effects of morphine-like analgesics and other drugs that act on chemoreceptor trigger zone. Mild alpha-adrenergic blocking activity and direct vasodilator effect may cause hypotension. Acts primarily at subcortical level to produce sedation.
THERAPEUTIC EFFECTS Sedative property reduces anxiety and motor activity without necessarily inducing sleep; client remains responsive. Potentiates other CNS depressants. Also has antiemetic properties.

USES To produce tranquilizing effect and to reduce nausea and vomiting during surgical and diagnostic procedures. Also for premedication, during induction, and as adjunct in maintenance of general or regional anesthesia. Principally used in fixed combination with the potent narcotic analgesic fentanyl (Innovar) to produce neuroleptanalgesia (quiescence, reduced motor activity, and indifference to pain and environmental stimuli) to permit carrying out of a variety of diagnostic and minor surgical procedures.
UNLABELED USES IV antiemetic in cancer chemotherapy; IM tranquilizer and antiaggression.

CONTRAINDICATIONS Known intolerance to droperidol. Safe use during pregnancy (category C), lactation, or in children <2 y is not established.
CAUTIOUS USE Older adult, debilitated, and other poor-risk clients; Parkinson's disease; hypotension; liver, kidney, cardiac disease; cardiac bradyarrhythmias.

ROUTE & DOSAGE

Premedication

Adult: **IV/IM** 2.5–10 mg 30–60 min preoperatively
Child: **IV/IM** *2–12 y,* 0.088–0.165 mg/kg 30–60 min preoperatively

Maintenance of General Anesthesia

Adult: **IV/IM** *Induction,* 0.22–0.275 mg/kg; *Maintenance,* 1.25–2.5 mg
Child: **IV/IM** *2–12 y,* 0.088–0.165 mg/kg

ADMINISTRATION

Intramuscular

- Give deep IM into a large muscle.

Intravenous

IV administration to infants and children: Verify correct rate of IV injection with prescriber.

PREPARE **Direct:** Give undiluted.

ADMINISTER **Direct:** Give at a rate of 10 mg or fraction thereof over 30–60 sec.

INCOMPATIBILITIES **Solution/Additive: Fluorouracil, furosemide, heparin, leucovorin, methotrexate, pentobarbital. Y-site: Fluorouracil, furosemide, heparin, leucovorin, methotrexate, nafcillin.**

- Store at 15°–30° C (59°–86° F), unless otherwise directed by manufacturer. Protect from light.

ADVERSE EFFECTS (≥1%) **CNS:** *Postoperative drowsiness, extrapyramidal symptoms:* dystonia, akathisia, oculogyric crisis; dizziness, restlessness, anxiety, hallucinations, mental depression. **CV:** *Hypotension, tachycardia,* irregular heartbeats *(prolonged QTc interval even at low doses).* **Other:** Chills, shivering, laryngospasm, bronchospasm.

PHARMACOKINETICS Onset: 3–10 min. **Peak:** 30 min. **Duration:** 2–4 h; may persist up to 12 h. **Distribution:** Crosses placenta. **Metabolism:** Metabolized in liver. **Elimination:** Excreted in urine and feces.

NURSING IMPLICATIONS

Assessment & Drug Effects

- Monitor ECG throughout therapy. Report immediately prolongation of QTc interval.
- Monitor vital signs closely. Hypotension and tachycardia are common adverse effects.
- Exercise care when moving medicated clients because of possibility of severe orthostatic hypotension. Avoid abrupt changes in position.
- Observe clients carefully for signs of impending respiratory depression when they are receiving a concurrent narcotic analgesic.
- Note: EEG patterns are slow to return to normal.
- Observe carefully and report promptly to prescriber early signs of acute dystonia: Facial grimacing, restlessness, tremors,

torticollis, oculogyric crisis. Extrapyramidal symptoms may occur within 24–48 h of use.

- Note: Droperidol may aggravate symptoms of acute depression.

Client & Family Education

- Do not breast feed while taking this drug without consulting prescriber.

HALAZEPAM

(hal-az′e-pam)

Paxipam

Classifications: CENTRAL NERVOUS SYSTEM AGENT; ANXIOLYTIC; SEDATIVE-HYPNOTIC; BENZODIAZEPINE

Pregnancy Category: D

Controlled Substance: Schedule IV

AVAILABILITY 20 mg, 40 mg tablets

ACTIONS Psychotropic drug that shares antianxiety action with other short-term benzodiazepine derivatives. Effects (anxiolytic, sedative, hypnotic, and skeletal muscle relaxant) are mediated by the inhibitory neurotransmitter GABA.

THERAPEUTIC EFFECTS Clinically it produces a dose-related CNS depressant effect ranging from mild improvement of psychomotor activity to decreased anxiety to sedative-hypnotic effects.

USES To manage anxiety disorders or for short-term relief of anxiety symptoms.

CONTRAINDICATIONS Hypersensitivity to halazepam or other benzodiazepines; psychosis, anxiety-free psychiatric disorders; acute narrow-angle glaucoma.

CAUTIOUS USE Abnormal kidney or liver function. Safe use during pregnancy (category D), lactation, or in children <8 y is not established.

ROUTE & DOSAGE

Anxiety

Adult: **PO** 20–40 mg t.i.d. or q.i.d.
Geriatric: **PO** 20 mg 1–2 times daily

ADMINISTRATION

Oral

- Note: Clients with renal or hepatic impairment may require lower doses. Consult prescriber.
- Store at 2°–30° C (36°–86° F) unless directed otherwise.

ADVERSE EFFECTS (≥1%) **CNS:** *Drowsiness, sedation,* headache, confusion, ataxia, paresthesia, motion sickness. **CV:** Hypotension, tachycardia, bradycardia. **GI:** Dry mouth, increased salivation, nausea, vomiting, constipation, abnormal liver values. **Special Senses:** Visual disturbances, **Urogenital:** GU distress. **Respiratory:** Respiratory disturbances.

INTERACTIONS Drug: Cimetidine, disulfiram, ORAL CONTRACEPTIVES may increase effects of halazepam; **alcohol,** other CNS DEPRESSANTS compound CNS depression. **Herbal: Kava-kava, valerian** may potentiate sedation.

PHARMACOKINETICS Absorption: Readily absorbed from GI tract. **Peak:** 1–3 h. **Distribution:** Crosses placenta; distributed into breast milk. **Metabolism:** Metabolized in liver to active form. **Elimination:** Excreted in urine. **Half-Life:** 30–200 h (active metabolite).

NURSING IMPLICATIONS

Assessment & Drug Effects

- Monitor for adverse effects. Ataxia, confusion, or oversedation may be symptoms of overdosage and can occur at relatively low dosage in older adults or debilitated clients.
- Reassess response to halazepam periodically.

Client & Family Education

- Expectations of medication's effectiveness should be aligned with therapeutic goals. Discuss with prescriber and therapist.
- Discuss with prescriber desirability of discontinuing drug because of its potential hazard to the fetus if you become or plan to become pregnant.
- Do not stop taking drug suddenly; dose needs to be slowly decreased. Barbiturate-like withdrawal symptoms may occur (dysphoria, insomnia, abdominal and muscle cramps, vomiting, sweating, tremors, convulsions).
- Note: Smoking decreases sedative effects of halazepam.
- Take a missed dose as soon as possible unless it is almost time for your next dose.

- Dry mouth can be alleviated with frequent mouth care, hard candies, or chewing gum.
- Do not drive or engage in other potentially hazardous activities until response to drug is known.
- Be aware that alcohol or other CNS depressants can produce additive effects.
- Do not breast feed while taking this drug without consulting prescriber.

HYDROXYZINE HYDROCHLORIDE

(hye-drox′i-zeen)

Atarax, Hyzine-50, Quiess, Vistacon, Vistaject-25 & -50, Vistaril IM

HYDROXYZINE PAMOATE

Hy-Pam, Vamate, Vistaril Oral

Classifications: ANTIHISTAMINE; ANTIPRURITIC
Pregnancy Category: C

AVAILABILITY Hydroxyzine HCl 10 mg, 25 mg, 50 mg, 100 mg tablets; 10 mg/5 mL syrup; 25 mg/ 5 mL oral suspension; 25 mg/mL, 50 mg/mL injection **Hydroxyzine Pamoate** 25 mg, 50 mg, 100 mg capsules

ACTIONS Piperazine derivative structurally and pharmacologically related to other cyclizines (e.g., buclizine, chlorcyclizine). In common with such agents, it causes CNS depression.
THERAPEUTIC EFFECTS Its tranquilizing (ataractic) effect is produced primarily by depression of hypothalamus and brain-stem reticular formation, rather than cortical areas. In addition, it is an effective agent for pruritus.

USES Emotional or psychoneurotic states characterized by anxiety, tension, or psychomotor agitation; to relieve anxiety, control nausea and emesis, and reduce narcotic requirements before or after surgery or delivery. Also used in management of pruritus due to allergic conditions, e.g., chronic urticaria, atopic and contact dermatoses, and in treatment of acute and chronic alcoholism with withdrawal symptoms or delirium tremens.

CONTRAINDICATIONS Known hypersensitivity to hydroxyzine; use as sole treatment in psychoses or depression. Safe use during early pregnancy (category C) or lactation is not established.
CAUTIOUS USE History of allergies; older adults.

ROUTE & DOSAGE

Anxiety

Adult: **PO** 25–100 mg t.i.d. or q.i.d. **IM** 25–100 mg q4–6h
Child: **PO** <*6 y,* 50 mg/d in divided doses; >*6 y,* 50–100 mg/d in divided doses **IM** 1.1 mg/kg q4–6h

Pruritus

Adult: **PO** 25 mg t.i.d. or q.i.d. **IM** 25 mg q4–6h
Geriatric: **PO** 10 mg 3–4 times daily
Child: **PO** <*6 y,* 50 mg/d in divided doses; >*6 y,* 50–100 mg/d in divided doses **IM** 1.1 mg/kg q4–6h

Nausea

Adult: **IM** 25–100 mg q4–6h
Child: **IM** 1.1 mg/kg q4–6h

ADMINISTRATION

Oral

- Tablets may be crushed and taken with fluid of client's choice. Capsules may be emptied and contents swallowed with water or mixed with food. Liquid formulations are available.

Intramuscular

- Give deep into body of a relatively large muscle. The Z-track technique of injection is recommended to prevent SC infiltration.
- Recommended site: In adults, the gluteus maximus or vastus lateralis; in children, the vastus lateralis.
- Protect all forms from light. Store at 15°–30° C (59°–86° F) unless otherwise specified.

INCOMPATIBILITIES **Solution/Additive: Aminophylline, amobarbital, chloramphenicol, dimenhydrinate, penicillin G, pentobarbital, phenobarbital.**

ADVERSE EFFECTS (≥1%) **CNS:** *Drowsiness* (usually transitory), sedation,dizziness, headache. **CV:** Hypotension. **GI:** *Dry mouth.* **Body as a Whole:** Urticaria, dyspnea, chest tightness, wheezing, involuntary motor activity (rare). **Hematologic:** Phlebitis, hemolysis, thrombosis. **Skin:** Erythematous macular eruptions, erythema multiforme, digital gangrene from inadvertent IV or intra-arterial injection, injection site reactions.

DIAGNOSTIC TEST INTERFERENCE Possibility of false-positive ***urinary 17-hydroxycorticosteroid*** determinations (modified ***Glenn-Nelson*** technique).

INTERACTIONS Drug: Alcohol and CNS DEPRESSANTS add to CNS depression; TRICYCLIC ANTIDEPRESSANT and other ANTICHOLINERGICS have additive anticholinergic effects; may inhibit pressor effects of **epinephrine.**

PHARMACOKINETICS Absorption: Readily absorbed from GI tract. **Onset:** 15–30 min PO. **Duration:** 4–6 h. **Distribution:** Not known if it crosses placenta or is distributed into breast milk. **Metabolism:** Metabolized in liver. **Elimination:** Probably excreted in bile.

NURSING IMPLICATIONS

Assessment & Drug Effects

- Evaluate alertness. Drowsiness may occur and usually disappears with continued therapy or following reduction of dosage.
- Monitor condition of oral membranes daily when client is on high dosage of hydroxyzine.
- Reevaluate usefulness of drug periodically.
- Reduce dosage of the depressant up to 50% when CNS depressants are prescribed concomitantly.

Client & Family Education

- Do not drive or engage in other potentially hazardous activities until response to drug is known.
- Do NOT take alcohol and hydroxyzine at the same time.
- Notify prescriber immediately if you become pregnant.
- Relieve dry mouth by frequent warm water rinses, increasing fluid intake, and use of a salivary substitute (e.g., Moi-Stir, Xero-Lube).
- Give teeth scrupulous care. Avoid irritation or abrasion of gums and other oral tissues.
- Consult prescriber before self-dosing with OTC medications.
- Do not breast feed while taking this drug without consulting prescriber.

LORAZEPAM

(lor-a′ze-pam)

Ativan

Classifications: CENTRAL NERVOUS SYSTEM AGENT; ANXIOLYTIC; SEDATIVE-HYPNOTIC; BENZODIAZEPINE

Pregnancy Category: D

Controlled Substance: Schedule IV

AVAILABILITY 0.5 mg, 1 mg, 2 mg tablets; 2 mg/mL oral solution; 2 mg/mL, 4 mg/mL injection

ACTIONS Most potent of the available benzodiazepines. Effects (anxiolytic, sedative, hypnotic, and skeletal muscle relaxant) are mediated by the inhibitory neurotransmitter GABA. Acts on the thalamic, hypothalamic, and limbic levels of CNS.

THERAPEUTIC EFFECTS Antianxiety agent that also causes mild suppression of REM sleep, while increasing total sleep time.

USES Management of anxiety disorders and for short-term relief of symptoms of anxiety. Also used for preanesthetic medication to produce sedation and to reduce anxiety and recall of events related to day of surgery; for management of status epilepticus.

UNLABELED USES Chemotherapy-induced nausea and vomiting.

CONTRAINDICATIONS Known sensitivity to benzodiazepines; acute narrow-angle glaucoma; primary depressive disorders or psychosis; children <12 y (PO preparation); coma, shock, acute alcohol intoxication; pregnancy (category D), and lactation.

CAUTIOUS USE Renal or hepatic impairment; organic brain syndrome; myasthenia gravis; narrow-angle glaucoma; suicidal tendency; GI disorders; older adults and debilitated clients; limited pulmonary reserve.

ROUTE & DOSAGE

Antianxiety

Adult: **PO** 2–6 mg/d in divided doses (max 10 mg/d)
Geriatric: **PO** 0.5–1 mg/d (max 2 mg/d)
Child: **PO/IV** 0.05 mg/kg q4–8h (max 2 mg/dose)

Insomnia

Adult: **PO** 2–4 mg at bedtime
Geriatric: **PO** 0.5–1 mg h.s.

Premedication

Adult: **IM** 2–4 mg (0.05 mg/kg) at least 2 h before surgery
IV 0.044 mg/kg up to 2 mg 15–20 min before surgery
Child: **PO/IV/IM** 0.05 mg/kg (range: 0.02–0.09 mg/kg)

Status Epilepticus

Adult: **IV** 4 mg injected slowly at 2 mg/min; may repeat dose once if inadequate response after 10 min
Child: **IV** 0.1 mg/kg slow IV over 2–5 min (max 4 mg/dose); may repeat with 0.05 mg in 10–15 min if needed
Neonate: **IV** 0.05 mg/kg over 2–5 min; may repeat in 10–15 min

ADMINISTRATION

Oral

- Increase the evening dose when higher oral dosage is required, before increasing daytime doses.

Intramuscular

- Injected undiluted, deep into a large muscle mass.

Intravenous

- IV administration to neonates, infants, children: Verify correct IV concentration and rate of infusion with prescriber.
- Clients >50 y may have more profound and prolonged sedation with IV lorazepam (usual max initial dose: 2 mg).

PREPARE **Direct:** Prepare lorazepam immediately before use. Dilute with an equal volume of sterile water, D5W, or NS.
ADMINISTER **Direct:** Inject directly into vein or into IV infusion tubing at rate not to exceed 2 mg/min and with repeated aspiration to confirm IV entry. Take extreme precautions to PREVENT intra-arterial injection and perivascular extravasation.
INCOMPATIBILITY **Y-site: Idarubicin, omeprazole, ondansetron, sargramostim, sufentanil, TPN with albumin.**

- Keep parenteral preparation in refrigerator; do not freeze.
- Do not use a discolored solution or one with a precipitate.

ADVERSE EFFECTS (≥1%) **Body as a Whole:** Usually disappear with continued medication or with reduced dosage. **CNS:** Anterograde amnesia, *drowsiness, sedation,* dizziness, weakness, unsteadiness, disorientation, depression, sleep disturbance, restlessness, confusion, hallucinations. **CV:** Hypertension or hypotension. **Special Senses:** Blurred vision, diplopia; depressed hearing. **GI:** Nausea, vomiting, abdominal discomfort, anorexia.

INTERACTIONS Drug: Alcohol, CNS DEPRESSANT, ANTICONVULSANTS potentiate CNS depression; **cimetidine** increases lorazepam plasma levels, increases toxicity; lorazepam may decrease antiparkinsonian effects of **levodopa;** may increase **phenytoin** levels; smoking decreases sedative and antianxiety effects. **Herbal: Kava-kava, valerian** may potentiate sedation.

PHARMACOKINETICS Absorption: Readily absorbed from GI tract. **Onset:** 1–5 min IV; 15–30 min IM. **Peak:** 60–90 min IM; 2 h PO. **Duration:** 12–24 h. **Distribution:** Crosses placenta; distributed into breast milk. **Metabolism:** Not metabolized in liver. **Elimination:** Excreted in urine. **Half-Life:** 10–20 h.

NURSING IMPLICATIONS

Assessment & Drug Effects

- Have equipment for maintaining patent airway immediately available before starting IV administration.
- IM or IV lorazepam injection of 2–4 mg is usually followed by a depth of drowsiness or sleepiness that permits client to respond to simple instructions whether client appears to be asleep or awake.
- Supervise ambulation of older adult clients for at least 8 h after lorazepam injection to prevent falling and injury.
- Lab tests: Assess CBC and liver function tests periodically for clients on long-term therapy.
- Supervise clients who exhibit depression with anxiety closely; the possibility of suicide exists, particularly when there is apparent improvement in mood.

Client & Family Education

- Expectations of medication's effectiveness should be aligned with therapeutic goals. Discuss with prescriber and therapist.
- Do not drive or engage in other hazardous activities for a least 24–48 h after receiving IM injection of lorazepam.
- Do not drink large volumes of coffee. Anxiolytic effects of lorazepam can be significantly altered by caffeine.
- Do not consume alcoholic beverages for at least 24–48 h after an injection and avoid when taking an oral regimen.
- Notify prescriber if daytime psychomotor function is impaired; a change in regimen or drug may be needed.

- Terminate regimen gradually over a period of several days. Do not stop long-term therapy abruptly; withdrawal may be induced with feelings of panic, tonic-clonic seizures, tremors, abdominal and muscle cramps, sweating, vomiting.
- Do not self-medicate with OTC drugs; seek prescriber guidance.
- Discuss discontinuation of drug with prescriber if you wish to become pregnant.
- Do not breast feed while taking this drug.

MEPROBAMATE

(me-proe-ba′mate)

Equanil, Meprospan, Miltown

Classifications: CENTRAL NERVOUS SYSTEM AGENT; PSYCHOTHERAPEUTIC; CARBAMATE; ANXIOLYTIC; SEDATIVE-HYPNOTIC

Pregnancy Category: D

Controlled Substance: Schedule IV

AVAILABILITY 200 mg, 400 mg, 600 mg tablets

ACTIONS Propanediol carbamate derivative structurally and pharmacologically related to carisoprodol. CNS depressant actions similar to those of barbiturates. Acts on multiple sites in CNS and appears to block corticothalamic impulses. No effect on medulla, reticular activating system, or autonomic nervous system.

THERAPEUTIC EFFECTS Antianxiety agent. Hypnotic doses suppress REM sleep.

USES To relieve anxiety and tension of psychoneurotic states and as adjunct in disease states associated with anxiety and tension. Also used to promote sleep in anxious, tense clients.

CONTRAINDICATIONS History of hypersensitivity to meprobamate or related carbamates such as carisoprodol and tybamate; history of acute intermittent porphyria; pregnancy (category D), lactation, children <6 y.

CAUTIOUS USE Impaired kidney or liver function; convulsive disorders; history of alcoholism or drug abuse; clients with suicidal tendencies.

ROUTE & DOSAGE

Sedative

Adult: **PO** 1.2–1.6 g/d in 3–4 divided doses (max 2.4 g/d)
Child: **PO** 100–200 mg b.i.d. or t.i.d.

Hypnotic

Adult: **PO** 400–800 mg
Geriatric: **PO** 200 mg 2–3 times/d
Child: **PO** 200 mg

ADMINISTRATION

Oral

- Give with food to minimize gastric distress.
- Treat physical dependence by gradual drug withdrawal over 1–2 wk to prevent onset of withdrawal symptoms.
- Store at 15°–30° C (59°–86° F) unless otherwise specified by manufacturer.

ADVERSE EFFECTS (≥1%) **Body as a Whole:** Allergy or idiosyncratic reactions (itchy, urticarial, or erythematous maculopapular rash; exfoliative dermatitis, petechiae, purpura, ecchymoses, eosinophilia, peripheral edema, angioneurotic edema, adenopathy, fever, chills, proctitis, bronchospasm, oliguria, anuria, Stevens-Johnson syndrome); anaphylaxis. **CNS:** *Drowsiness and ataxia,* dizziness, vertigo, slurred speech, headache, weakness, paresthesias, impaired visual accommodation, paradoxic euphoria and rage reactions, seizures in epileptics, panic reaction, rapid EEG activity. **CV:** Hypotensive crisis, syncope, palpitation, tachycardia, arrhythmias, transient ECG changes, circulatory collapse (toxic doses). **GI:** Anorexia, nausea, vomiting, diarrhea. **Hematologic:** Aplastic anemia (rare): leukopenia, agranulocytosis, thrombocytopenia. Exacerbation of acute intermittent porphyria. **Respiratory:** Respiratory depression.

DIAGNOSTIC TEST INTERFERENCE Meprobamate may cause falsely high ***urinary steroid*** determinations. ***Phentolamine*** tests may be falsely positive; meprobamate should be withdrawn at least 24 h and preferably 48–72 h before the test.

INTERACTIONS Drug: Alcohol, entacapone, TRICYCLIC ANTIDEPRESSANTS, ANTIPSYCHOTICS, OPIATES, SEDATING ANTIHISTAMINES, **pentazocine, tramadol,** MAOIS, SEDATIVE-HYPNOTICS, ANIXIOLYTICS may potentiate CNS depression. **Herbal: Kava-kava, valerian** may potentiate sedation.

PHARMACOKINETICS Absorption: Well absorbed from GI tract. **Peak:** 1–3 h. **Onset:** 1 h. **Distribution:** Uniformly distributed throughout body; crosses placenta. **Metabolism:** Rapidly metabolized in liver. **Elimination:** Renally excreted; excreted in breast milk. **Half-Life:** 10–11 h.

NURSING IMPLICATIONS

Assessment & Drug Effects

- Supervise ambulation, if necessary. Older adults and debilitated clients are prone to oversedation and to the hypotensive effects, especially during early therapy.
- Utilize safety precautions for hospitalized clients. Hypnotic doses may cause increased motor activity during sleep.
- Consult prescriber if daytime psychomotor function is impaired. A change in regimen or drug may be indicated.
- Withdraw gradually in physically dependent clients to prevent preexisting symptoms or withdrawal reactions within 12–48 h: Vomiting, ataxia, muscle twitching, mental confusion, hallucinations, convulsions, trembling, sleep disturbances, increased dreaming, nightmares, insomnia. Symptoms usually subside within 12–48 h.

Client & Family Education

- Take drug as prescribed. Psychological or physical dependence may occur with long-term use of high doses.
- Be aware that tolerance to alcohol will be lowered.
- Make position changes slowly, especially from lying down to upright; dangle legs for a few minutes before standing.
- Avoid driving or engaging in hazardous activities until response to drug is known.
- Report immediately onset of skin rash, sore throat, fever, bruising, unexplained bleeding.
- Do not breast feed while using this drug.

OXAZEPAM

(ox-a′ze-pam)

Ox-Pam ♣, Serax, Zapex ♣

Classifications: CENTRAL NERVOUS SYSTEM AGENT; ANXIOLYTIC; SEDATIVE-HYPNOTIC; BENZODIAZEPINE

Pregnancy Category: C

Controlled Substance: Schedule IV

AVAILABILITY 10 mg, 15 mg, 30 mg capsules; 15 mg tablets

ACTIONS Benzodiazepine derivative related to lorazepam. Effects are mediated by the inhibitory neurotransmitter GABA. Acts on the thalamic, hypothalamic, and limbic levels of CNS.
THERAPEUTIC EFFECTS Has anxiolytic, sedative, hypnotic, and skeletal muscle relaxant effects.

USES Management of anxiety and tension associated with a wide range of emotional disturbances. Also to control acute withdrawal symptoms in chronic alcoholism.

CONTRAINDICATIONS Hypersensitivity to oxazepam and other benzodiazepines; psychoses, pregnancy (category C), lactation, children <12 y; acute-angle glaucoma, acute alcohol intoxication.
CAUTIOUS USE Older adult and debilitated clients; impaired kidney and liver function; addiction-prone clients; COPD; mental depression.

ROUTE & DOSAGE

Anxiety
Adult: **PO** 10–30 mg t.i.d. or q.i.d.
Acute Alcohol Withdrawal
Adult: **PO** 15–30 mg t.i.d. or q.i.d.

ADMINISTRATION

Oral
- Give with food if GI upset occurs.
- Store in tightly closed container at 15°–30° C (59°–86° F) unless otherwise specified.

ADVERSE EFFECTS (≥1%) **CNS:** *Drowsiness,* dizziness, mental confusion, vertigo, ataxia, headache, lethargy, syncope, tremor, slurred speech, paradoxic reaction (euphoria, excitement). **GI:** Nausea, xerostomia, jaundice. **Skin:** Skin rash, edema. **CV:** Hypotension, edema. **Hematologic:** Leukopenia. **Urogenital:** Altered libido.

INTERACTIONS Drug: Alcohol, CNS DEPRESSANTS, ANTICONVULSANTS potentiate CNS depression; **cimetidine** increases oxazepam plasma levels, increasing its toxicity; may decrease antiparkinsonian effects of **levodopa;** may increase **phenytoin** levels; smoking decreases sedative and antianxiety effects. **Herbal: Kava-kava, valerian** may potentiate sedation.

PHARMACOKINETICS Absorption: Readily absorbed from GI tract. **Peak:** 2–3 h. **Distribution:** Crosses placenta; distributed into breast milk. **Metabolism:** Metabolized in liver. **Elimination:** Primarily excreted in urine, some in feces. **Half-Life:** 2–8 h.

NURSING IMPLICATIONS

Assessment & Drug Effects

- Observe older adult clients closely for signs of overdosage. Report to prescriber if daytime psychomotor function is depressed.
- Lab tests: Perform liver function and white blood cell counts on a regular planned basis.
- Note: Excessive and prolonged use may cause physical dependence.

Client & Family Education

- Report promptly any mild paradoxic stimulation of affect and excitement with sleep disturbances that may occur within the first 2 wk of therapy. Dosage reduction is indicated.
- Do not change dose or dose schedule and refrain from using drug to treat a self-diagnosed condition.
- Consult prescriber before self-medicating with OTC drugs.
- Do not drive or engage in potentially hazardous activities until response to drug is known.
- Do not drink alcoholic beverages while taking oxazepam. The CNS depressant effects of each agent may be intensified.
- Contact prescriber if you intend to or do become pregnant during therapy about discontinuing the drug.
- Withdraw drug slowly following prolonged therapy to avoid precipitating withdrawal symptoms (seizures, mental confusion, nausea, vomiting, muscle and abdominal cramps, tremulousness, sleep disturbances, unusual irritability, hyperhidrosis).
- Do not breast feed while taking this drug.

ANTICONVULSANTS/MOOD STABILIZERS AND ANTIAGGRESSION AGENTS

Note: See Antipsychotics section for further agents indicated for treatment of bipolar illness.

CARBAMAZEPINE

(kar-ba-maz′e-peen)

Apo-Carbamazepine ♣, Carbatrol, Epitol, Mazepine ♣, PMS-Carbamazepine ♣, Tegretol, Tegretol-XR

Classifications: CENTRAL NERVOUS SYSTEM AGENT; ANTICONVULSANT

Pregnancy Category: D

AVAILABILITY 100 mg chewable tablets; 200 mg tablets; 100 mg, 200 mg, 400 mg sustained-release tablets; 200 mg, 300 mg sustained-release capsules; 100 mg/5 mL suspension

ACTIONS Structurally related to tricyclic antidepressants (TCAs) but lacks antidepressant properties. Anticonvulsant actions appear qualitatively similar to those of phenytoin. Like phenytoin, provides relief in trigeminal neuralgia by reducing synaptic transmission within trigeminal nucleus. Also has sedative, anticholinergic, antidepressant, and muscle relaxant (by inhibition of neuromuscular transmission) effects and slight analgesic actions.

THERAPEUTIC EFFECTS Effective anticonvulsant for a range of seizure disorders, and as an adjuvant reduces depressive signs and symptoms and stabilizes mood. It is effective for pain and other symptoms associated with neurologic disorders.

USES Alone or concomitantly with other anticonvulsants in treatment of grand mal and psychomotor or temporal lobe epilepsy and mixed seizures in clients who have not responded satisfactorily to other agents. Also used for symptomatic treatment of trigeminal (tic douloureux) and glossopharyngeal neuralgias and for pain and paroxysmal symptoms associated with multiple sclerosis and other neurologic disorders.

UNLABELED USES Certain psychiatric disorders including prophylaxis and treatment of bipolar disorder, treatment of schizoaffective illness, treatment-resistant schizophrenia, depression, dyscontrol syndrome; for management of alcohol withdrawal, rage outbursts, and for antidiuretic effect in diabetes insipidus.

CONTRAINDICATIONS Hypersensitivity to carbamazepine and to TCAs; history of myelosuppression or hematologic reaction to other drugs; increased IOP; SLE; cardiac, hepatic, or renal disease; coronary artery disease; hypertension; pregnancy (category D), lactation. Safe use in children <6 mo not established.
CAUTIOUS USE The older adult; history of cardiac disease.

ROUTE & DOSAGE

Epilepsy

Adult: **PO** 200 mg b.i.d., gradually increased to 800–1200 mg/d in 3–4 divided doses. Tegretol-XR dosed b.i.d.
Child: **PO** *<6 y,* 10–20 mg/kg/d; may gradually increase weekly; recommended max 35 mg/kg/d in 3–4 divided doses; *6–12 y,* 100 mg b.i.d., gradually increased to 400–800 mg/d in 3–4 divided doses (max 1 g/d)

Trigeminal Neuralgia

Adult: **PO** 100 mg b.i.d., gradually increased by 100 mg increments q12h until relief; usual dose 200–800 mg/d in 3–4 divided doses (max 1.2 g/d). Tegretol-XR dosed b.i.d.

ADMINISTRATION

Oral

- Do not administer within 14 d of client receiving a MAO inhibitor.
- Give with a meal to increase absorption.
- Ensure that chewable tablets are chewed or crushed before being swallowed with a liquid.
- Ensure that sustained-release form of drug is not chewed or crushed. It must be swallowed whole.
- Do not administer carbamazepine suspension simultaneously with other liquid medications; a precipitate may form in the stomach.

ADVERSE EFFECTS (≥1%) **Body as a Whole:** Myalgia, arthralgia, leg cramps, carbamazepine-induced SLE. **CV:** Edema, syncope, arrhythmias, heart block. **GI:** Nausea, vomiting, anorexia, abdominal pain, diarrhea, constipation, dry mouth and pharynx, abnormal liver function tests, hepatitis, cholestatic and hepatocellular jaundice, pancreatitis. **Endocrine:** Hypothyroidism, SIADH. **Hematologic:** Aplastic anemia, *leukopenia* (transient), leukocytosis, agranulocytosis, eosinophilia, thrombocytopenia. **CNS:** Dizziness, vertigo, drowsiness, disturbances of coordination, ataxia, confusion, headache, fatigue, listlessness, speech difficulty, development of minor motor seizures, hyperreflexia, akathisia, involuntary movements, tremors, visual hallucinations; activation of latent psychosis, aggression; agitation, respiratory depression. **Skin:** Skin rashes, urticaria, petechiae, erythema multiforme, Stevens-Johnson syndrome, photosensitivity reactions, altered skin pigmentation, exfoliative dermatitis, alopecia. **Special Senses:** Abnormal hearing acuity, scotomas, conjunctivitis, blurred vision, transient diplopia, oculomotor disturbances, oscillopsia, nystagmus. **Urogenital:** Urinary frequency or retention, oliguria, impotence.

DIAGNOSTIC TEST INTERFERENCE False-negative ***pregnancy test*** results with tests involving ***human chorionic gonadotropin.***

INTERACTIONS Drug: Serum concentrations of other ANTICONVULSANTS may decrease because of increased metabolism; **verapamil, erythromycin, ketoconazole, nefazadone** may increase carbamazepine levels; decreases hypoprothrombinemic effects of ORAL ANTICOAGULANTS; increases metabolism of ESTROGENS, thus decreasing effectiveness of ORAL CONTRACEPTIVES. **Herbal: Ginkgo** may decrease anticonvulsant effectiveness.

PHARMACOKINETICS Absorption: Slowly absorbed from GI tract. **Peak:** 2–8 h. **Distribution:** Widely distributed; high concentrations in CSF; crosses placenta; distributed into breast milk. **Metabolism:** Metabolized in liver; can induce liver microsomal enzymes. **Elimination:** Excreted in urine and feces. **Half-Life:** 14–16 h (decreases with long-term use).

NURSING IMPLICATIONS

Assessment & Drug Effects

- Lab tests: Baseline and periodic CBCs including platelets, reticulocytes, serum electrolytes and serum iron, liver function tests, BUN, and complete urinalysis.
- At least 3 mo into therapy, it is recommended that prescriber attempt dosage reduction or termination of drug therapy, if possible, in clients with trigeminal neuralgia. Some clients develop tolerance to the effects of carbamazepine.
- Tegretol suspension should not be taken with other liquid medicines or diluted with other liquids. Such mixtures cause stool with green-yellow masses that could be unabsorbed Tegretol suspension.

- Monitor for the following reactions, which commonly occur during early therapy: Drowsiness, dizziness, light-headedness, ataxia, gastric upset. If these symptoms do not subside within a few days, dosage adjustments may be indicated.
- Withhold drug and notify prescriber if any of the following signs of myelosuppression occur: RBC <4 million/mm^3, Hct $<32\%$, Hgb <11 g/dL, WBC $<4000/mm^3$, platelet count $<100{,}000/mm^3$, reticulocyte count $<20{,}000/mm^3$, serum iron >150 mg/dL.
- Monitor for toxicity, which can develop when serum concentrations are even slightly above the therapeutic range.
- Monitor I&O ratio and vital signs during period of dosage adjustment. Report oliguria, signs of fluid retention, changes in I&O ratio, and changes in BP or pulse patterns.
- Cardiac syncope may resemble epileptic seizures. Therefore, it is recommended that clients who experience an apparent increase in frequency of seizures or a change in their character should be checked by continuous ECG monitoring for 24 h.
- Doses higher than 600 mg/d may precipitate arrhythmias in clients with heart disease.
- Confusion and agitation may be aggravated in the older adult; therefore, side rails and supervision of ambulation may be indicated.

Client & Family Education

- Bipolar disorder is easier to stabilize when medication is taken consistently over long periods of time.
- Discontinue drug and notify prescriber immediately if early signs of toxicity or a possible hematologic problem appear (e.g., anorexia, fever, sore throat or mouth, malaise, unusual fatigue, tendency to bruise or bleed, petechiae, ecchymoses, bleeding gums, nosebleeds).
- Avoid hazardous tasks requiring mental alertness and physical coordination until reaction to drug is known, because dizziness, drowsiness, and ataxia are common adverse effects.
- Remain under close medical supervision throughout therapy.
- Avoid excessive sunlight, because photosensitivity reactions have been reported. Apply a sunscreen (if allowed) with SPF of 12 or above.
- Carbamazepine may cause breakthrough bleeding and may also affect the reliability of oral contraceptives.
- Be aware that abrupt withdrawal of any anticonvulsant drug may precipitate seizures or even status epilepticus, even if the client is not being treated for seizures.
- Do not breast feed while taking this drug.

CLORAZEPATE DIPOTASSIUM

(klor-az_e-pate)

Novoclopate, Tranxene, Tranxene-SD (*See* Antianxiety Agents)

FELBAMATE

(fel'ba-mate)

Felbatol

Classifications: CENTRAL NERVOUS SYSTEM AGENT; ANTICONVULSANT

Pregnancy Category: C

AVAILABILITY 400 mg, 600 mg tablets; 600 mg/5 mL suspension

ACTIONS Anticonvulsant mechanism has not been identified. Blocks repetitive firing of neurons and increases seizure threshold; prevents seizure spread. Less potent than phenytoin.

THERAPEUTIC EFFECTS Increases seizure threshold and prevents seizure spread.

USES Treatment of Lennox-Gastaut syndrome and partial seizures.

UNLABELED USES Prophylaxis and treatment of bipolar disorder. Monotherapy or in combination with other anticonvulsants for the treatment of generalized tonic-clonic seizures.

CONTRAINDICATIONS Hypersensitivity to felbamate or other carbamates; history of blood dyscrasia or hepatic dysfunction.

CAUTIOUS USE Pregnancy (category C), lactation, older adults. Safety and effectiveness in children other than those with Lennox-Gastaut syndrome are not established.

ROUTE & DOSAGE

Partial Seizures

Adult: **PO** Initiate with 1200 mg/d in 3–4 divided doses, may increase by 600 mg/d q2wk (max 3600 mg/d); when converting to monotherapy, reduce dose of concomitant anticonvulsants by 1/3 when initiating felbamate, then continue to decrease other anticonvulsants by 1/3 with each increase in felbamate q2wk; when using as adjunctive therapy, decrease other anticonvulsants by 20% when initiating felbamate and note that further reductions in other anticonvulsants may be required to minimize side effects and drug interactions

Lennox-Gastaut Syndrome

Child: **PO** Start at 15 mg/kg/d in 3 or 4 divided doses, reduce concurrent antiepileptic drugs by 20%; further reductions may be required to minimize side effects due to drug interactions; may increase felbamate by 15 mg/kg/d at weekly intervals (max 45 mg/kg/d)

ADMINISTRATION

Oral

- Do not give this drug to anyone with a history of blood dyscrasia or hepatic dysfunction.
- Titrate dose under close clinical supervision.
- Shake suspension well before giving a dose.
- Store in airtight container at room temperature, 15°–30° C (59°–86° F).

ADVERSE EFFECTS (≥1%) **CNS:** Mild tremors, headache, dizziness, ataxia, diplopia, blurred vision; agitation, aggression, hallucinations, fatigue, psychological disturbances. **Endocrine:** Slight elevation of serum cholesterol, hyponatremia, hypokalemia, weight gain and loss. **GI:** *Nausea and vomiting,* anorexia, constipation, hiccup, taste disturbance, indigestion, esophagitis, increased appetite, acute liver failure. **Hematologic:** *Aplastic anemia.*

INTERACTIONS Drug: Felbamate reduces serum **carbamazepine** levels by a mean of 25%, but increases levels of its active metabolite, increases serum **phenytoin** levels approximately 20%, and increases **valproic acid** levels. **Herbal: Gingko** may decrease anticonvulsant effectiveness.

PHARMACOKINETICS Absorption: 90% absorbed from GI tract. Absorption of tablet not affected by food. **Onset:** Therapeutic effect approximately 14 d. **Peak:** Peak plasma levels at 1–6 h. **Distribution:** 20–25% protein bound, readily crosses the blood–brain barrier. **Metabolism:** Metabolized in the liver via the cytochrome P-450 system. **Elimination:** 40–50% excreted unchanged in urine, rest excreted in urine as metabolites. **Half-Life:** 20–23 h.

NURSING IMPLICATIONS

Assessment & Drug Effects

- Lab tests: Obtain baseline values for liver function and complete hematologic studies before initiating therapy, repeat frequently during therapy, and for a lengthy period after discontinuation of felbamate. Monitor serum sodium and potassium levels periodically because hyponatremia and hypokalemia have been reported.

- Report immediately any hematologic abnormalities.
- Monitor results of hepatic function tests throughout therapy.
- Note: When used concomitantly with either phenytoin or carbamazepine, carefully monitor serum levels of these drugs when felbamate is added, when adjustments in felbamate dosing are made, or when felbamate is discontinued.
- Note: A reduction in phenytoin of 10–40% is usually needed when felbamate is added to the regimen.
- Monitor weight, because both weight gain and loss have been reported.
- Monitor for S&S of drug toxicity including GI distress and CNS toxicity.

Client & Family Education

- Bipolar disorder is easier to stabilize when medication is taken consistently over long periods of time.
- Note: It is highly recommended that patients and prescribers review the indication for treatment, risks associated with the drug, and the importance of undergoing regular blood monitoring.
- Report unusual changes (e.g., blurred vision, dysplopia) to prescriber.
- Report to prescriber S&S of hypersensitivity including pruritus, urticaria, and (rarely) photosensitivity allergic reaction.
- Learn adverse effects and report these to prescriber immediately.
- Do not breast feed while taking this drug.

GABAPENTIN

(gab-a-pen′tin)

Neurontin

Classifications: CENTRAL NERVOUS SYSTEM AGENT; ANTICONVULSANT

Pregnancy Category: C

AVAILABILITY 100 mg, 300 mg, 400 mg capsules; 600 mg, 800 mg tablets; 250 mg/5 mL solution.

ACTIONS Gabapentin is a GABA neurotransmitter analog; however, it does not interact with GABA receptors, and it does not

 Common adverse effects in *italic*; life-threatening effects underlined; generic names in **bold**; drug classifications in SMALL CAPS; ♣ Canadian drug name.

inhibit GABA uptake or degradation. Mechanism of action is unknown. An effect of gabapentin on central serotonin metabolism has been postulated.
THERAPEUTIC EFFECTS Gabapentin is used in conjunction with other anticonvulsants to control certain types of seizures in clients with epilepsy.

USES Adjunctive therapy for partial seizures with or without secondary generalization in adults, post-herpetic neuralgia.
UNLABELED USES Pain management, mood stabilization in bipolar disorder; may be useful as a treatment for people with antipsychotic-induced tardive dyskinesia. Add-on therapy for generalized seizures.

CONTRAINDICATIONS Hypersensitivity to gabapentin; pregnancy (category C), lactation.
CAUTIOUS USE Status epilepticus, renal impairment, older adults. Safety and efficacy in children <3 y are not established.

ROUTE & DOSAGE

Adjunctive Therapy for Seizure Disorder

Adult/Child: **PO** *>12 y,* Initiate with 300 mg on day 1, 300 mg b.i.d. on day 2, 300 mg t.i.d. on day 3, and continue to increase over a week to an initial total dose of 400 mg t.i.d. (1200 mg/d); may increase to 1800–2400 mg/d depending on response (most clients receive 600–1800 mg/d in 3 divided doses) 400 mg t.i.d. (1200 mg/d); may increase to 1800–2400 mg/d depending on response (most clients receive 600–1800 mg/d in 3 divided doses) *Child:* **PO** *3–12 y,* Initiate with 10–15 mg/kg/d in 3 divided doses, titrate q3d to target dose of 40 mg/kg/d in pts 3–4 y or 25–35 mg/kg/d in pts ≥5 y in 3 divided doses

Post-Herpetic Neuralgia

Adult: **PO** Initiate with 300 mg day 1, 300 mg b.i.d. day 2, and 300 mg t.i.d. day 3; may increase up to 600 mg t.i.d. if needed

Renal Impairment

Cl_{cr} >60 mL/min: 400 mg t.i.d; 30–60 mL/min: 300 mg b.i.d.; 15–30 mL/min: 300 mg q.d.; <15 mL/min: 300 mg q.o.d.; hemodialysis: 200–300 mg following dialysis

ADMINISTRATION

Oral

- Adjust dosage for clients with creatinine clearance of 60 mL/min or less. See manufacturer's recommendations.
- Separate doses of gabapentin and antacids by 2 h.
- Withdraw drug gradually over 1 wk; abrupt discontinuation may cause status epilepticus.
- Store at 15°–30° C (59°–86° F); protect from heat, moisture, and direct light.

ADVERSE EFFECTS (≥1%) **CNS:** *Drowsiness, fatigue,* dizziness, tremor, slurred speech, impaired concentration, headache, increased frequency of partial seizures. **Endocrine:** Weight gain. **GI:** Nausea, gastric upset, vomiting. **Special Senses:** Blurred vision, nystagmus. **Skin:** Rash, eczema.

INTERACTIONS Drug: Increase in **phenytoin** levels at higher doses (300–600 mg/d gabapentin). Does not appear to affect serum levels of other ANTICONVULSANTS. ANTACIDS reduce absorption of gabapentin about 20%. **Herbal: Ginkgo** may decrease anticonvulsant effectiveness.

PHARMACOKINETICS Absorption: 50–60% absorbed from GI tract. **Peak:** Peak level 1–3 h; peak effect 2–4 wk. **Distribution:** Crosses the blood–brain barrier comparable to other anticonvulsants; readily passes into cerebrospinal fluid; is not bound to plasma proteins; highest concentrations (in animal studies) found in pancreas and kidneys. **Metabolism:** Does not appear to be metabolized. **Elimination:** 76–81% excreted unchanged in 96 h; 10–23% recovered in feces. **Half-Life:** 5–6 h.

NURSING IMPLICATIONS

Assessment & Drug Effects

- Monitor for therapeutic effectiveness; may not occur until several weeks following initiation of therapy.
- Gabapentin is sometimes effective for patients with mood disorders who have failed to respond to antidepressants or mood stabilizers.
- Gabapentin has been successful in controlling rapid cycling and mixed bipolar states in a few people who have not received adequate relief from carbamazepine and/or valproate.
- Gabapentin has significantly more antianxiety and antiagitation potency than some other mood-stabilizing anticonvulsants.

- Assess frequency of seizures: In rare cases, the drug has increased the frequency of partial seizures.
- Assess safety: Vision, concentration, and coordination may be impaired by gabapentin.

Client & Family Education

- Bipolar disorder is easier to stabilize when medication is taken consistently over long periods of time.
- Learn potential adverse effects of drug.
- Notify prescriber immediately if any of the following occur: Visual changes, unusual bruising or bleeding.
- Do not drive or engage in other potentially hazardous activities until response to drug is known.
- Do not abruptly discontinue use of drug; do not take drug within 2 h of an antacid.
- Do not breast feed while taking this drug.

LAMOTRIGINE

(la-mo′tri-geen)

Lamictal

Classifications: CENTRAL NERVOUS SYSTEM AGENT; ANTICONVULSANT

Pregnancy Category: C

AVAILABILITY 25 mg, 100 mg, 150 mg, 200 mg tablets; 5 mg, 25 mg chewable tablets

ACTIONS Anticonvulsant. The exact mechanism of action is not known; thought to act by inhibiting the release of glutamate, an excitatory neurotransmitter, at voltage-sensitive sodium channels. **THERAPEUTIC EFFECTS** Stabilizes neuronal membranes and inhibits neurotransmitter release (i.e., glutamate) in brain tissue.

USES Long-term maintenance treatment for bipolar disorder in adults (clinically noted especially for use in bipolar depressive phase). Adjunctive therapy for partial seizures in adults (>16 y). Generalized tonic–clonic, absence, or myoclonic seizures in adults.

CONTRAINDICATIONS Hypersensitivity to lamotrigine, lactation. **CAUTIOUS USE** Renal insufficiency, concomitant administration of other anticonvulsants, pregnancy (category C), cardiac or liver function impairment. Safety and efficacy in children <16 y are not established. Fatal rash has been reported in children <16 y.

ROUTE & DOSAGE

Partial Seizures, Clients Receiving Anticonvulsants Other Than Valproic Acid

Adult: **PO** Start with 50 mg q.d. for 2 wk, then 50 mg b.i.d. for 2 wk; may titrate up to 300–500 mg/d in 2 divided doses (max 700 mg/d)
Child: **PO** *2–16 y,* 1 mg/kg b.i.d. times 2 wk, then 2.5 mg/kg b.i.d. times 2 wk, then 5 mg/kg b.i.d. (max 15 mg/kg/d or 400 mg/d)

Partial Seizures, Clients Receiving Valproic Acid

Adult: **PO** Start with 25 mg q.o.d. for 2 wk, then 25 mg q.d. for 2 wk; may titrate up to 150 mg/d in 2 divided doses (max 200 mg/d)
Child: **PO** *2–16 y,* 0.2 mg/kg/d times 2 wk, then 0.5 mg/kg/d × 2 wk, then 1 mg/kg/d (max 5 mg/kg/d or 250 mg/d)

ADMINISTRATION

Oral

- Note: Reduced dose may be warranted with renal and hepatic impairment.
- Ensure that chewable tablets are chewed or crushed before being swallowed with a liquid.
- When discontinued, drug should be tapered off gradually over a 2-wk period, unless client safety is at risk.

ADVERSE EFFECTS (≥1%) **CNS:** *Dizziness, ataxia, somnolence, headache,* aphasia, vertigo, confusion, slurred speech, irritability, depression, incoordination, hostility. **GI:** *Nausea,* vomiting, anorexia, abdominal pain, diarrhea, dyspepsia, constipation. **Urogenital:** Hematuria, dysmenorrhea, vaginitis. **Special Senses:** *Diplopia, blurred vision.* **Musculoskeletal:** Peripheral neuropathy, chills, tremor, arthralgia. **Skin:** Rash (<u>including Stevens-Johnson syndrome, toxic epidermal necrolysis</u>), urticaria, pruritus, alopecia, acne. **Respiratory:** *Rhinitis,* pharyngitis, cough.

INTERACTIONS Drug: Carbamazepine, phenobarbital, primidone, phenytoin, fosphenytoin may decrease lamotrigine levels. **Valproic acid** may increase lamotrigine levels. Lamotrigine may decrease serum levels of **valproic acid. Herbal: Ginkgo** may decrease anticonvulsant effectiveness.

PHARMACOKINETICS Absorption: Readily absorbed from GI tract; 98% reaches systemic circulation. **Onset:** 12 wk. **Peak:** 1–4 h. **Distribution:** 55% protein bound; crosses placenta; distributed into breast milk. **Metabolism:** Metabolized in liver to inactive metabolite. **Elimination:** Can induce own metabolism; excreted in urine. **Half-Life:** 25–30 h.

NURSING IMPLICATIONS

Assessment & Drug Effects

- Withhold drug if rash develops and immediately report to prescriber.
- Monitor the plasma levels of lamotrigine and other anticonvulsants when given concomitantly.
- Monitor for adverse reactions when lamotrigine is used with other anticonvulsants, especially valproic acid.
- Be aware of drug interactions and closely monitor when interacting drugs are added or discontinued.

Client & Family Education

- Bipolar disorder is easier to stabilize when medication is taken consistently over long periods of time.
- Notify prescriber for any of the following: skin rash, ataxia, blurred vision or diplopia, fever or flu-like symptoms.
- Do not drive or engage in other potentially hazardous activities until response to the drug is known.
- Use protection from sunlight or ultraviolet light until tolerance is known; drug increases photosensitivity.
- Schedule periodic ophthalmologic exams with long-term use.
- Do not discontinue lamotrigine abruptly.
- Do not breast feed while taking this drug.

LEVETIRACETAM

(lev-e-tir′a-ce-tam)

Keppra

Classifications: CENTRAL NERVOUS SYSTEM AGENT; ANTICONVULSANT

Pregnancy Category: C

AVAILABILITY 250 mg, 500 mg, 750 mg tablets

ACTIONS The precise mechanism of antiepileptic effects is unknown. It is a broad-spectrum antiepileptic agent, which does not involve GABA inhibition.

THERAPEUTIC EFFECTS Inhibits complex partial seizures and prevents epileptic and seizure activity.

USES Adjunctive therapy for partial onset seizures in adults.
UNLABELED USES Add-on therapy for mood stabilization

CONTRAINDICATIONS Hypersensitivity to levetiracetam; labor and delivery.
CAUTIOUS USE Renal impairment; older adults; pregnancy (category C), lactation; suicidal tendencies. Safety and efficacy in children <16 y are not established.

ROUTE & DOSAGE

Partial Onset Seizures

Adult: **PO** 500 mg b.i.d.; may increase by 500 mg b.i.d. q2wk (max 3000 mg/d)

Renal Impairment

Cl_{cr} 50–80 mL/min: 500–1000 mg q12h; 30–50 mL/min: 250–750 mg q12h; <30 mL/min: 250–500 mg q12h; hemodialysis: 500–1000 mg q24h

ADMINISTRATION

Oral

- Reduced doses are indicated when creatinine clearance is 80 mL/min.
- Make dosage increment changes at 2-wk intervals.
- Taper dose if discontinued.
- Give supplemental doses to dialysis clients after dialysis.
- Store at 15°–30° C (59°–86° F).

ADVERSE EFFECTS (≥1%) **Body as a Whole:** *Asthenia, headache, infection,* pain. **CNS:** *Somnolence,* amnesia, anxiety, ataxia, depression, dizziness, emotional lability, hostility, nervousness, vertigo. **GI:** Anorexia. **Respiratory:** Cough, pharyngitis, rhinitis, sinusitis. **Special Senses:** Diplopia.

INTERACTIONS No clinically significant interactions established.

PHARMACOKINETICS **Absorption:** Rapidly and almost completely absorbed. **Peak:** 1 h; steady state 2 d. **Distribution:** <10% protein bound. **Metabolism:** Minimal hepatic metabolism. **Elimination:** Renally eliminated. **Half-Life:** 7.1 h (9.6 h in older adults).

NURSING IMPLICATIONS

Assessment & Drug Effects

- Monitor and notify prescriber of difficulty with gait or coordination.
- Lab tests: Periodic CBC with differential, Hct & Hgb, LFTs.
- Monitor for changes in phenytoin blood levels with coadministered drugs.

Client & Family Education

- Bipolar disorder is easier to stabilize when medication is taken consistently over long periods of time.
- Do not drive or engage in potentially hazardous activities until response to drug is known.
- Do not abruptly discontinue drug. MUST use gradual dose reduction/taper.
- Notify prescriber of intention to become pregnant.
- Do not breast feed while taking this drug without consulting prescriber.

LITHIUM CARBONATE

(li'thee-um)

Eskalith, Eskalith CR, Lithane, Lithobid, Lithonate, Lithotabs

LITHIUM CITRATE

Cibalith-S

Classifications: CENTRAL NERVOUS SYSTEM AGENT; PSYCHOTHERAPEUTIC AGENT; ANTIMANIC

Pregnancy Category: D

AVAILABILITY **Lithium Carbonate** 150 mg, 300 mg, 600 mg capsules; 300 mg tablets; 300 mg, 450 mg sustained-release tablets **Lithium Citrate** 300 mg/5 mL syrup

ACTIONS The lithium ion behaves in the body much like the sodium ion, but its exact mechanism of action is unclear. Competes with various physiologically important cations: Na^+, K^+, Ca^{2+}, Mg^{2+}; therefore, it affects cell membranes, body water, and neurotransmitters. At the synapse, it accelerates catecholamine destruction, inhibits the release of neurotransmitters, and decreases sensitivity of postsynaptic receptors.

THERAPEUTIC EFFECTS Inhibits neurotransmitters; decreases overactivity of receptors involved in stimulating manic states. Response evidenced by changed facial affect, improved posture, assumption of self-care, improved ability to concentrate, improved sleep pattern.

USES Control and prophylaxis of acute mania and the acute manic phase of mixed bipolar disorder.
UNLABELED USES Acute and recurrent depression (unipolar affective disorder), schizophrenic disorders, disorders of impulse control, alcohol dependence, antineoplastic drug-induced neutropenia, aplastic anemia, SIADH, cyclic neutropenia.

CONTRAINDICATIONS Significant cardiovascular or kidney disease, brain damage, severe debilitation, dehydration or sodium depletion; clients on low-salt diet or receiving diuretics; pregnancy, especially first trimester (category D), lactation, children <12 y.
CAUTIOUS USE Older adults; thyroid disease; epilepsy; concomitant use with haloperidol and other antipsychotics; parkinsonism; diabetes mellitus; severe infections; urinary retention.

ROUTE & DOSAGE

Mania

Adult: **PO Loading Dose** 600 mg t.i.d. or 900 mg sustained-release b.i.d. or 30 mL (48 mEq) of solution t.i.d. **PO Maintenance Dose** 300 mg t.i.d. or q.i.d. or 15–20 mL (24–32 mEq) solution in 2–4 divided doses (max 2.4 g/d)
Child: **PO** 15–60 mg/kg/d in divided doses

ADMINISTRATION

Oral

- Give with meals.
- Ensure that sustained-release tablets are not chewed or crushed; must be swallowed whole.
- Protect from light and moisture.

ADVERSE EFFECTS (≥1%) **CNS:** Dizziness, *headache, lethargy,* drowsiness, *fatigue,* slurred speech, psychomotor retardation, giddiness, incontinence, restlessness, seizures, confusion, blackout spells, disorientation, *recent memory loss,* stupor, coma, EEG changes. **CV:** Arrhythmias, hypotension, vasculitis, <u>peripheral circulatory collapse</u>, ECG changes. **Special Senses:** Impaired vision, transient scotomas, tinnitus. **Endocrine:** Diffuse thyroid enlargement, hypothyroidism, *nephrogenic diabetes insipidus,* transient hyperglycemia, glycosuria, hyponatremia. **GI:** *Nausea, vomiting, anorexia, abdominal pain, diarrhea, dry mouth,* metallic taste. **Musculoskeletal:** *Fine hand tremors,* coarse tremors, choreoathetotic movements; fasciculations, clonic movements, incoordination including ataxia, *muscle weakness,* hyperreflexia, encephalopathic syndrome (weakness, lethargy, fever, tremors, confusion, extrapyramidal symptoms). **Skin:** Thought to be toxicity rather than allergy: Pruritus, maculopapular rash, hyperkeratosis, chronic folliculitis, transient acneiform papules (face, neck, intertriginous areas), anesthesia of skin, cutaneous ulcers, drying and thinning of hair, allergic vasculitis. **Hematologic:** *Reversible leukocytosis* (14,000 to 18,000/mm^3). **Urogenital:** Albuminuria, oliguria, urinary incontinence, polyuria, polydipsia, increased uric acid excretion. **Body as a Whole:** Edema, weight gain (common) or loss, exacerbation of psoriasis; flu-like symptoms.

INTERACTIONS Drug: Carbamazepine, haloperidol, PHENOTHIAZINES increase risk of neurotoxicity, extrapyramidal effects, and tardive dyskinesias; DIURETICS, NSAIDS, **methyldopa, probenecid,** TETRACYCLINES decrease renal clearance of lithium, increasing pharmacologic and toxic effects; THEOPHYLLINES, **urea, sodium bicarbonate, sodium or potassium citrate** increase renal clearance of lithium, decreasing its pharmacologic effects.

PHARMACOKINETICS Absorption: Readily absorbed from GI tract. **Peak:** 0.5–3 h carbonate; 15–60 min citrate. **Distribution:** Crosses blood–brain barrier and placenta; distributed into breast milk. **Metabolism:** Not metabolized. **Elimination:** 95% excreted in urine, 1% in feces, 4–5% in sweat. **Half-Life:** 20–27 h.

NURSING IMPLICATIONS

Assessment & Drug Effects

- Monitor response to drug. Usual lag of 1–2 wk precedes response to lithium therapy. Keep prescriber informed of progress.
- Monitor lithium level: Generally dosage regimen is designed to maintain serum lithium levels of 1.0–1.5 mEq/L in acute mania and 0.6–1.6 mEq/L during maintenance treatment; blood sample to determine serum lithium level is drawn prior to next dose (8–12 h after last dose) when lithium level is fairly stable.

- Monitor for S&S of lithium toxicity, often when lithium levels are 1.5–2.0 mEq/L (e.g., vomiting, diarrhea, lack of coordination, drowsiness, muscular weakness, slurred speech). Withhold one dose and call prescriber. Drug should not be stopped abruptly.
- When lithium levels are above 2.0 mEq/L, symptoms may include ataxia, blurred vision, giddiness, tinnitus, muscle twitching or coarse tremors, and a large output of dilute urine.
- Weigh client daily; check ankles, tibiae, and wrists for edema. Report changes in I&O ratio, sudden weight gain, or edema.
- Polydipsia and polyuria, apparently not dose related, are common early adverse effects, particularly in older adults. Symptoms may lessen but reappear after several months or even years of maintenance.
- Report early signs of extrapyramidal reactions promptly to prescriber. The encephalopathic syndrome may be induced when lithium is given concomitantly with haloperidol or with other antipsychotic medication, particularly in older adults.
- Keep prescriber informed of all presenting S&S. The fine tremor of hand or jaw, polyuria, mild thirst, transient mild nausea, and general discomfort that may occur in early treatment of mania sometimes persist throughout therapy. Usually, however, symptoms subside with temporary reduction of dose. If symptoms persist, drug is withdrawn.
- Monitor thyroid function periodically. Be alert to and report symptoms of hypothyroidism.
- Neonates born of mothers who took lithium during pregnancy may have high serum lithium level manifested by flaccidity, poor reflexes, cardiac dysrhythmia, and chronic twitching.
- Lithane contains tartrazine, which may cause an allergic-type reaction in susceptible clients.
- Monitor older adults carefully to prevent toxicity, which may occur at serum levels ordinarily tolerated by other clients.

Client & Family Education

- Bipolar disorder is easier to stabilize when medication is taken consistently over long periods of time.
- Be alert to increased output of dilute urine and persistent thirst. Dose reduction may be indicated.
- Contact prescriber if diarrhea or fever develops. Avoid practices that may encourage dehydration: Hot environment, excessive caffeine beverages (diuresis).
- Drink plenty of liquids (2–3 L/d) during stabilization period and at least 1.5 L/d during ongoing therapy.

- Avoid self-prescribed low-salt regimen and high-sodium foods (e.g., prepared meats and diet soda); avoid self-dosing with Rolaids, Soda-mints, or other sodium antacids. Avoid also crash diets or diet pills that reduce appetite and food, salt, and fluid intake.
- Reduced intake of fluid and sodium can accelerate lithium retention with subsequent toxicity. Conversely, marked increase in sodium intake can increase lithium excretion and reduce drug effect.
- Do not drive or engage in other potentially hazardous activities until response to drug is known. Lithium may impair both physical and mental ability.
- Use effective contraceptive measures during lithium therapy. If therapy is continued during pregnancy, serum lithium levels must be closely monitored to prevent toxicity. Kidney clearance of lithium increases during pregnancy but reverts to lower rate immediately after delivery; dosage is reduced to prevent toxicity.
- Follow a regular clinical evaluation schedule on serum lithium levels to ensure safe and effective treatment. It is important to you and your family to keep all clinic appointments.
- Do not breast feed while taking this drug.

OLANZAPINE

(o-lan'za-peen)

FLUOXETINE HYDROCHLORIDE

(flu'ox-e-tine)

Symbyax (SIMM-bee-ax)

See Antipsychotics, Olanzapine and Antidepressants, Selective Serotonin-Reuptake Inhibitors, Fluoxetine Hydrochloride for details in all categories about the individual medications that make up this compound.

Classifications: CENTRAL NERVOUS SYSTEM AGENT; PSYCHOTHERAPEUTIC; NEUROLEPTIC AGENT; ATYPICAL; SEROTONIN-REUPTAKE INHIBITOR (SSRI); MOOD STABILIZER

Pregnancy Category: C

AVAILABILITY Available in four dosage option capsules (olanzapine/fluoxetine HCl): 6 mg/25 mg, 6 mg/50 mg, 12 mg/25 mg, 12 mg/50 mg

ACTIONS Although the exact mechanism of Symbyax is unknown, it has been proposed that the activation of three monoaminergic neural systems (serotonin, norepinephrine, and dopamine) is responsible for its enhanced antidepressant effect. This is supported by animal studies in which the olanzapine/fluoxetine combination has been shown to produce synergistic increases in norepinephrine and dopamine release in the prefrontal cortex compared with either component alone, as well as increases in serotonin.

THERAPEUTIC EFFECTS Produces antipsychotic, antidepressant, and anticholinergic activity.

USE Treatment for bipolar depression. Symbyax is a combination of **olanzapine** (the active ingredient in Zyprexa) and **fluoxetine** (the active ingredient in Prozac) indicated for the treatment of depressive episodes associated with bipolar disorder.

CONTRAINDICATIONS Hypersensitivity to olanzapine; pregnancy (category C), lactation. Hypersensitivity to fluoxetine (category B) or other SSRI drugs. Symbyax should not be administered until at least 2 wk have passed since discontinuing an MAOI, and an MAOI is contraindicated for at least 5 wk after discontinuation with Symbyax. **Thioridazine** should not be administered with Symbyax or within a minimum of 5 wk after discontinuing Symbyax. Symbyax should be discontinued immediately if rash or other possible allergic phenomena appear for which an alternative explanation cannot be identified. Concomitant use with NSAIDs, ASA, or other drugs that affect coagulation.

CAUTIOUS USE Known cardiovascular disease, cerebrovascular disease. Although Symbyax is not approved for elderly patients with dementia it is important to note that the label for Symbyax includes a warning for patients in this population. The warning states that strokes or mini-strokes (also called transient ischemic attacks or TIAs), including fatalities, were reported in elderly patients with dementia-related psychosis participating in clinical trials for olanzapine, an active ingredient in Symbyax. In fact, Symbyax has not been studied in elderly patients with dementia, nor do we expect Symbyax to be used to treat these patients.

In conditions that predispose to hypotension (i.e., dehydration, hypovolemia), history of syncope; Symbyax may induce orthostatic hypotension (a drop in blood pressure when standing up), associated with dizziness, speeding or slowing of heart rate, and in some patients, fainting, especially during initial therapy.

Symbyax prescribing should be consistent with the need to minimize the risk of neuroleptic malignant syndrome, tardive dyskinesia, and orthostatic hypotension. Hepatic impairment, concurrent use of hepatotoxic drugs. Hyperglycemia and diabetes mellitus should be monitored regularly for worsening glucose control. Safety and effectiveness in children <18 y are not established.

ROUTE & DOSAGE

Psychotic Disorders

Adult: **PO** Start with the 6 mg/25 mg capsule once daily in the evening; may increase through the dosage options to 12 mg/50 mg capsule until desired response
Geriatric: **PO** Start with 5 mg once daily

Bipolar Mania

Adult: **PO** 6 mg/25 mg capsule once daily in the evening. Dose escalation with caution.

ADMINISTRATION

Oral

- Store at 25° C (77° F). Keep tightly closed and protect from moisture.

ADVERSE EFFECTS (≥1%) **Body as a Whole:** *Weight gain, swelling,* prescribe to minimize risk of neuroleptic malignant syndrome and tardive dyskinesia, hyponatremia. **CNS:** *Drowsiness,* somnolence, *difficulty concentrating, tremor.* **CV:** Orthostatic hypotension, associated with dizziness, speeding or slowing of heart rate, and in some patients, fainting, especially during initial therapy. **GI:** *Increased appetite, sore throat,* abdominal pain, constipation, dry mouth, increased appetite, increased salivation, nausea, vomiting, elevated liver function tests. *Nausea, diarrhea,* anorexia, dyspepsia, abnormal bleeding, dysphagia. **Special Senses:** *Feeling weak,* disruption of body's ability to reduce core body temperature, hyperprolactinemia. **Endocrine:** Hyperglycemia, in some cases associated with ketoacidosis, coma, or death, has been reported in patients treated with atypical antipsychotics, including olanzapine, and concomitant olanzapine and fluoxetine. Assessment of the relationship between atypical antipsychotic use and glucose abnormalities is complicated by the possibility of an increased background risk of diabetes mellitus in patients with schizophrenia and the increasing incidence of diabetes mellitus in the general population. The available data are insufficient to provide reliable estimates of differences in hyperglycemia-related adverse-event risk among the marketed atypical antipsychotics. All patients taking atypicals should be monitored for symptoms of hyperglycemia. Persons with diabetes who are started on atypicals should be monitored regularly for worsening of glucose control; those with risk factors for diabetes should undergo baseline and periodic fasting blood-glucose testing. Patients who develop symptoms of hyperglycemia during treatment should undergo fasting blood-glucose testing.

INTERACTIONS Drug: Symbyax should not be administered until at least 2 wk have passed since discontinuing an MAOI, and an MAOI is contraindicated for at least 5 wk after discontinuation with Symbyax. **Thioridazine** should not be administered with Symbyax or within a minimum of 5 wk after discontinuing Symbyax. Symbyax should be discontinued immediately if rash or other possible allergic phenomena appear for which an alternative explanation cannot be identified. Because of olanzapine's potential to induce hypotension, Symbyax may enhance hypotensive effects of ANTIHYPERTENSIVES. The olanzapine component of Symbyax may antagonize the effects of levadopa and DOPAMINE AGONISTS. May enhance effects of other CNS ACTIVE DRUGS, **alcohol. Diazepam** with olanzapine potentiated the orthostatic hypotension observed with olanzapine. **Diazepam** with fluoxetine prolonged the half-life of diazepam in some patients. **Alprazolam** with fluoxetine increased alprazolam plasma concentrations. **Carbamazepine, omeprazole, rifampin** may increase metabolism and clearance of olanzapine. **Fluvoxamine** may inhibit metabolism and clearance of olanzapine. Elevation of blood levels of **clozapine, haloperidol, phenytoin** seen with fluoxetine. **Herbal: St. John's wort** may cause **serotonin** syndrome (headache, dizziness, sweating, agitation).

PHARMACOKINETICS The pharmacokinetics of the individual components is expected to reasonably characterize the overall pharmacokinetics of the combination. **Absorption:** Effect of food on absorption and bioavailability of the medications in combination has not been evaluated, but is unlikely. **Peak:** Olanzapine and fluoxetine 4 and 6 h, respectively. **Distribution:** The *in vitro* binding to human plasma proteins of the olanzapine/fluoxetine combination is similar to the binding of the individual components. **Metabolism:** Steady state concentrations of norfluoxetine were similar to those seen with fluoxetine in the therapeutic dose range. The complexity of the metabolism of fluoxetine has several consequences that may potentially affect the clinical use of Symbyax. About 7% of the population has reduced activity of CYP2D6 and are therefore poor metabolizers. See DRUG INTERACTIONS. **Elimination:** Fluoxetine has a relatively slow elimination. **Half-Life:** Fluoxetine 1–3 d after acute administration, 4–6 d after chronic administration; norfluoxetine 4–16 d after acute and chronic administration. Active drug substance will persist in the body for weeks. The pharmacokinetics of Symbyax may be altered in geriatric patients (elimination half-life approximately 1.5 times greater in elderly).

NURSING IMPLICATIONS

Assessment & Drug Effects

- Due to the cyclical nature of bipolar disorder, patients should be monitored for the signs of mania and hypomania during treatment with Symbyax.
- Patients should inform their prescribers if they are taking Zyprexa, Prozac, Sarafem, or fluoxetine.
- Patients at high risk for suicide should be closely monitored. Prescribe smallest quantity for management to reduce risk of overdosage.
- Withhold drug and immediately report S&S of neuroleptic malignant syndrome; assess for and report S&S of tardive dyskinesia.
- Lab tests: Periodically monitor ALT, especially in those with hepatic dysfunction or being treated with other potentially hepatotoxic drugs.
- Monitor BP and HR periodically. Monitor temperature, especially under conditions such as strenuous exercise, extreme heat, or treatment with other anticholinergic drugs.
- Monitor for seizures, especially in older adults and persons with cognitive impairments.
- Monitor for diabetes, worsening of glucose control; those with risk factors should undergo fasting glucose testing at baseline and periodically throughout treatment.
- Use with caution in the older adult patient or patient with impaired renal or hepatic function (may need lower dose).
- Check that patient is not self-treating with **St. John's wort** because it is a botanical MAOI.
- Report significant weight change to prescriber.
- Observe for and promptly report rash or urticaria and S&S of fever, leukocytosis, arthralgias, carpal tunnel syndrome, edema, respiratory distress, and proteinuria. Drug may have to be

discontinued or adjunctive therapy instituted with steroids or antihistamines.
- Observe for dizziness and drowsiness and employ safety measures (assistance, up with side rails, etc.) as indicated.
- Monitor for and report increased anxiety, nervousness, or insomnia; may need modification of drug dose.
- Monitor for seizures in patients with a history of seizures. Use appropriate safety precautions.
- Supervise patients closely who are high suicide risks; especially during initial therapy.
- Monitor patients with hepatic or renal impairment carefully for S&S of toxicity (e.g., agitation, restlessness, nausea, vomiting, seizures).

Client & Family Education
- Notify prescriber of intent to become pregnant.
- Notify prescriber of any rash; possible sign of a serious group of adverse effects.
- Do not self-treat with **St. John's wort** because it is a botanical MAOI and cannot be combined with this medication.
- Monitor blood glucose for loss of glycemic control if diabetic.
- Note: Drug may increase seizure activity in those with history of seizure.
- Do not drive or engage in potentially hazardous activities until response to drug is known; drug increases risk of orthostatic hypotension and cognitive impairment.
- Learn healthy eating habits, exercise reasonably, and monitor for weight gain.
- Take drug as prescribed for continued mood stabilization.
- Learn common adverse effects and possible drug interactions.
- Avoid alcohol and do not take additional medications without informing prescriber.
- Do not become overheated; avoid conditions leading to dehydration.
- Do not breast feed while taking this drug.

OXCARBAZEPINE
(oc-car′ba-ze-peen)
Trileptal
Classifications: CENTRAL NERVOUS SYSTEM AGENT; ANTICONVULSANT
Pregnancy Category: C

AVAILABILITY 150 mg, 300 mg, 600 mg tablets; 300 mg/5 mL suspension

ACTIONS Structurally related to tricyclic antidepressants (TCAs) but lacks antidepressant properties. Anticonvulsant properties may result from blockage of voltage-sensitive sodium channels, which results in stabilization of hyperexcited neural membranes.
THERAPEUTIC EFFECTS Inhibits repetitive neuronal firing, and decreased propagation of neuronal impulses.

USES Monotherapy or adjunctive therapy in the treatment of partial seizures in adults and children age 4–16.
UNLABELED USES Therapy for mood stabilization, treatment for eating disorders.

CONTRAINDICATIONS Hypersensitivity to oxcarbazepine; pregnancy (category C), lactation; children <4 y.
CAUTIOUS USE Older adults; renal impairment; children <8 y; infertility, hyponatremia, SIADH, and drugs associated with SIADH as an adverse effect.

ROUTE & DOSAGE

Partial Seizures

Adult: **PO** Start with 300 mg b.i.d. and increase by 600 mg/d qwk to 2400 mg/d in 2 divided doses for monotherapy or 1200 mg/d as adjunctive therapy
Child: **PO** *4–16 y,* Initiate with 8–10 mg/kg/d divided b.i.d. (max 600 mg/d), gradually increase weekly to target dose (divided b.i.d.) based on weight: *20–29 kg,* 900 mg/d; *29.1–39 kg,* 1200 mg/d; *>39 kg,* 1800 mg/d

Renal Impairment

Cl_{cr} <30 mL/min: Initiate at 1/2 usual starting dose (300 mg b.i.d.)

ADMINISTRATION

Oral

- Initiate therapy at one-half the usual starting dose (300 mg/d) if creatinine clearance <30 mL/min.
- Do not abruptly stop this medication; withdraw drug gradually when discontinued to minimize seizure potential.
- Store preferably at 25° C (77° F), but room temperature permitted. Keep container tightly closed.

ADVERSE EFFECTS (≥1%) **Body as a Whole:** *Fatigue,* asthenia, peripheral edema, generalized edema, chest pain, weight gain. **CV:** Hypotension. **GI:** *Nausea, vomiting, abdominal pain,* diarrhea, dyspepsia, constipation, gastritis, anorexia, dry mouth. **Hematologic:** Lymphadenopathy. **Metabolic:** Hyponatremia. **Musculoskeletal:** Muscle weakness. **CNS:** *Headache, dizziness, somnolence, ataxia, nystagmus, abnormal gait,* insomnia, tremor, nervousness, agitation, abnormal coordination, speech disorder, confusion, abnormal thinking, aggravation of convulsions, emotional lability. **Respiratory:** Rhinitis, cough, bronchitis, pharyngitis. **Skin:** Acne, hot flushes, purpura. **Special Senses:** *Diplopia, vertigo, abnormal vision,* abnormal accommodation, taste perversion, earache. **Urogenital:** Urinary tract infection, micturition frequency, vaginitis.

INTERACTIONS Drug: Carbamazepine, phenobarbital, phenytoin, valproic acid, verapamil may decrease oxcarbazepine levels; may increase levels of **phenobarbital, phenytoin;** may decrease levels of **felodipine,** ORAL CONTRACEPTIVES. **Herbal: Ginkgo** may decrease anticonvulsant effectiveness.

PHARMACOKINETICS Absorption: Rapidly and completely absorbed from GI tract. **Peak:** Steady state levels reached in 2–3 d. **Distribution:** 40% protein bound. **Metabolism:** Extensively metabolized in liver to active 10-monohydroxy metabolite (MHD). **Elimination:** 95% excreted in kidneys. **Half-Life:** 2 h, MHD 9 h.

NURSING IMPLICATIONS

Assessment & Drug Effects

- Monitor for and report S&S of hyponatremia (e.g., nausea, malaise, headache, lethargy, confusion), CNS impairment (e.g., somnolence, excessive fatigue, cognitive deficits, speech or language problems, incoordination, gait disturbances).
- Monitor phenytoin levels when administered concurrently.
- Lab tests: Periodic serum sodium, T_4 level.

Client & Family Education

- Bipolar disorder is easier to stabilize when medication is taken consistently over long periods of time.
- Notify prescriber of the following: Dizziness, excess drowsi-

ness, frequent headaches, malaise, double vision, lack of coordination, or persistent nausea.
- Exercise special caution with concurrent use of alcohol or CNS depressants.
- Use caution with potentially hazardous activities and driving until response to drug is known.
- Use or add barrier contraceptive since drug may render hormonal contraceptive methods ineffective.
- Do not breast feed while taking this drug.

TIAGABINE HYDROCHLORIDE

(ti-a′ ga-been)

Gabitril Filmtabs

Classifications: CENTRAL NERVOUS SYSTEM AGENT; ANTICONVULSANT; GABA INHIBITOR

Pregnancy Category: C

AVAILABILITY 2 mg, 4 mg, 12 mg, 16 mg, 20 mg tablets

ACTIONS GABA inhibitor for the treatment of partial epilepsy. Potent and selective inhibitor of GABA uptake into presynaptic neurons; allows more GABA to bind to the surfaces of postsynaptic neurons in the CNS.

THERAPEUTIC EFFECTS Effectiveness indicated by reduction in seizure activity.

USES Adjunctive therapy for partial seizures.

UNLABELED USES Therapy for mood stabilization.

CONTRAINDICATIONS Hypersensitivity to tiagabine; pregnancy (category C).

CAUTIOUS USE Liver function impairment; lactation; history of spike and wave discharge on EEG; status epilepticus.

ROUTE & DOSAGE

Seizures

Adult: **PO** Start with 4 mg q.d.; may increase dose by 4–8 mg/d qwk (max 56 mg/d in 2–4 divided doses)

Adolescent: **PO** *12–18 y,* Start with 4 mg q.d., after 2 wk may increase dose by 4–8 mg/d qwk (max 32 mg/d in 2–4 divided doses)

ADMINISTRATION

Oral

- Give with food.
- Make dosage increases, when needed, at weekly intervals.
- Store at 15°–30° C (59°–86° F) in a tightly closed container and protect from light.

ADVERSE EFFECTS (≥1%) **Body as a Whole:** Infection, flu-like syndrome, pain, myasthenia, allergic reactions, chills, malaise, arthralgia. **CNS:** *Dizziness, asthenia, tremor, somnolence, nervousness,* difficulty concentrating, ataxia, depression, insomnia, abnormal gait, hostility, confusion, speech disorder, difficulty with memory, paresthesias, emotional lability, agitation, dysarthria, euphoria, hallucinations, hyperkinesia, hypertonia, hypotonia, myoclonus, twitching, vertigo. **CV:** Vasodilation, hypertension, palpitations, tachycardia, syncope, edema, peripheral edema. **GI:** Abdominal pain, diarrhea, nausea, vomiting, increased appetite, mouth ulcers. **Respiratory:** Pharyngitis, cough, bronchitis, dyspnea, epistaxis, pneumonia. **Skin:** Rash, pruritus, alopecia, dry skin, sweating, ecchymoses. **Special Senses:** Amblyopia, nystagmus, tinnitus. **Urogenital:** Dysmenorrhea, dysuria, metrorrhagia, incontinence, vaginitis, UTI.

INTERACTIONS Drug: Carbamazepine, phenytoin, phenobarbital decrease levels of tiagabine. **Herbal: Ginkgo** may decrease anticonvulsant effectiveness.

PHARMACOKINETICS Absorption: Rapidly absorbed; 90% bioavailability. **Peak:** 45 min. **Distribution:** 96% protein bound. **Metabolism:** Metabolized in liver, probably by cytochrome P-450 3A isoform. **Elimination:** 25% excreted in urine, 63% excreted in feces. **Half-Life:** 7–9 h (4–7 h with other enzyme-inducing drugs).

NURSING IMPLICATIONS

Assessment & Drug Effects

- Lab tests: Measure plasma levels of tiagabine before and after changes are made in the drug regimen.
- Be aware that concurrent use of other anticonvulsants may decrease effectiveness of tiagabine or increase the potential for adverse effects.
- Monitor carefully for S&S of CNS depression.

Client & Family Education

- Do not stop taking drug abruptly; may cause sudden onset of seizures.
- Bipolar disorder is easier to stabilize when medication is taken consistently over long periods of time.
- Exercise caution while engaging in potentially hazardous activities because drug may cause dizziness.
- Use caution when taking other prescription or OTC drugs that can cause drowsiness.
- Report any of the following to the prescriber: Rash or hives; red, peeling skin; dizziness; drowsiness; depression; GI distress; nervousness or tremors; difficulty concentrating or talking.
- Do not breast feed while taking this drug without consulting prescriber.

TOPIRAMATE

(to-pir'a-mate)

Topamax

Classifications: CENTRAL NERVOUS SYSTEM AGENT; ANTICONVULSANT

Pregnancy Category: C

AVAILABILITY 25 mg, 100 mg, 200 mg tablets; 15 mg, 25 mg, 50 mg capsules

ACTIONS Sulfamate-substituted monosaccharide with a broad spectrum of anticonvulsant activity. Its precise mechanism of action is unknown. Exhibits sodium channel blocking action, as well as enhancing the ability of GABA to induce a flux of chloride ions into the neurons, thus potentiating the activity of this inhibitory neurotransmitter (GABA).

THERAPEUTIC EFFECTS Indicated by a decrease in seizure activity. Effectively controls partial-onset seizures in adults and children by inhibiting GABA.

USE Adjunctive therapy for partial-onset seizures in adults and in children age 2–16 y.

UNLABELED USE Adjunctive mood stabilizer for pharmacotherapy in bipolar disorder.

CONTRAINDICATIONS Hypersensitivity to topiramate. Effect on labor and delivery is unknown.

CAUTIOUS USE Renal impairment, hepatic impairment; pregnancy (category C), lactation. While topiramate has been studied in patients 2–17 y of age, safety and effectiveness in children are not established.

ROUTE & DOSAGE

Partial-Onset Seizures

Adult: **PO** Initiate with 25 mg b.i.d., increase by 50 mg/wk to efficacy **PO Maintenance Dose** 200–400 mg/d divided b.i.d. (max 1600 mg/d)
Child: **PO** *2–16 y,* Initiate with 1–3 mg/kg h.s. times 1 wk, then increase by 1–3 mg/kg/d in 2 divided doses q1–2wk to a target range of 5–9 mg/kg/d

Renal Impairment

Cl_{cr} <70 mL/min: decrease dose by 50%

ADMINISTRATION

Oral

- Make dosage increments of 50 mg at weekly intervals to the recommended dose, usually 400 mg/d.
- Do not break tablets unless absolutely necessary because of bitter taste.
- Store at 15°–30° C (59°–86° F) in a tightly closed container. Protect from light and moisture.

ADVERSE EFFECTS (≥1%) **Body as a Whole:** *Fatigue, speech problems,* weight loss. **CNS:** *Somnolence, dizziness, ataxia, psychomotor slowing, confusion, nystagmus, paresthesia, memory difficulty, difficulty concentrating, nervousness,* depression, anxiety, tremor. **GI:** Anorexia. **Special Senses:** Oligohidrosis (decreased sweating) and hyperthermia—especially in hot weather—have been added to the warning on topiramate labeling; angle-closure glaucoma (rare).

INTERACTIONS Drug: Increased CNS depression with **alcohol** and other CNS DEPRESSANTS; may increase **phenytoin** concentrations; may decrease ORAL CONTRACEPTIVE, **valproate** concentrations; may increase risk of kidney stone formation with other CARBONIC ANHYDRASE INHIBITORS. **Carbamazepine, phenytoin, valproate** may decrease topiramate concentrations. **Herb: Ginkgo** may decrease anticonvulsant effectiveness.

PHARMACOKINETICS Absorption: Rapidly absorbed from GI tract; 80% bioavailability. **Peak:** 2 h. **Distribution:** 13–17% protein

Common adverse effects in *italic;* life-threatening effects underlined; generic names in **bold;** drug classifications in SMALL CAPS; ♣ Canadian drug name.

bound. **Metabolism:** Minimally metabolized in the liver. **Elimination:** Excreted primarily in urine, therefore much less likely to cause drug interactions via modulation of the P-450 enzymes in the liver. **Half-Life:** 21 h.

NURSING IMPLICATIONS

Assessment & Drug Effects

- Monitor mental status and report significant cognitive impairment.
- Monitor lithium levels because they can be increased by topiramate (occurs outside the P-450 metabolic system.
- Lab tests: Periodically monitor CBC with Hgb and Hct.

Client & Family Education

- Do not stop drug abruptly; discontinue gradually to minimize seizures.
- Bipolar disorder is easier to stabilize when medication is taken consistently over long periods of time.
- Minimize risk of kidney stones—drink at least 6–8 full glasses of water each day.
- Weight loss from decreased appetite may occur. Please monitor.
- Exercise caution with potentially hazardous activities. Sedation is common, especially with concurrent use of alcohol or other CNS depressants.
- Observe for hyperthermia, an elevation of body temperature, and decreased sweating especially in hot weather.
- Use or add barrier contraceptive if using hormonal contraceptives.
- Be aware that psychomotor slowing and speech/language problems may develop while on topiramate therapy.
- Report adverse effects that interfere with activities of daily living.
- Do not breast feed while taking this drug without consulting prescriber.

VALPROIC ACID (DIVALPROEX SODIUM, SODIUM VALPROATE)

(val-proe′ic)

Depacon, Depakene, Depakote, Depakote ER, Depakote Sprinkle, Epival ♣

Classifications: CENTRAL NERVOUS SYSTEM AGENT; ANTICONVULSANT; GABA INHIBITOR

Pregnancy Category: D

AVAILABILITY: 250 mg capsules; 125 mg sprinkle capsules; 125 mg, 250 mg, 500 mg delayed-release tablets; 500 mg sustained-release tablets; 250 mg/5 mL syrup; 100 mg/mL injection

ACTIONS Anticonvulsant unrelated chemically to other drugs used to treat seizure disorders. Mechanism of action unknown; may be related to increased bioavailability of the inhibitory GABA neurotransmitter to brain neurons. Inhibits secondary phase of platelet aggregation.

THERAPEUTIC EFFECTS Depresses abnormal neuron discharges in the CNS, thus decreasing seizure activity.

USES Alone or with other anticonvulsants in management of absence (petit mal) and mixed seizures; mania; migraine headache prophylaxis.

UNLABELED USES Therapy for mood stabilization, status epilepticus refractory to IV diazepam, petit mal variant seizures, febrile seizures in children, other types of seizures including psychomotor (temporal lobe), myoclonic, akinetic and tonic-clonic seizures, photosensitivity seizures, and those refractory to other anticonvulsants.

CONTRAINDICATIONS Patient with bleeding disorders or liver dysfunction or disease, pregnancy (category D), lactation.

CAUTIOUS USE History of kidney disease; adjunctive treatment with other anticonvulsants.

ROUTE & DOSAGE

Management of Seizures, Mania

Adult/Child: **PO/IV** 15 mg/kg/d in divided doses when total daily dose >250 mg, increase at 1-wk intervals by 5–10 mg/kg/d until seizures are controlled or adverse effects develop (max 60 mg/kg/d)

Migraine Headache Prophylaxis

Adult: **PO** 250 mg b.i.d. (max 1000 mg/d) or **Depakote ER** 500 mg q.d. times 1 wk, may increase to 1000 mg q.d.

Mania

Adult: **PO** 250 mg t.i.d. (max 60 mg/kg/d)

ADMINISTRATION

Oral

- Give tablets and capsules whole; instruct patient to swallow whole and to not chew. Instruct to swallow capsules whole or sprinkle entire contents on teaspoonful of soft food, and instruct to not chew food.

- Avoid using a carbonated drink as diluent for the syrup because it will release drug from delivery vehicle; free drug painfully irritates oral and pharyngeal membranes.
- Reduce gastric irritation by administering drug with food because serious GI adverse effects can lead to discontinuation of therapy. Enteric-coated tablet or syrup formulation is usually well tolerated.

Intravenous

PREPARE **IV Infusion:** Dilute each dose in 50 mL or more of D5W, NS, or RL.

ADMINISTER **IV Infusion:** Give a single dose over at least 60 min ($\leq$20 mg/min). Avoid rapid infusion.

INCOMPATIBILITIES **Solution/Additive:** No compatibility data available. Should avoid mixing with other drugs.

ADVERSE EFFECTS ($\geq$1%) **CNS:** Breakthrough seizures, *sedation, drowsiness,* dizziness, increased alertness, hallucinations, emotional upset, aggression; <u>deep coma, death (with overdose)</u>. **GI:** *Nausea, vomiting, indigestion (transient),* hypersalivation, anorexia with weight loss, increased appetite with weight gain, abdominal cramps, diarrhea, constipation, <u>liver failure, pancreatitis</u>. **Hematologic:** *Prolonged bleeding time,* leukopenia, lymphocytosis, thrombocytopenia, hypofibrinogenemia, bone marrow depression, anemia. **Skin:** Skin rash, photosensitivity, transient hair loss, curliness or waviness of hair. **Endocrine:** Irregular menses, secondary amenorrhea. **Metabolic:** Hyperammonemia (usually asymptomatic), hyperammonemic encephalopathy in patients with urea cycle disorders. **Respiratory:** Pulmonary edema (with overdose).

DIAGNOSTIC TEST INTERFERENCE Valproic acid produces false-positive results for ***urine ketones,*** elevated ***AST, ALT, LDH,*** and ***serum alkalinephosphatase,*** prolonged ***bleeding time,*** altered ***thyroidfunction tests.***

INTERACTIONS Drug: Alcohol and other CNS DEPRESSANTS potentiate depressant effects; other ANTICOVULSANTS, BARBITURATES increase or decrease anticonvulsant and barbiturate levels; **haloperidol, loxapine, maprotiline,** MAOIS, PHENOTHIAZINES, THIOXANTHENES, TRICYCLIC ANTIDEPRESSANTS can increase CNS depression or lower seizure threshold; **aspirin, dipyridamole, warfarin** increase risk of spontaneous bleeding and decrease clotting; **clonazepam** may precipitate absence seizures; SALICYLATES, **cimetidine** may increase valproic acid levels and toxicity. **Mefloquine** can decrease valproic acid levels; **isoniazid** may increase valproic acid levels and hepatotoxicity; **meropenem** may decrease valproic acid levels; **cholestyramine** may decrease absorption. **Herbal: Ginkgo** may decrease anticonvulsant effectiveness.

PHARMACOKINETICS Absorption: Readily absorbed from GI tract. **Peak:** 1–4 h valproic acid; 3–5 h divalproex. **Therapeutic Range:** 50–100 g/mL. **Distribution:** Crosses placenta; distributed into breast milk. **Metabolism:** Metabolized in liver. **Elimination:** Excreted primarily in urine; small amount excreted in feces and expired air. **Half-Life:** 5–20 h.

NURSING IMPLICATIONS

Assessment & Drug Effects

- Monitor for therapeutic effectiveness achieved with serum levels of valproic acid at 50–100 mcg/mL.
- Monitor patient alertness especially with multiple drug therapy for seizure control. Evaluate plasma levels of the adjunctive anticonvulsants periodically as indicators of possible neurologic toxicity.
- Monitor patient carefully during dose adjustments and promptly report presence of adverse effects. Increased dosage is associated with frequency of adverse effects.
- Lab tests: Perform baseline platelet counts, bleeding time, and serum ammonia, then repeat at least q2mo, especially during the first 6 mo of therapy.
- Multiple drugs for seizure control increase the risk of hyperammonemia, marked by lethargy, anorexia, asterixis, increased seizure frequency, and vomiting. Report such symptoms promptly to prescriber. If they persist with decreased dosage, the drug will be discontinued.

Client & Family Education

- Do not discontinue therapy abruptly; such action could result in seizures. Consult prescriber before you stop or alter dosage regimen.
- Bipolar disorder is easier to stabilize when medication is taken consistently over long periods of time.
- Note to diabetic patients: Drug may cause a false-positive test for urine ketones. Notify prescriber if this occurs; a differential diagnostic blood test may be indicated.

- Notify prescriber promptly if spontaneous bleeding or bruising occurs (e.g., petechiae, ecchymotic areas, otorrhagia, epistaxis, melena).
- Withhold dose and notify prescriber for following symptoms: Visual disturbances, rash, jaundice, light-colored stools, protracted vomiting, diarrhea. Fatal liver failure has occurred in patients receiving this drug.
- Avoid alcohol and self-medication with other depressants during therapy.
- Consult prescriber before using any OTC drugs during anticonvulsant therapy. Combination drugs containing aspirin, sedatives, and medications for hay fever or other allergies are particularly UNSAFE.
- Do not drive or engage in potentially hazardous activities until response to drug is known.
- Inform doctor or dentist before any kind of surgery that you are taking valproic acid.
- Carry medical identification card at all times. It needs to indicate medical diagnosis, medication(s), prescriber's name, address, and telephone number.
- Do not breast feed while taking this drug.

ZONISAMIDE

(zon-i′sa-mide)

Zonegran

Classifications: CENTRAL NERVOUS SYSTEM AGENT; ANTICONVULSANT; SULFONAMIDE

Pregnancy Category: C

AVAILABILITY 100 mg capsules

ACTIONS Anticonvulsant effective against a variety of seizure types. A sulfonamide derivative and a broad-spectrum anticonvulsant that does not potentiate the activity of GABA in the synapses of the neurons. It does, however, facilitate dopaminergic and serotonergic neurotransmission.
THERAPEUTIC EFFECTS Suppresses focal spike discharges and electroshock seizures.

USES Adjunctive therapy for partial seizures in adults.
UNLABELED USES Therapy for mood stabilization.

CONTRAINDICATIONS Hypersensitivity to sulfonamides or zonisamide; pregnancy (category C), lactation.

CAUTIOUS USE Children <6 y; renal or hepatic insufficiency, concomitant administration of drugs that induce or inhibit CYP3A4; older adults.

ROUTE & DOSAGE

Partial Seizures

Adult: **PO** start at 100 mg q.d.; may increase after 2 wk to 200 mg/d; may then increase q2wk, if necessary (max 400 mg/d in 1–2 divided doses)

ADMINISTRATION

Oral

- Do not crush or break capsules; ensure capsules are swallowed whole with adequate fluid.
- Withdraw drug gradually when discontinued to minimize seizure potential.
- Store at 25° C (77° F); room temperature permitted. Protect from light and moisture.

ADVERSE EFFECTS (≥1%) **Body as a Whole:** Flu-like syndrome, weight loss. **CNS:** Agitation, irritability, anxiety, ataxia, confusion, depression, difficulty concentrating, difficulty with memory, *dizziness,* fatigue, *headache,* insomnia, mental slowing, nervousness, nystagmus, paresthesia, schizophrenic behavior, *somnolence,* tiredness, tremor, convulsion, abnormal gait, hyperesthesia, incoordination. **GI:** Abdominal pain, *anorexia,* constipation, diarrhea, dyspepsia, nausea, dry mouth, flatulence, gingivitis, gum hyperplasia, gastritis, stomatitis, cholelithiasis, glossitis, melena, rectal hemorrhage, ulcerative stomatitis, ulcer, dysphagia. **Metabolic:** Oligohidrosis, sometimes resulting in heat stroke and hyperthermia in children. **Respiratory:** Rhinitis, pharyngitis, cough. **Skin:** Ecchymosis, rash, pruritus. **Special Senses:** Difficulties in verbal expression, diplopia, speech abnormalities, taste perversion, amblyopia, tinnitus. **Urogenital:** Kidney stones.

INTERACTIONS Drug: Phenytoin, carbamazepine, phenobarbital, valproic acid may decrease half-life of zonisamide.

PHARMACOKINETICS Peak: 2–6 h. **Distribution:** 40% protein bound, extensively binds to erythrocytes. **Metabolism:** Acetylated in liver by CYP3A4. **Elimination:** Excreted primarily in urine. **Half-Life:** 63–105 h.

Common adverse effects in *italic;* life-threatening effects underlined; generic names in **bold;** drug classifications in SMALL CAPS; ♣ Canadian drug name.

NURSING IMPLICATIONS

Assessment & Drug Effects

- Withhold drug and notify prescriber if an unexplained rash or S&S of hypersensitivity appear.
- Monitor for and report S&S of CNS impairment (somnolence, excessive fatigue, cognitive deficits, speech or language problems, incoordination, gait disturbances), oligohidrosis (lack of sweating), and hyperthermia in pediatric patients.
- Lab tests: Periodic BUN and serum creatinine, and CBC with differential.

Client & Family Education

- Do not abruptly stop taking this medication.
- Bipolar disorder is easier to stabilize when medication is taken consistently over long periods of time.
- Increase daily fluid intake to minimize risk of renal stones. Notify prescriber immediately of S&S of renal stones: Sudden back or abdominal pain, and blood in urine.
- Report any of the following: Dizziness, excess drowsiness, frequent headaches, malaise, double vision, lack of coordination, persistent nausea, sore throat, fever, mouth ulcers, or easy bruising.
- Exercise special caution with concurrent use of alcohol or CNS depressants.
- Do not drive or engage in other potentially hazardous activities until response to drug is known.
- Do not breast feed while taking this drug.

ANTIDEPRESSANTS

BUPROPION HYDROCHLORIDE

(byoo-pro'pi-on)

Wellbutrin, Wellbutrin SR, Zyban

Classification: CENTRAL NERVOUS SYSTEM AGENT; ANTIDEPRESSANT

Pregnancy Category: B

AVAILABILITY 75 mg, 100 mg tablets; 100 mg, 150 mg, 200 mg sustained-release tablets

ACTIONS The neurochemical mechanism of bupropion is unknown. It does not inhibit monoamine oxidase. Compared to

tricyclic antidepressants (TCA), it is a weak blocker of neural uptake of serotonin and norepinephrine.
THERAPEUTIC EFFECTS Its antidepressive effect is related to CNS stimulant effects.

USES Indicated for mental depression; since it has been associated with increased risk of seizures, it is not the agent of first choice; adjunct for smoking cessation.
UNLABELED USES Cyclic mood disorders, schizoaffective disorders.

CONTRAINDICATIONS Hypersensitivity to bupropion; history of seizure disorder; current or prior diagnosis of bulimia or anorexia nervosa; concurrent administration of a MAOI; head trauma; CNS tumor; recent MI; lactation.
CAUTIOUS USE Renal or hepatic function impairment; drug abuse or dependence; pregnancy (category B).

ROUTE & DOSAGE

Depression

Adult: **PO** 75–100 mg t.i.d.; start with 75 mg t.i.d. or 100 mg b.i.d. and increase dose q3d to 300 mg/d; doses >450 mg/d are associated with an increased risk of adverse reactions including seizures
Geriatric: **PO** 50–100 mg/d; may increase by 50–100 mg q3–4d (max 150 mg/dose)

Smoking Cessation

Adult: **PO** Start with 150 mg once daily times 3 d, then increase to 150 mg b.i.d. (max 300 mg/d) for 7–12 wk

ADMINISTRATION

Oral

- Give with meals to decrease incidence of nausea and vomiting.
- Ensure that sustained-release tablets are not cut, chewed, or crushed. They must be swallowed whole.
- Note: Increases in dosage should not exceed 100 mg/d over a 3-d period. Greater increments increase the seizure potential.
- Store away from heat, direct light, and moisture.

ADVERSE EFFECTS (≥1%) **Body as a Whole:** Weight loss, weight gain. **CNS:** Seizures. The risk of seizure appears to be strongly associated with dose (especially >450 mg/d) and may be increased by predisposing factors (e.g., head trauma, CNS tumor) or a history of prior seizure; *agitation, insomnia, dry mouth, blurred vision, headache, dizziness, tremor.* **GI:** *Nausea, vomiting, constipation.* **CV:** Tachycardia. **Skin:** Rash.

INTERACTIONS Drug: May increase metabolism of **carbamazepine, cimetidine, phenytoin, phenobarbital,** decreasing their effect; may increase incidence of adverse effects of **levodopa,** MAOI.

PHARMACOKINETICS Absorption: Readily absorbed from GI tract. **Onset:** 3–4 wk. **Peak:** 1–3 h. **Metabolism:** Metabolized in liver (including first-pass metabolism) to active metabolites. **Elimination:** 80% excreted in urine as inactive metabolites **Half-Life:** 8–24 h.

NURSING IMPLICATIONS

Assessment & Drug Effects

- Monitor for therapeutic effectiveness. The full antidepressant effect of drug may not be realized for 4 or more weeks.
- Use extreme caution when administering drug to patient with history of seizures, cranial trauma, or other factors predisposing to seizures; during sudden and large increments in dose, seizure potential is increased.
- Report significant restlessness, agitation, anxiety, and insomnia. Symptoms may require treatment or discontinuation of drug.
- Monitor for and report delusions, hallucinations, psychotic episodes, confusion, and paranoia.
- Lab tests: Monitor hepatic and renal function tests while patient is taking this drug.

Client & Family Education

- Take drug at the same time each day.
- Monitor your weight at least weekly. Report significant changes in weight (±5 lb) to prescriber.
- Minimize or avoid alcohol because it increases the risk of seizures.
- Do not drive or engage in potentially hazardous activities until response to drug is known because judgment or motor and cognitive skills may be impaired.
- Do not abruptly discontinue drug. Gradual dosage reduction may be necessary to prevent adverse effects.
- Do not take any OTC drugs without consulting prescriber.
- Do not breast feed while taking this drug.

NEFAZODONE

(nef-a-zo′done)

Serzone

Classifications: CENTRAL NERVOUS SYSTEM AGENT; PSYCHOTHERAPEUTIC; SEROTONIN-REUPTAKE INHIBITOR (SSRI); ANTIDEPRESSANT

Pregnancy Category: C

AVAILABILITY 50 mg, 100 mg, 150 mg, 200 mg, 250 mg tablets

ACTIONS Antidepressant with a dual mechanism of action. Inhibits neuronal serotonin ($5\text{-}HT_1$) reuptake and also possesses $5\text{-}HT_2$ antagonist properties. It is unrelated to tricyclic, MAOI, or other antidepressants.

THERAPEUTIC EFFECTS Antidepressant effects with minimal cardiovascular effects, fewer anticholinergic effects, less sedation, and less sexual dysfunction than other antidepressants.

USE Treatment of depression.

CONTRAINDICATIONS Hypersensitivity to nefazodone or alcohol.

CAUTIOUS USE Older adults, women; history of seizure disorders; renal or hepatic impairment; pregnancy (category C), lactation. Safety and efficacy in children <18 y are not established.

ROUTE & DOSAGE

Depression

Adult: **PO** 50–100 mg b.i.d., may need to increase up to 300–600 mg/d in 2–3 divided doses
Geriatric: **PO** Start with 50 mg b.i.d.

ADMINISTRATION

Oral

- Do not give within 14 d of discontinuation of an MAOI.
- Store at 15°–30° C (59°–86° F).

ADVERSE EFFECTS (≥1%) **CNS:** *Headache, dizziness, drowsiness,* asthenia, tremor, insomnia, agitation, anxiety. **GI:** Dry mouth, constipation, nausea, liver toxicity, liver failure (1 in 250,000–300,000 patient-years of nefazodone treatment). **Special Senses:** Visual disturbances, blurred vision, scotomata.

Body as a Whole: Anaphylactic reactions, angioedema. **Endocrine:** Galactorrheas, gynecomastia, serotonin syndrome. **Skin:** Stevens-Johnson syndrome.

INTERACTIONS Drug: May cause confusion, delirium, coma, seizures or hyperthermia with MAOIS; may increase plasma levels of some BENZODIAZEPINES, including **alprazolam** and **triazolam.** May decrease plasma levels and effects of **propranolol.** May increase levels and toxicity of **buspirone, carbamazepine, cilostazol, digoxin;** reports of QTc prolongation and ventricular arrhythmias with **astemizole, cisapride, pimozide;** increased risk of rhabdomyolysis with **lovastatin, simvastatin;** may cause **serotonin** syndrome with other SSRIs. **Herbal: St. John's wort** may cause **serotonin** syndrome (headache, dizziness, sweating, agitation).

PHARMACOKINETICS Onset: 1 wk. **Peak:** 3–5 wk. **Metabolism:** Metabolized in liver to at least two active metabolites. **Half-Life:** Nefazodone 3.5 h, metabolites 2–33 h.

NURSING IMPLICATIONS

Assessment & Drug Effects

- Evaluate concurrent drugs for possible interactions.
- Monitor patients with a history of seizures for increased activity.
- Assess safety, because dizziness and drowsiness are common adverse effects.
- Lab tests: Monitor liver function and CBC periodically during long-term therapy. Increased serum AST or serum ALT levels three times normal limit indicate hepatocellular injury and client should be removed from nefazodone treatment.
- Canada withdrew this medication from the market in 2003 due to liver-related adverse effects.

Client & Family Education

- Be aware that significant improvement in mood may not occur for several weeks following initiation of therapy.
- Do not drive or engage in potentially hazardous activities until response to the drug is known.
- Be alert for jaundice, anorexia, unusually dark urine, unusual tiredness and weakness, GI complaints, and malaise and report to prescriber immediately.
- Report changes in visual acuity.
- Do not breast feed while taking this drug without consulting prescriber.

TRAZODONE HYDROCHLORIDE

(tray'zoe-done)

Desyrel, Desyrel Dividose

Classifications: CENTRAL NERVOUS SYSTEM AGENT; PSYCHOTHERAPEUTIC; ANTIDEPRESSANT

Pregnancy Category: C

AVAILABILITY 50 mg, 100 mg, 150 mg, 300 mg tablets

ACTIONS Centrally acting triazolopyridine derivative antidepressant chemically and structurally unrelated to tricyclic, tetracyclic, or other antidepressants. Potentiates serotonin effects by selectively blocking serotonin reuptake at presynaptic membranes in CNS. Does not stimulate CNS and causes fewer anticholinergic genitourinary and neurologic effects as compared with other antidepressants. Produces varying degrees of sedation in normal and mentally depressed patients.

THERAPEUTIC EFFECTS Increases total sleep time, decreases number and duration of awakenings in depressed patient, and decreases REM sleep. Has anxiolytic effect in severely depressed patient.

USES Both inpatient and outpatient with major depression with or without prominent anxiety.

UNLABELED USES Adjunctive treatment of alcohol dependence, anxiety neuroses, drug-induced dyskinesias.

CONTRAINDICATIONS Initial recovery phase of MI; ventricular ectopy; electroshock therapy. Safety during pregnancy (category C) or in children <8 y is not established.

CAUTIOUS USE Patient with suicidal ideation; cardiac arrhythmias or disease; lactation.

ROUTE & DOSAGE

Depression

Adult: **PO** 150 mg/d in divided doses. May increase by 50 mg/d q3–4d (max 400–600 mg/d)
Geriatric: **PO** 25–50 mg h.s., may increase q3–7d to usual range of 75–150 mg/d
Child: **PO** *6–18 y,* 1.5–2 mg/kg/d in divided doses, increase q3–4d prn (max 6 mg/kg/d)

ADMINISTRATION

Oral

- Give drug with food; increases amount of absorption by 20% and appears to decrease incidence of dizziness or light-headedness. Maintain the same schedule for food-drug intake throughout treatment period to prevent variations in serum concentration.
- Store in tightly closed, light-resistant container at 15°–30° C (59°–86° F).

ADVERSE EFFECTS (≥1%) **CNS:** *Drowsiness,* light-headedness, tiredness, dizziness, insomnia, headache, agitation, impaired memory and speech, disorientation. **CV:** *Hypotension (including orthostatic hypotension),* hypertension, syncope, shortness of breath, chest pain, tachycardia, palpitations, bradycardia, PVCs, ventricular tachycardia (short episodes of 3–4 beats). **Special Senses:** Nasal and sinus congestion, blurred vision, eye irritation, sweating or clamminess, tinnitus. **GI:** *Dry mouth,* anorexia, constipation, abdominal distress, nausea, vomiting, dysgeusia, flatulence, diarrhea. **Urogenital:** Hematuria, increased frequency, delayed urine flow, early or absent menses, male priapism, ejaculation inhibition. **Hematologic:** Anemia. **Musculoskeletal:** Skeletal aches and pains, muscle twitches. **Skin:** Skin eruptions, rash, pruritus, acne, photosensitivity. **Body as a Whole:** Weight gain or loss.

INTERACTIONS Drug: ANTIHYPERTENSIVE AGENTS may potentiate hypotensive effects; **alcohol** and other CNS DEPRESSANTS add to depressant effects; may increase **digoxin** or **phenytoin** levels; MAOIS may precipitate hypertensive crisis.

PHARMACOKINETICS Absorption: Readily absorbed from GI tract. **Onset:** 1–2 wk. **Peak:** 1–2 h. **Distribution:** Distributed into breast milk. **Metabolism:** Metabolized in liver. **Elimination:** 75% excreted in urine, 25% in feces. **Half-Life:** 5–9 h.

NURSING IMPLICATIONS

Assessment & Drug Effects

- Monitor pulse rate and regularity before administration if patient has preexisting cardiac disease.
- Note: Adverse effects generally are mild and tend to decrease and disappear after the first few weeks of treatment.
- Observe patient's level of activity. If it appears to be increasing toward sleeplessness and agitation with changes in reality orientation, report to prescriber. Manic episodes have been reported.

- Check patient for symptoms of hypotension. If orthostatic hypotension is troublesome, suggest measures to reduce danger of falling and help patient to tolerate the effects. Discuss with prescriber; reduction of dose or discontinuation of the drug may be prescribed.
- Male patient should report inappropriate or prolonged penile erections (priapism). The drug may be discontinued.
- Be aware that overdose is characterized by an extension of common adverse effects: Vomiting, lethargy, drowsiness, and exaggerated anticholinergic effects. Seizures or arrhythmias are unusual.

Client & Family Education

- Expect therapeutic response to begin in 1 wk; may require 2–4 wk to reach maximum levels. Adhere to regimen.
- Do not alter dose or intervals between doses.
- Consult prescriber if drowsiness becomes a distressing adverse effect. Dose regimen may be changed so that largest dose is at bedtime.
- Limit or abstain from alcohol use. The depressant effects of CNS depressants and alcohol may be potentiated by this drug.
- Do not self-medicate with OTC drugs for colds, allergy, or insomnia treatment without advice of prescriber. Many of these drugs contain CNS depressants.
- Keep follow-up appointments to permit dose adjustment or discontinuation, as indicated.
- Alert dentist, surgeon, or emergency personnel that drug is being used. Trazodone is discontinued as long as possible prior to elective surgery.
- Do not breast feed while taking this drug without consulting prescriber.

ANTIDEPRESSANTS, MONOAMINE OXIDASE INHIBITORS

ISOCARBOXAZID

(eye-soe-kar-box'a-zid)

Marplan

Classifications: CENTRAL NERVOUS SYSTEM AGENT; PSYCHOTHERAPEUTIC; ANTIDEPRESSANT; MONOAMINE OXIDASE INHIBITOR (MAOI)

Pregnancy Category: C

AVAILABILITY 10 mg tablets

ACTIONS MAOI of the hydrazine group. Inhibits monoamine oxidase, the enzyme involved in the catabolism of catecholamine neurotransmitters and serotonin.

THERAPEUTIC EFFECTS Marplan increases concentration of catecholamine neurotransmitters as well as serotonin and dopamine within presynaptic neurons and at receptor sites, the proposed basis for the antidepressant effect of MAOIS.

USES Symptomatic treatment of depressed patients refractory to or intolerant of TCAs or electroconvulsive therapy.

CONTRAINDICATIONS Hypersensitivity to MAOIS; pheochromocytoma; CHF; children (<16 y); older adults (>60 y) or debilitated patients; severe renal or hepatic impairment. Safe use during pregnancy (category C) or lactation is not established.

CAUTIOUS USE Hypertension, hyperthyroidism, parkinsonism, cardiac arrhythmias, epilepsy, suicidal risks.

ROUTE & DOSAGE

Refractory Depression

Adult: **PO** 10–30 mg/d in 1–3 divided doses (max 30 mg/d)

ADMINISTRATION

Oral

- Note: Dosage is individualized on the basis of patient response. Lowest effective dosage should be used.
- Store in a tight, light-resistant container.

ADVERSE EFFECTS (≥1%) **CNS:** Dizziness, light-headedness, tiredness, weakness, *drowsiness,* vertigo, headache, *overactivity,* hyperreflexia, muscle twitching, tremors, mania, hypomania, *insomnia,* confusion, memory impairment. **CV:** *Orthostatic hypotension,* paradoxical hypertension, palpitation, tachycardia, other arrhythmias. **Special Sense:** *Blurred vision,* nystagmus, glaucoma. **GI:** Increased appetite, weight gain, *nausea,* diarrhea, *constipation, anorexia,* black tongue, *dry mouth,* abdominal pain. **Urogenital:** Dysuria, *urinary retention,* incontinence, sexual disturbances. **Body as a Whole:** Peripheral edema, excessive sweating, chills, skin rash, hepatitis, jaundice.

INTERACTIONS Drug: TRICYCLIC ANTIDEPRESSANTS, **fluoxetine,** AMPHETAMINES, **ephedrine, phenylpropanolamine, reserpine, guanethidine, buspirone, methyldopa, dopamine,**

levodopa, tryptophan may precipitate hypertensive crisis, headache, or hyperexcitability; **alcohol** and other CNS DEPRESSANTS compound CNS depressant effects; **meperidine** can cause fatal cardiovascular collapse; ANESTHETICS exaggerate hypotensive and CNS depressant effects; **metrizamide** increases risk of seizures; compounds hypotensive effects of DIURETICS and other ANTIHYPERTENSIVE AGENTS. **Food:** All **tyramine**-containing foods, which include foods that have been aged, pickled, fermented, or smoked (aged cheeses, processed cheeses, sour cream, wine, champagne, beer, pickled herring, anchovies, caviar, shrimp, liver, dry sausage, figs, raisins, overripe bananas or avocados, chocolate, soy sauce, bean curd, yeast extracts, yogurt, papaya products, meat tenderizers, broad beans) may precipitate hypertensive crisis. **Herbal: Ginseng, ephedra, ma huang, St. John's wort** may precipitate hypertensive crisis.

PHARMACOKINETICS Duration: Up to 2 wk. **Metabolism:** Metabolized in liver.

NURSING IMPLICATIONS

Assessment & Drug Effects

- Note: Toxic symptoms from overdosage or from ingestion of contraindicated substances (e.g., foods high in tyramine) may occur within hours.
- Note: Toxic symptoms from ingestion of contraindicated substances (e.g., foods high in tyramine) may occur up to 2 wk following discontinuing medication.
- Monitor for therapeutic effectiveness: May be apparent within 1 wk or less, but in some patients there may be a time lag of 3–4 wk before improvement occurs.
- Monitor BP. Monitor for orthostatic hypotension by evaluating BP with patient recumbent and standing.
- Check for peripheral edema daily and monitor weight several times weekly.
- Monitor I&O and bowel elimination patterns.

Client & Family Education

- Avoid alcohol and excessive caffeine-containing beverages and tryptophan- and tyramine-containing foods including cheeses, yeast, meat extracts, smoked or pickled meat, poultry, or fish, fermented sausages, and overripe fruit.
- Do not breast feed while taking this drug without consulting prescriber.

- Make position changes slowly and in stages; lie down or sit down if faintness occurs.
- Use caution when performing potentially hazardous activities.
- Consult prescriber before self-medicating with OTC agents (e.g., cough, cold, hay fever, or diet medications).

PHENELZINE SULFATE

(fen'el-zeen)

Nardil

Classifications: CENTRAL NERVOUS SYSTEM AGENT; PSYCHOTHERAPEUTIC; ANTIDEPRESSANT; MONAMINE OXIDASE INHIBITOR (MAOI)

Pregnancy Category: C

AVAILABILITY 15 mg tablets

ACTIONS Potent hydrazine MAOI. Precise mode of action is not known. Antidepressant and diverse effects believed to be due to irreversible inhibition of MAO, thereby permitting increased concentrations of endogenous epinephrine, norepinephrine, serotonin, and dopamine within presynaptic neurons and at receptor sites. Also thought to inhibit hepatic microsomal drug metabolizing enzymes; thus it may intensify and prolong the effects of many drugs.

THERAPEUTIC EFFECTS Antidepressant utilization of the drug is limited to individuals who do not respond well to other classes of antidepressants. Termination of drug action depends on regeneration of MAO, which occurs 2–3 wk after discontinuation of therapy.

USES Management of endogenous depression, depressive phase of manic-depressive psychosis, and severe exogenous (reactive) depression not responsive to more commonly used therapy.

CONTRAINDICATIONS Hypersensitivity to MAOIS; pheochromocytoma; hyperthyroidism; CHF, cardiovascular or cerebrovascular disease; impaired kidney function, hypernatremia; atonic colitis; glaucoma; history of frequent or severe headaches; history of liver disease, abnormal liver function tests; older adult or debilitated patients; paranoid schizophrenia. Safety during pregnancy (category C), lactation, or in children <6 y of age is not established.

CAUTIOUS USE Epilepsy; pyloric stenosis; diabetes; depression accompanying alcoholism or drug addiction; manic-depressive states; agitated patients; suicidal tendencies; chronic brain syndromes; history of angina pectoris.

ROUTE & DOSAGE

Depression

Adult: **PO** 15 mg t.i.d., rapidly increase to at least 60 mg/d; may need up to 90 mg/d

ADMINISTRATION

Oral

- Discontinue at least 10 d before elective surgery to allow time for recovery from MAO before anesthetics are given.
- Avoid rapid withdrawal of MAOIS, particularly after high dosage, because a rebound effect may occur (e.g., headache, excitability, hallucinations, and possibly depression).
- Store in tightly covered containers away from heat and light.

ADVERSE EFFECTS ($\geq$1%) **Body as a Whole:** Dizziness or vertigo, headache, *orthostatic hypotension,* drowsiness or *insomnia,* weakness, fatigue, edema, tremors, twitching, akathisia, ataxia, hyperreflexia, faintness, hyperactivity, marked agitation, anxiety, seizures, trismus, opisthotonos, respiratory depression, coma. **CNS:** Mania, hypomania, confusion, memory impairment, delirium, hallucinations, euphoria, acute anxiety reaction, toxic precipitation of schizophrenia, convulsions, peripheral neuropathy. **CV:** Hypertensive crisis (intense occipital headache, palpitation, marked hypertension, stiff neck, nausea, vomiting, sweating, fever, photophobia, dilated pupils, bradycardia or tachycardia, constricting chest pain, intracranial bleeding), hypotension or hypertension, circulatory collapse. **GI:** *Constipation, dry mouth, nausea,* vomiting, *anorexia,* weight gain. **Hematologic:** Normocytic and normochromic anemia, leukopenia. **Skin:** Hyperhidrosis, skin rash, photosensitivity. **Special Senses:** Blurred vision.

DIAGNOSTIC TEST INTERFERENCE Phenelzine may cause a slight false increase in ***serum bilirubin.***

INTERACTIONS Drug: TRICYCLIC ANTIDEPRESSANTS may cause hyperpyrexia, seizures; **fluoxetine, sertraline, paroxetine** may cause hyperthermia, diaphoresis, tremors, seizures, delirium; SYMPATHOMIMETIC AGENTS (e.g., **amphetamine, phenylephrine,**

phenylpropanolamine), **guanethidine,** and **reserpine** may cause hypertensive crisis; CNS DEPRESSANTS have additive CNS depressive effects; OPIATE ANALGESICS (especially **meperidine**) may cause hypertensive crisis and circulatory collapse; **buspirone,** hypertension; GENERAL ANESTHETICS, prolonged hypotensive and CNS depressant effects; hypertension, headache, hyperexcitability reported with **dopamine, methyldopa, levodopa, tryptophan; metrizamide** may increase risk of seizures; HYPOTENSIVE AGENTS and DIURETICS have additive hypotensive effects. **Food:** Foods containing tyramine, including foods that have been aged, pickled, fermented, or smoked. Aged meats or aged cheeses, protein extracts, sour cream, alcohol, anchovies, liver, sausages, overripe figs, bananas, avocados, chocolate, soy sauce, bean curd, natural yogurt, fava beans—**tyramine**-containing foods—may precipitate hypertensive crisis. **Herbal: Ginseng, ephedra, ma huang, St. John's wort** may cause hypertensive crisis.

PHARMACOKINETICS Absorption: Readily absorbed from GI tract. **Onset:** 2 wk. **Metabolism:** Rapidly metabolized. **Elimination:** 79% of metabolites excreted in urine in 96 h.

NURSING IMPLICATIONS

Assessment & Drug Effects

- Evaluate patient's BP in standing and recumbent positions prior to initiation of treatment.
- Lab tests: Perform baseline CBC and liver function tests. Also perform periodic CBC and liver function tests during prolonged or high-dose therapy.
- Monitor BP and pulse between doses when titrating initial dosages. Observe closely for evidence of adverse drug effects. Thereafter, monitor at regular intervals throughout therapy.
- Report immediately if hypomania (exaggeration of feelings, ideas, and self-worth) occurs as depression improves. This reaction may also appear at higher than recommended doses or with long-term therapy.
- Observe for and report therapeutic effectiveness of drug: Improvement in sleep pattern, appetite, physical activity, interest in self and surroundings, as well as lessening of anxiety and bodily complaints.
- Observe patient with diabetes closely for S&S of hypoglycemia. Patients on prolonged therapy should be checked periodically for altered color perception, changes in fundi or visual fields.

Changes in red-green vision may be the first indication of eye damage.

Client & Family Education

- Do not consume foods and beverages containing tyramine or tryptophan or drugs containing a pressor agent. These can cause severe hypertensive reactions. Typically includes foods that have been aged, pickled, fermented, or smoked. Get a list from your care provider.
- Note: Toxic symptoms from ingestion of contraindicated substances (e.g., foods high in tyramine) may occur up to 2 wk following discontinuing medication.
- Avoid drinking excessive caffeine beverages (e.g., coffee, tea, cocoa, or cola).
- Avoid self-medication. OTC preparations containing dextromethorphan, sympathomimetic agents, or antihistamines (e.g., cough, cold, and hay fever remedies, appetite suppressants) can precipitate severe hypertensive reactions if taken during therapy or within 2–3 wk after discontinuation of an MAOI.
- Drug is usually discontinued if no therapeutic response occurs after 3 or 4 wk. Maximum antidepressant effects generally appear in 2–6 wk and persist several weeks after drug withdrawal.
- Report immediately to prescriber the onset of headache and palpitation, prodromal symptoms of hypertensive crisis, or any other unusual effects that may indicate need to discontinue therapy.
- Discuss with prescriber wearing elastic stockings and elevating legs when sitting to minimize hypotensive effects of drug.
- Make position changes slowly, especially from recumbent to upright posture, and dangle legs over bed a few minutes before rising to walk. Avoid standing still for prolonged periods. Also avoid hot showers and baths (resulting vasodilatation may potentiate hypotension); lie down immediately if feeling lightheaded or faint.
- Check weight 2 or 3 times per week and report unusual gain.
- Report jaundice. Hepatotoxicity is believed to be a hypersensitivity reaction unrelated to dosage or duration of therapy.
- Avoid overexertion while taking this drug. MAOIS may suppress anginal pain that would otherwise serve as a warning sign of myocardial ischemia.
- Do not breast feed while taking this drug without consulting prescriber.

TRANYLCYPROMINE SULFATE

(tran-ill-sip′roe-meen)

Parnate

Classifications: CENTRAL NERVOUS SYSTEM AGENT; PSYCHOTHERAPEUTIC; ANTIDEPRESSANT; MAOI

Pregnancy Category: C

AVAILABILITY 10 mg tablets

ACTIONS Potent nonhydrazine MAOI structurally similar to amphetamine. Actions and toxicity similar to those of hydrazine MAOI but also has rapid and direct amphetamine-like CNS stimulatory action, is less likely to cause hepatotoxicity and does not produce prolonged MAO inhibition (reversible binding).

THERAPEUTIC EFFECTS Drug of last choice for severe depression unresponsive to other MAOIS.

USES Severe depression.

CONTRAINDICATIONS Pregnancy (category C); patients >60 y; confirmed or suspected cerebrovascular defect, cardiovascular disease, hypertension, pheochromocytoma, history of severe or recurrent headaches; lactation.

ROUTE & DOSAGE

Severe Depression

Adult: **PO** 30 mg/d in 2 divided doses (20 mg in a.m., 10 mg in p.m.); may increase by 10 mg/d at 3 wk intervals (max: 60 mg/d)

ADMINISTRATION

Oral

- Crush tablet and give with fluid or mix with food if patient cannot swallow pill.
- Note: Usually not given in the evening because of possibility of insomnia.

ADVERSE EFFECTS (≥1%) **CNS:** Vertigo, dizziness, tremors, muscle twitching, headache, blurred vision. **CV:** *Orthostatic hypotension,* arrhythmias, <u>hypertensive crisis</u>. **GI:** Dry mouth, anorexia, constipation, diarrhea, abdominal discomfort. **Skin:** Rash. **Urogenital:** Impotence. **Body as a Whole:** Peripheral edema, sweating.

INTERACTIONS Drug: TRICYCLIC ANTIDEPRESSANTS, **fluoxetine,** AMPHETAMINES, **ephedrine, phenylpropanolamine, reserpine, guanethidine, buspirone, methyldopa, dopamine, levodopa, tryptophan** may precipitate hypertensive crisis, headache, or hyperexcitability; **alcohol** and other CNS DEPRESSANTS add to CNS depressant effects; **meperidine** can cause fatal cardiovascular collapse; ANESTHETICS exaggerate hypotensive and CNS depressant effects; **metrizamide** increases risk of seizures; DIURETICS and other ANTIHYPERTENSIVE AGENTS add to hypotensive effects. **Food: Tyramine**-containing foods, including foods that have been aged, pickled, fermented, or smoked, may precipitate hypertensive crisis (e.g., aged cheeses, processed cheeses, sour cream, wine, champagne, beer, pickled herring, anchovies, caviar, shrimp, liver, dry sausage, figs, raisins, overripe bananas or avocados, chocolate, soy sauce, bean curd, yeast extracts, yogurt, papaya products, meat tenderizers, broad beans). **Herbal: Ginseng, ephedra, ma huang, St. John's wort** may lead to hypertensive crisis; **ginseng** may lead to manic episodes.

PHARMACOKINETICS Absorption: Completely absorbed from GI tract. **Onset:** 10 d. **Metabolism:** Rapidly metabolized in liver to active metabolite. **Elimination:** Primarily excreted in urine. **Half-Life:** 2.5 h (but may take 120 h for urinary tryptamine levels to return to normal).

NURSING IMPLICATIONS

Assessment & Drug Effects

- Monitor BP closely. Incidence of severe hypertensive reactions appears to be greater with tranylcypromine than with other MAOIS.
- Expect therapeutic response within 3 d, but full antidepressant effects may not be obtained until 2–3 wk of drug therapy.

Client & Family Education

- Do not eat tyramine-containing foods (see INTERACTIONS, FOOD).
- Be aware that excessive use of caffeine-containing beverages (chocolate, coffee, tea, cola) can contribute to development of rapid heartbeat, arrhythmias, and hypertension.
- Note: Toxic symptoms from ingestion of contraindicated substances (e.g., foods high in tyramine) may occur up to 2 wk following discontinuing medication.

- Make position changes slowly, particularly from recumbent to upright posture.
- Avoid potentially hazardous activities until response to drug is known.
- Avoid alcohol or other CNS depressants because of their possible additive effects.
- Do not breast feed while taking this drug.

ANTIDEPRESSANTS, SELECTIVE NOREPINEPHRINE- AND SEROTONIN-REUPTAKE INHIBITOR

VENLAFAXINE

(ven-la-fax′een)

Effexor, Effexor XR

Classifications: CENTRAL NERVOUS SYSTEM AGENT; PSYCHOTHERAPEUTIC; ANTIDEPRESSANT; SELECTIVE SEROTONIN-REUPTAKE INHIBITOR (SSRI), SELECTIVE NOREPINEPHRINE-REUPTAKE INHIBITOR

Pregnancy Category: C

AVAILABILITY 25 mg, 37.5 mg, 50 mg, 75 mg, 100 mg tablets; 37.5 mg, 75 mg, 150 mg sustained-release capsules

ACTIONS Selectively inhibits neuronal uptake of serotonin, norepinephrine, and dopamine in decreasing order of potency. A bicyclic "second-generation" antidepressant, drug is chemically unrelated to tricyclic, tetracyclic, or other antidepressants.

THERAPEUTIC EFFECTS Antidepressant effect is presumed to be linked to its inhibition of CNS presynaptic neuronal uptake of serotonin. Drug does not cause anticholinergic, sedative, or cardiovascular effects.

USES Depression, generalized anxiety disorder.

UNLABELED USES Obsessive-compulsive disorder.

CONTRAINDICATIONS Hypersensitivity to venlafaxine, concurrent administration with MAOIS.

CAUTIOUS USE Renal and hepatic impairment, anorexia, history of mania, suicidal ideations, cardiac disorders, recent MI. Safety during pregnancy (category C), lactation, and in children <18 y is not established.

ROUTE & DOSAGE

Depression

Adult: **PO** 25–125 mg t.i.d.
Geriatric: **PO** Start with lower doses in older adults

Anxiety

Adult: **PO** Start with 37.5 mg sustained release q.d and increase to 75–225 mg sustained release per day

Renal Impairment

Cl_{cr} 10–70 mL/min: Reduce total daily dose by 25–50%; <10 mL/min: Reduce total daily dose by 50%

ADMINISTRATION

Oral

- Give with food. Sustained-release capsules must be swallowed whole, must not be opened or chewed.
- Dosage increments of up to 75 mg/d are usually made at 4 d or longer intervals.
- Allow 14-d interval after discontinuing an MAOI before starting venlafaxine.
- Do not abruptly withdraw drug after 1 wk or more of therapy.
- Store at room temperature, 15°–30° C (59°–86° F).

ADVERSE EFFECTS (≥1%) **CV:** *Increased blood pressure and heart rate,* palpitations. **CNS:** *Dizziness,* fatigue, headache, anxiety, insomnia, *somnolence.* **Endocrine:** Small but statistically significant increase in serum cholesterol, weight loss (approximately 3 lb). **GI:** *Nausea, vomiting, dry mouth,* constipation. **Urogenital:** Sexual dysfunction, erectile failure, delayed orgasm, anorgasmia, impotence, abnormal ejaculation. **Special Senses:** Blurred vision. **Body as a Whole:** *Sweating,* asthenia.

INTERACTIONS Drug: Cimetidine, MAOIS, **desipramine, haloperidol** may increase venlafaxine levels and toxicity. Should not use in combination with MAOIS; do not start until >14 d after stopping MAOI; do not start MAOI until 7 d after stopping venlafaxine. **Trazodone** may lead to **serotonin** syndrome. **Herbal: St. John's wort** may cause **serotonin** syndrome.

PHARMACOKINETICS Absorption: Well absorbed from GI tract. **Onset:** 2 wk. **Peak:** Venlafaxine 1–2 h; metabolite 3–4 h. **Duration:** Approximately 30% protein bound, but extensively tissue bound. **Metabolism:** Undergoes substantial first-pass metabolism to its major active metabolite, *O*-desmethylvenlafaxine, with similar activity to venlafaxine. **Elimination:** Approximately 60% excreted in urine as parent compound and metabolites. **Half-Life:** Venlafaxine 3–4 h, *O*-desmethylvenlafaxine 10 h.

NURSING IMPLICATIONS

Assessment & Drug Effects

- Monitor cardiovascular status periodically with measurements of HR and BP.
- Lab tests: Periodic lipid profile.
- Monitor neurologic status and report excessive anxiety, nervousness, and insomnia.
- Check that patient is not self-treating with **St. John's wort** because it is a botanical MAOI.
- Monitor weight periodically and report excess weight loss.
- Assess safety; dizziness and sedation are common.

Client & Family Education

- Be aware of potential adverse effects and notify prescriber of those that are bothersome.
- Do not drive or engage in potentially hazardous activities until response to drug is known.
- Avoid using alcohol while on venlafaxine.
- Do not use herbal medications without consulting prescriber, **St. John's wort** in particular, because it is a botanical MAOI.
- Do not breast feed while taking this drug without consulting prescriber.

ANTIDEPRESSANTS, SELECTIVE SEROTONIN-REUPTAKE INHIBITORS

CITALOPRAM HYDROBROMIDE

(cit-a-lo′pram)

Celexa

Classifications: CENTRAL NERVOUS SYSTEM AGENT; PSYCHOTHERAPEUTIC; SELECTIVE SEROTONIN-REUPTAKE INHIBITOR (SSRI)

Pregnancy Category: C

AVAILABILITY 20 mg, 40 mg tablets; 10 mg/5 mL oral solution

ACTIONS Selective serotonin-reuptake inhibitor (SSRI) in the CNS. Antidepressant effect is presumed to be linked to its inhibition of CNS presynaptic neuronal uptake of serotonin, which results in antidepressant activity. Does not produce any sympathomimetic response or anticholinergic activity.

THERAPEUTIC EFFECTS Does not inhibit MAO. Selective serotonin-reuptake inhibition mechanism results in the antidepressant activity of citalopram.

USE Depression.

CONTRAINDICATIONS Hypersensitivity to citalopram; concurrent use of MAOIS or use within 14 d of discontinuing MAOIS; pregnancy (category C); volume depleted; lactation; children <18 y.

CAUTIOUS USE Hypersensitivity to other SSRIs; renal or hepatic insufficiency; older adults; concurrent use of diuretics, cardiovascular disease (e.g., dysrhythmias, conduction defects, myocardial ischemia); history of seizure disorders or suicidal tendencies.

ROUTE & DOSAGE

Depression

Adult: **PO** Start at 20 mg q.d.; may increase to 40 mg q.d. if needed
Geriatric: **PO** 20 mg q.d.

ADMINISTRATION

Oral

- Do not begin this drug within 14 d of stopping a MAOI.
- Check that patient is not self-treating with **St. John's wort** because it is a botanical MAOI.
- Reduced doses are advised for the older adult and those with hepatic or renal impairment.
- Dose increments should be separated by at least 1 wk.
- Store at 15°–30° C (59°–86° F) in tightly closed container and protect from light.

ADVERSE EFFECTS (≥1%) **Body as a Whole:** Asthenia, fatigue, fever, arthralgia, myalgia. **CV:** Tachycardia, postural hypotension, hypotension. **GI:** *Nausea,* vomiting, diarrhea, dyspepsia, abdominal pain, *dry mouth,* anorexia, flatulence. **CNS:** Dizziness, *insomnia, somnolence,* agitation, tremor, anxiety, paresthesia, migraine. **Respiratory:** URI, rhinitis, sinusitis. **Skin:** Increased sweating. **Urogenital:** Dysmenorrhea, decreased libido, ejaculation disorder, impotence.

INTERACTIONS Drug: Combination with MAOIS could result in hypertensive crisis, hyperthermia, rigidity, myoclonus, autonomic instability; **cimetidine** may increase citalopram levels. **Herbal: St. John's wort** is a botanical MAOI and cannot be combined with an SSRI; may cause **serotonin** syndrome.

PHARMACOKINETICS Absorption: Rapidly absorbed from GI tract; approximately 80% reaches systemic circulation. **Peak:** Steady state serum concentrations in 1 wk; peak blood levels at 4 h. **Distribution:** 80% protein bound; crosses placenta; distributed into breast milk. **Metabolism:** Metabolized in liver by cytochrome P-450 3A4 and cytochrome P-450 2C9 enzymes. **Elimination:** 20% excreted in urine, 80% in bile. **Half-Life:** 35 h.

NURSING IMPLICATIONS

Assessment & Drug Effects

- Monitor for therapeutic effectiveness: Indicated by elevation of mood; 1–4 wk may be needed before improvement is noted.
- Lab tests: Monitor periodically hepatic functions, CBC, serum sodium, and lithium levels when the two drugs are given concurrently.
- Monitor periodically HR and BP, and carefully monitor complete cardiac status in person with known or suspected cardiac disease.
- Monitor closely older adult patients for adverse effects especially with doses >20 mg/d.

Client & Family Education

- Do not engage in hazardous activities until reaction to this drug is known.
- Avoid using alcohol while taking citalopram.
- Inform prescriber of commonly used OTC drugs because there is potential for drug interactions.
- Do not self-treat with **St. John's wort** because it is a botanical MAOI and cannot be combined with this medication
- Report distressing adverse effects including any changes in sexual functioning or response.
- Some side effects experienced may subside within 3 wk without changes to dose or schedule.
- Periodic ophthalmology exams are advised with long-term treatment.
- Do not breast feed while taking this drug.

ESCITALOPRAM OXALATE

(es-ci-tal′o-pram)

Lexapro

Classifications: CENTRAL NERVOUS SYSTEM AGENT; PSYCHOTHERAPEUTIC; SELECTIVE SEROTONIN-REUPTAKE INHIBITOR (SSRI)

Pregnancy Category: C

AVAILABILITY 5 mg, 10 mg, 20 mg tablets

ACTIONS Selective serotonin-reuptake inhibitor (SSRI) in the CNS. Antidepressant effect is presumed to be linked to its inhibition of CNS presynaptic neuronal uptake of serotonin, which results in antidepressant activity. Does not produce any sympathomimetic response or anticholinergic activity.

THERAPEUTIC EFFECTS Does not inhibit MAO. Selective serotonin-reuptake inhibition mechanism results in the antidepressant activity of citalopram.

USES Depression.

CONTRAINDICATIONS Hypersensitivity to citalopram; concurrent use of MAOIS or use within 14 d of discontinuing MAOIS; pregnancy (category C); volume depleted; lactation; children <18 y.

CAUTIOUS USE Hypersensitivity to other SSRIs; renal or hepatic insufficiency; older adults; concurrent use of diuretics, cardiovascular disease (e.g., dysrhythmias, conduction defects, myocardial ischemia); history of seizure disorders or suicidal tendencies.

ROUTE & DOSAGE

Depression

Adult: **PO** 10 q.d.; may increase to 20 mg q.d. if needed after 1 wk
Geriatric: **PO** 10 mg q.d.

Hepatic Impairment

Adult: **PO** 10 q.d.

ADMINISTRATION

Oral

- Do not begin this drug within 14 d of stopping an MAOI.
- Check that patient is not self-treating with **St. John's wort** because it is a botanical MAOI.

- Reduced doses are advised for the older adult and those with hepatic or renal impairment.
- Dose increments should be separated by at least 1 wk.
- Store at 15°–30° C (59°–86° F) in tightly closed container and protect from light.

ADVERSE EFFECTS (≥1%) **Body as a Whole:** Fatigue, fever, arthralgia, myalgia. **CV:** Palpitation, hypertension. **GI:** *Nausea,* diarrhea, dyspepsia, abdominal pain, dry mouth, vomiting, flatulence, reflux. **CNS:** Dizziness, *insomnia, somnolence,* paresthesia, migraine, tremor, vertigo. **Metabolic:** Increased or decreased weight. **Respiratory:** URI, rhinitis, sinusitis. **Skin:** Increased sweating. **Urogenital:** Dysmenorrhea, decreased libido, ejaculation disorder, impotence, menstrual cramps.

INTERACTIONS Drug: Combination with MAOIS could result in hypertensive crisis, hyperthermia, rigidity, myoclonus, autonomic instability; **cimetidine** may increase escitalopram levels. **Herbal: St. John's wort** may cause **serotonin** syndrome; is a botanical MAOI and cannot be coadministered with an SSRI.

PHARMACOKINETICS Absorption: Rapidly absorbed from GI tract. **Onset:** Approximately 1 wk. **Peak:** 3 h. **Distribution:** 80% protein bound; crosses placenta; distributed into breast milk. **Metabolism:** Metabolized in liver by CYP3A4, 2C19, and 2D6 enzymes. **Elimination:** 20% excreted in urine, 80% in bile. **Half-Life:** 25 h.

NURSING IMPLICATIONS

Assessment & Drug Effects

- Monitor for therapeutic effectiveness: Indicated by elevation of mood; 1–4 wk may be needed before improvement is noted.
- Lab tests: Monitor periodically hepatic functions, CBC, serum sodium, and lithium levels when the two drugs are given concurrently.
- Monitor periodically HR and BP, and carefully monitor complete cardiac status in person with known or suspected cardiac disease.
- Monitor closely older adult patients for adverse effects, especially with doses >20 mg/d.

Client & Family Education

- Do not engage in hazardous activities until reaction to this drug is known.
- Avoid using alcohol while taking escitalopram.

- Inform prescriber of commonly used OTC drugs because there is potential for drug interactions.
- Do not self-treat with **St. John's wort** because it is a botanical MAOI and cannot be combined with this medication.
- Report distressing adverse effects including any changes in sexual functioning or response.
- Some side effects experienced may subside within 3 wk without changes to dose or schedule.
- Periodic ophthalmology exams are advised with long-term treatment.
- Do not breast feed while taking this drug.

FLUOXETINE HYDROCHLORIDE

(flu'ox-e-tine)

Prozac, ProzacWeekly, Sarafem

Classifications: CENTRAL NERVOUS SYSTEM AGENT; PSYCHOTHERAPEUTIC; SELECTIVE SEROTONIN-REUPTAKE INHIBITOR (SSRI)

Pregnancy Category: B

AVAILABILITY 10 mg tablets; 10 mg, 20 mg capsules; 20 mg/5 mL solution; 90 mg sustained-release capsules (Prozac Weekly)

ACTIONS Oral antidepressant chemically unrelated to tricyclic, tetracyclic, MAOI, or other available antidepressants. Antidepressant effect is presumed to be linked to its inhibition of CNS neuronal uptake of serotonin, a neurotransmitter.

THERAPEUTIC EFFECTS Effectiveness may take from several days to 5 wk to develop fully. Drug has antidepressant, antiobsessive-compulsive, and antibulimic actions.

USES Depression, geriatric depression, obsessive-compulsive disorder, bulimia nervosa, premenstrual dysphoric disorder, pediatric major depressive disorder.

UNLABELED USES Obesity.

CONTRAINDICATIONS Hypersensitivity to fluoxetine or other SSRI drugs.

CAUTIOUS USE Hepatic and renal impairment, anorexia, hyponatremia, diabetes, patients with history of suicidal ideations. Older adults may require dose adjustments. Safety in pregnancy (category B), lactation, and in children is not established.

ROUTE & DOSAGE

Depression, Obsessive-Compulsive Disorder

Adult: **PO** 20 mg/d in a.m.; may increase by 20 mg/d at weekly intervals (max 80 mg/d); 20 mg/d in a.m.; when stable may switch to 90 mg sustained-release capsule qwk (max 90 mg/wk)
Geriatric: **PO** Start with 10 mg/d

Premenstrual Dysphoric Disorder

Adult: **PO** 10–20 mg q.d. (max 60 mg/d)

Bulimia Nervosa

Adult: **PO** 60 mg q.d.

ADMINISTRATION

Oral

- Give as a single dose in morning. Give in two divided doses; one in a.m. and one at noon to prevent insomnia, when more than 20 mg/d prescribed.
- Provide suicidal or potentially suicidal patient with small quantities of prescription medication.
- Store at 15°–25° C (59°–77° F).

ADVERSE EFFECTS (>1%) **CNS:** *Headache, nervousness, anxiety, insomnia,* drowsiness, fatigue, tremor, dizziness. **CV:** Palpitations, hot flushes, chest pain. **GI:** *Nausea, diarrhea,* anorexia, dyspepsia, increased appetite, dry mouth. **Skin:** Rash, pruritus, sweating, hypersensitivity reactions. **Special Senses:** Blurred vision. **Body as a Whole:** Myalgias, arthralgias, flu-like syndrome, hyponatremia. **Urogenital:** Sexual dysfunction, menstrual irregularities.

INTERACTIONS Drug: Concurrent use of **tryptophan** may cause agitation, restlessness, and GI distress; MAOIS, **selegiline** may increase risk of severe hypertensive reaction and death; increases half-life of **diazepam;** may increase toxicity of TRICYCLIC ANTIDEPRESSANTS; AMPHETAMINES, **cilostazol, nefazodone, pentazocine, propafenone, sibutramine, tramadol, venlafaxine** may increase risk of serotonin syndrome; may inhibit metabolism of **carbamazepine, phenytoin, ritonavir. Herbal: St. John's wort** may cause **serotonin** syndrome.

PHARMACOKINETICS Absorption: 60–80% absorbed from GI tract. **Onset:** 1–3 wk. **Peak:** 4–8 h. **Distribution:** Widely distributed, including CNS. **Metabolism:** Metabolized in liver to active metabolite, norfluoxetine. **Elimination:** >80% excreted in urine; 12% in feces. **Half-Life:** Fluoxetine 2–3 d, norfluoxetine 8–10 d. **Geriatric** (≥65) **Half-Life:** (females retain longer half-life than males) fluoxetine 5–7 d, norfluoxetine 14–16 d.

NURSING IMPLICATIONS

Assessment & Drug Effects

- Use with caution in the older adult patient or patient with impaired renal or hepatic function (may need lower dose).
- Check that patient is not self-treating with **St. John's wort** because it is a botanical MAOI.
- Use with caution in patient with anorexia, because weight loss is a possible side effect.
- Thus far, this is the only SSRI deemed effective for pediatric MDD.
- Monitor for S&S of anaphylactoid reaction.
- Lab tests: Periodic serum electrolytes; monitor closely plasma glucose in diabetes.
- Monitor serum sodium level for development of hyponatremia, especially in patients who are taking diuretics or are otherwise hypovolemic.
- Monitor diabetics for loss of glycemic control; hypoglycemia has occurred during initiation of therapy, and hyperglycemia during drug withdrawal.
- Monitor for S&S of improved affect. Requires approximately 2–3 wk for therapeutic effects to be felt.
- Weigh weekly to monitor weight loss, particularly in the older adult or nutritionally compromised patient. Report significant weight loss to prescriber.
- Observe for and promptly report rash or urticaria and S&S of fever, leukocytosis, arthralgias, carpal tunnel syndrome, edema, respiratory distress, and proteinuria. Drug may have to be discontinued or adjunctive therapy instituted with steroids or antihistamines.
- Observe for dizziness and drowsiness and employ safety measures (assistance, up with side rails, etc.) as indicated.
- Monitor for and report increased anxiety, nervousness, or insomnia; may need modification of drug dose.
- Monitor for seizures in patients with a history of seizures. Use appropriate safety precautions.
- Supervise patients closely who are high suicide risks; especially during initial therapy.

- Monitor patients with hepatic or renal impairment carefully for S&S of toxicity (e.g., agitation, restlessness, nausea, vomiting, seizures).

Client & Family Education

- Notify prescriber of intent to become pregnant.
- Notify prescriber of any rash; possible sign of a serious group of adverse effects.
- Some side effects experienced may subside within 3 wk without changes to dose or schedule.
- Do not self-treat with **St. John's wort** because it is a botanical MAOI and cannot be combined with this medication.
- Do not drive or engage in potentially hazardous activities until response to drug is known, especially if dizziness noted.
- Monitor blood glucose for loss of glycemic control if diabetic.
- Note: Drug may increase seizure activity in those with history of seizure.
- Do not breast feed while taking this drug without consulting prescriber.

FLUVOXAMINE

(flu-vox'a-meen)

Luvox

Classifications: CENTRAL NERVOUS SYSTEM AGENT; PSYCHOTHERAPEUTIC; SELECTIVE SEROTONIN-REUPTAKE INHIBITOR (SSRI)

Pregnancy Category: B

AVAILABILITY 25 mg, 50 mg, 100 mg tablets

ACTIONS Antidepressant with potent, selective, inhibitory activity on neuronal (5-HT) serotonin-reuptake; structurally unrelated to TCAs. Compared with TCAs, shows fewer anticholinergic effects and no severe cardiovascular effects.

THERAPEUTIC EFFECTS Effective as an antidepressant and for control of obsessive-compulsive disorders.

USES Treatment of depression and obsessive-compulsive disorders.

UNLABELED USES Chronic tension-type headaches, panic attacks.

CONTRAINDICATIONS Hypersensitivity to fluvoxamine or fluoxetine.

CAUTIOUS USE Pregnancy (category B), lactation, liver disease, renal impairment, history of seizures.

ROUTE & DOSAGE

Depression, Obsessive-Compulsive Disorder

Adult: **PO** Start with 50 mg q.d.; may increase slowly up to 300 mg/d given q.h.s. or divided b.i.d.
Child: **PO** *8–11 y,* Start with 25 mg q.h.s., may increase by 25 mg q4–7d (max 200 mg/d in divided doses)

ADMINISTRATION

Oral

- Give starting doses at bedtime to improve tolerance to nausea and vomiting; both are common early in therapy.
- Store at room temperature, 15°–30° C (59°–86° F), away from moisture and light.

ADVERSE EFFECTS (>1%) **CNS:** *Somnolence, headache, agitation, insomnia, dizziness,* seizures. **CV:** Orthostatic hypotension, slight bradycardia. **GI:** *Nausea, vomiting, dry mouth, constipation, anorexia.* **Urogenital:** Sexual dysfunction. **Skin:** Stevens-Johnson syndrome, toxic epidermal necrolysis (rare).

DIAGNOSTIC TEST INTERFERENCE ***Gamma-glutamyl transferase*** increased by more than threefold following 3 wk of therapy.

INTERACTIONS Drug: Fluvoxamine has been shown to significantly increase plasma levels of **amitriptyline, clomipramine,** and other TRICYCLIC ANTIDEPRESSANTS to mildly increase levels of their metabolites. May antagonize the blood pressure-lowering effects of **atenolol** and other BETA BLOCKERS. May increase levels and toxicity of **carbamazepine, mexiletine.** May increase **lithium** levels causing neurotoxicity, **serotonin** syndrome, somnolence, and mania. One report of increased **theophylline** levels with toxicity. Increases prothrombin time in patients on **warfarin. Herbal: Melatonin** may increase and prolong drowsiness; **St. John's wort** may cause **serotonin** syndrome.

PHARMACOKINETICS Absorption: Almost completely absorbed from GI tract. **Onset:** 4–7 d. **Distribution:** Approximately 77% bound to plasma proteins; excreted in human breast milk but in an amount that poses little risk to the nursing infant. **Metabolism:** Metabolized in liver. **Elimination:** Completely excreted in urine. **Half-Life:** 16–24 h.

NURSING IMPLICATIONS

Assessment & Drug Effects

- Monitor for significant nausea and vomiting, especially during initial therapy.
- Assess safety; drowsiness and dizziness are common adverse effects.
- Check that patient is not self-treating with **St. John's wort** because it is a botanical MAOI.
- Monitor PT and INR carefully with concurrent warfarin therapy; adjust warfarin as needed.

Client & Family Education

- Note: Nausea and vomiting are common in early therapy. Notify prescriber if these adverse effects last more than a few days.
- Some side effects experienced may subside within 3 wk without changes to dose or schedule.
- Do not self-treat with **St. John's wort** because it is a botanical MAOI and cannot be combined with this medication.
- Exercise caution with hazardous activity until response to the drug is known.
- Do not breast feed while taking this drug without consulting prescriber.

PAROXETINE

(par-ox′e-teen)

Asimia, Paxil, Paxil CR

Classifications: CENTRAL NERVOUS SYSTEM AGENT; PSYCHOTHERAPEUTIC; ANTIDEPRESSANT; SELECTIVE SEROTONIN-REUPTAKE INHIBITOR (SSRI)

Pregnancy Category: B

AVAILABILITY 10 mg, 20 mg, 30 mg, 40 mg tablets; 12.5 mg, 25 mg sustained-release tablets; 10 mg/5 mL suspension

ACTIONS Antidepressant structurally unrelated to other serotonin-reuptake inhibitors. Potent and highly selective inhibitor of serotonin reuptake by neurons in CNS.

THERAPEUTIC EFFECTS Efficacious in depression resistant to other antidepressants and in depression complicated by anxiety.

USES Depression, obsessive-compulsive disorders, panic attacks, excessive social anxiety disorder, generalized anxiety, post-traumatic stress disorder (PTSD).

UNLABELED USES Diabetic neuropathy, myoclonus, bipolar depression in conjunction with lithium, chronic headache, premature ejaculation, fibromyalgia.

CONTRAINDICATIONS Concomitant use of MAOIS.
CAUTIOUS USE Renal/hepatic impairment; older adult; history of metabolic disorders; pregnancy (category B), lactation. Safety and efficacy have not been established in children.

ROUTE & DOSAGE

Depression

Adult: **PO** 10–50 mg/d (max 80 mg/d); 25 mg sustained release q.d. in morning; may increase by 12.5 mg (max 62.5 mg/d); use lower starting doses for patients with renal or hepatic insufficiency and geriatric patients
Geriatric: **PO** Start with 10 mg/d (12.5 mg/d sustained release) [max 40 mg/d (50 mg/d sustained release)]

Obsessive-Compulsive Disorder

Adult: **PO** 20–60 mg/d

Panic Attacks

Adult: **PO** 40 mg/d

Social Anxiety Disorder

Adult: **PO** 20–60 mg/d

Generalized Anxiety, PTSD

Adult: **PO** Start with 10 mg q.d., may increase by 10 mg/d at weekly intervals if needed to target dose of 40 mg q.d. (max 60 mg/d)
Geriatric: **PO** Start with 10 mg PO once daily; may increase by 10 mg/d at weekly intervals if needed (max 40 mg/d)

ADMINISTRATION

Oral

- Recommended initial dose with older adult, debilitated, or those with severe renal or hepatic impairment is 10 mg/d.
- Ensure that sustained-release form is not cut, chewed, or crushed. Must be swallowed whole.
- Be aware that at least 14 d should elapse when switching a patient from/to a MAOI to/from paroxetine.

ADVERSE EFFECTS (≥1%) **CV:** Postural hypotension. **CNS:** *Headache,* tremor, agitation or nervousness, anxiety, paresthesias, dizziness, insomnia, *sedation*. **GI:** *Nausea,* constipation, vomiting, anorexia, diarrhea, dyspepsia, flatulence, increased appetite, taste aversion, *dry mouth*. **Urogenital:** Urinary hesitancy or frequency. **Hepatic:** Isolated reports of elevated liver enzymes. **Special Senses:** Blurred vision. **Skin:** Diaphoresis, rash, pruritus. **Metabolic:** Hyponatremia in older adult.

INTERACTIONS Drug: Activated charcoal reduces absorption of paroxetine. **Cimetidine** increases paroxetine levels. MAOIS, **selegiline** may cause an increased vasopressor response leading to hypertensive crisis or death. **Phenytoin** can cause liver enzyme induction, resulting in lower paroxetine levels and shorter half-life. **Warfarin** may increase risk of bleeding. May increase **thioridazine** levels and prolong QTc interval leading to heart block. **Herbal: St. John's wort** may cause **serotonin** syndrome (headache, dizziness, sweating, agitation).

PHARMACOKINETICS Absorption: 99% absorbed from GI tract. **Onset:** 2 wk. **Peak:** 5–8 h. **Distribution:** Very lipophilic; 95% protein bound. Distributes into breast milk. **Metabolism:** Extensively metabolized in the liver to inactive metabolites. **Elimination:** Less than 2% is excreted unchanged in urine. Approximately 65% of dose appears in urine as metabolites. Metabolites of paroxetine are also excreted in feces, presumably via bile. **Half-Life:** 24 h.

NURSING IMPLICATIONS

Assessment & Drug Effects

- Monitor for adverse effects, which include headache, weakness, sedation, dizziness, insomnia; nausea, constipation, or diarrhea; dry mouth; sweating; male ejaculatory disturbance. These occur in more than 10% of all patients and may result in poor compliance with drug regimen.
- Check that patient is not self-treating with **St. John's wort** because it is a botanical MAOI.
- Monitor older adult for fluid and sodium imbalances.
- Monitor for significant weight loss.
- Monitor patients with history of mania for reactivation of condition.
- Monitor patients with preexisting cardiovascular disease carefully because paroxetine may adversely affect hemodynamic status.

Client & Family Education

- Use caution when operating hazardous machinery or equipment until response to drug is known.

- Concurrent use of alcohol may increase risk of adverse CNS effects.
- Do not self-treat with **St. John's wort** because it is a botanical MAOI and cannot be combined with this medication.
- Adaptation to some adverse effects (especially dizziness and nausea) may occur over a period of 4–6 wk.
- Do not stop drug therapy after improvement in emotional status occurs.
- Notify prescriber of any distressing adverse effects.
- Do not breast feed while taking this drug without consulting prescriber.

SERTRALINE HYDROCHLORIDE

(ser′tra-leen)

Zoloft

Classifications: CENTRAL NERVOUS SYSTEM AGENT; PSYCHOTHERAPEUTIC; ANTIDEPRESSANT; SELECTIVE SEROTONIN-REUPTAKE INHIBITOR (SSRI)

Pregnancy Category: C

AVAILABILITY 25 mg, 50 mg, 100 mg tablets; 20 mg/mL liquid

ACTIONS Potent inhibitor of serotonin (5-HT) reuptake in the brain, and chemically unrelated to TCA, tetracyclic, or other available antidepressants. Chronic administration of sertraline results in down regulation of norepinephrine, a reaction found with other effective antidepressants. Sertraline does not inhibit MAO.

THERAPEUTIC EFFECTS Treats depression, obsessive-compulsive disorder, and panic disorder.

USES Major depression, obsessive-compulsive disorder, panic disorder, premenstrual dysphoric disorder, generalized anxiety, post-traumatic stress disorder.

CONTRAINDICATIONS Patients taking MAOIS or within 14 d of discontinuing MAOI; Antabuse.

CAUTIOUS USE Seizure disorders, major affective disorders, suicidal patients; liver dysfunction, renal impairment; pregnancy (category C). Unknown if sertraline is excreted in breast milk. Safety and effectiveness in children <6 y are not established.

ROUTE & DOSAGE

Depression, Anxiety

Adult: **PO** Begin with 50 mg/d, gradually increase every few weeks according to response (range: 50–200 mg)
Geriatric: **PO** Start with 25 mg/d

Premenstrual Dysphoric Disorder

Adult: **PO** Begin with 50 mg/d for first cycle; may titrate up to 150 mg/d

Obsessive-Compulsive Disorder

Adult: **PO** Begin with 50 mg/d; may titrate at weekly intervals up to 200 mg/d
Child: **PO** *6–12 y,* Begin with 25 mg/d; may increase by 50 mg/wk, as tolerated and needed, up to 200 mg/d

ADMINISTRATION

Oral

- Give in the morning or evening.
- Do not give concurrently with a MAOI or within 14 d of discontinuing a MAOI.

ADVERSE EFFECTS (≥1%) **CV:** Palpitations, chest pain, hypertension, hypotension, edema, syncope, tachycardia. **CNS:** *Agitation, insomnia, headache, dizziness, somnolence, fatigue,* ataxia, incoordination, vertigo, abnormal dreams, aggressive behavior, delusions, hallucinations, emotional lability, paranoia, suicidal ideation, depersonalization. **Endocrine:** Gynecomastia, male sexual dysfunction. **GI:** Nausea, vomiting, diarrhea, constipation, indigestion, anorexia, flatulence, abdominal pain, dry mouth. **Special Senses:** Exophthalmos, blurred vision, dry eyes, diplopia, photophobia, tearing, conjunctivitis, mydriasis. **Skin:** Rash, urticaria, acne, alopecia. **Respiratory:** Rhinitis, pharyngitis, cough, dyspnea, bronchospasm. **Body as a Whole:** Myalgia, arthralgia, muscle weakness. **Metabolic:** Hyponatremia in older adults.

DIAGNOSTIC TEST INTERFERENCE May cause asymptomatic elevations in ***liver function tests.*** Slight decrease in ***uric acid.***

INTERACTIONS Drug: MAOIS (e.g., **selegiline, phenelzine**) should be stopped 14 d before sertraline is started because of serious problems with other SEROTONIN-REUPTAKE INHIBITORS (shivering, nausea, diplopia, confusion, anxiety). **Sertraline** may increase levels and toxicity of **diazepam, pimozide, tolbutamide.** Use cautiously with other centrally acting CNS drugs. **Herbal: St. John's wort** may cause **serotonin** syndrome (headache, dizziness, sweating, agitation).

PHARMACOKINETICS Absorption: Slowly absorbed from GI tract. **Onset:** 2–4 wk. **Distribution:** 99% protein bound; not known if distributed into breast milk. **Metabolism:** Extensive first-pass metabolism in liver to inactive metabolites. **Elimination:** 40–45% excreted in urine, 40–45% in feces. **Half-Life:** 24 h.

NURSING IMPLICATIONS

Assessment & Drug Effects

- Supervise patients at risk for suicide closely during initial therapy.
- Check that patient is not self-treating with **St. John's wort** because it is a botanical MAOI.
- Monitor older adults for fluid and sodium imbalances.
- Monitor patients with a history of a seizure disorder closely.
- Lab tests: Monitor PT and INR with patients receiving concurrent warfarin therapy.

Client & Family Education

- Report diarrhea, nausea, dyspepsia, insomnia, drowsiness, dizziness, or persistent headache to prescriber.
- Do not self-treat with **St. John's wort** because it is a botanical MAOI and cannot be combined with this medication.
- Report signs of bleeding promptly to prescriber when taking concomitant warfarin.
- Some side effects experienced may subside within 3 wk without changes to dose or schedule.
- Do not breast feed while taking this drug without consulting prescriber.

ANTIDEPRESSANTS, TETRACYCLIC

MAPROTILINE HYDROCHLORIDE

(ma-proe'ti-leen)

Maprotiline HCl

Classifications: CENTRAL NERVOUS SYSTEM AGENT; PSYCHOTHERAPEUTIC; TETRACYCLIC ANTIDEPRESSANT

Pregnancy Category: B

AVAILABILITY 25 mg, 50 mg, 75 mg tablets

ACTIONS Tetracyclic antidepressant pharmacologically and therapeutically similar to the tricyclic antidepressants. Has significant sedative effect and less prominent anticholinergic action; may lower seizure threshold. Precise mechanism is unknown; however, it blocks the reuptake of norepinephrine at the neural membranes.
THERAPEUTIC EFFECTS Useful in depression associated with anxiety and sleep disturbances.

USES Treatment of major depressive disorder, dysthymic disorder, and bipolar illness, depressed type.

CONTRAINDICATIONS Patients <18 y; history of seizure disorder; pregnancy (category B), lactation.
CAUTIOUS USE History of seizure activity. Also see precautions under imipramine HCl.

ROUTE & DOSAGE

Mild to Moderate Depression

Adult: **PO** Start at 75 mg/d and gradually increase q2wk up to 150 mg/d in single or divided doses
Geriatric: **PO** Start with 25 mg h.s. and gradually increase to 50–75 mg/d

Severe Depression

Adult: **PO** Start at 100–150 mg/d and gradually increase up to 300 mg/d in single or divided doses if needed

ADMINISTRATION

Oral

- Give as single dose or in divided doses. Initiate therapy with low dosages to reduce risk of seizures.
- Store at 15°–30° C (59°–86° F) unless otherwise specified.

ADVERSE EFFECTS (≥1%) **CNS:** Seizures, exacerbation of psychosis, hallucinations, tremors, excitement, confusion, dizziness, *drowsiness*. **CV:** *Orthostatic hypotension,* hypertension, tachycardia. **Special Senses:** Accommodation disturbances, blurred vision, mydriasis. **GI:** Nausea, vomiting, epigastric distress, *constipation, dry mouth*. **Urogenital:** *Urinary retention,* frequency. **Skin:** Hypersensitivity reactions (skin rash, urticaria, photosensitivity).

INTERACTIONS Drug: May decrease some response to ANTIHYPERTENSIVES; CNS DEPRESSANTS, **alcohol,** HYPNOTICS, BARBITURATES, SEDATIVES potentiate CNS depression; may increase hypoprothrombinemic effect of ORAL ANTICOAGULANTS; transient delirium with **ethchlorvynol;** with **levodopa,** SYMPATHOMIMETICS (e.g., **epinephrine, norepinephrine**) there is possibility of sympathetic hyperactivity with hypertension and hyperpyrexia; with MAOIS there is possibility of severe reactions, toxic psychosis, cardiovascular instability; **methylphenidate** increases plasma TCA levels; THYROID DRUGS increase possibility of arrhythmias; **cimetidine** may increase plasma TCA levels.

PHARMACOKINETICS Absorption: Slowly absorbed from GI tract. **Peak:** 12 h. **Distribution:** Distributed chiefly to brain, lungs, liver, and kidneys. **Metabolism:** Metabolized in liver. **Elimination:** 70% excreted in urine, 30% in feces. **Half-Life:** 51 h.

NURSING IMPLICATIONS

Assessment & Drug Effects

- Monitor for therapeutic effectiveness; 2–3 wk are usually necessary for full effect.
- Assess level of sedative effect. If recovering patient becomes too lethargic to care for personal hygiene or to maintain food intake and interactions with others, report to prescriber.
- Monitor bowel elimination pattern and I&O ratio. Severe constipation and urinary retention are potential problems, especially in the older adult. Advise increased fluid intake (at least 1500 mL/d).
- Observe seizure precautions; risk of seizures appears to be high in those who consume moderate to high levels of ETOH.
- Bear in mind that if patient uses excessive amounts of ETOH, potentiated effects of maprotiline may increase the danger of overdosage or suicide attempt.

Client & Family Education

- Report symptoms of stomatitis and dry mouth when taking high doses. Sore or dry mouth can lead to lack of compliance.
- Use caution with tasks that require alertness and skill; ability may be impaired during early therapy.
- Do not change dose or dose schedule without consulting prescriber.
- Do not use OTC drugs unless approved by prescriber.

- Avoid alcohol; the effects of maprotiline are potentiated when both are used together and for 2 wk after maprotiline is discontinued.
- Do not breast feed while using this drug.

MIRTAZAPINE

(mir-taz′a-peen)

Remeron, Remeron SolTab

Classifications: CENTRAL NERVOUS SYSTEM AGENT; PSYCHOTHERAPEUTIC; TETRACYCLIC ANTIDEPRESSANT

Pregnancy Category: C

AVAILABILITY 15 mg, 30 mg, 45 mg tablets and orally disintegrating tablets

ACTIONS Tetracyclic antidepressant pharmacologically and therapeutically similar to the tricyclic antidepressants. Tetracyclics enhance central noradrenergic and serotonergic activity; thought to be due to normalizing of neurotransmission efficacy. Mirtazapine is a potent antagonist of $5\text{-}HT_2$ and $5\text{-}HT_3$ serotonin receptors.

THERAPEUTIC EFFECTS Acts as antidepressant. Effectiveness is indicated by mood elevation.

USES Treatment of depression.

CONTRAINDICATIONS Hypersensitivity to mirtazapine or mianserin; hypersensitivity to other antidepressants (e.g., tricyclic antidepressants and MAOI depressants).

CAUTIOUS USE History of cardiovascular or GI disorders; BPH; narrow-angle glaucoma; hepatic or renal impairment; older adults; pregnancy (category C), lactation. Safety and effectiveness in children are not established.

ROUTE & DOSAGE

Depression

Adult: **PO** 15 mg/d in single dose h.s.; may increase q1–2wk (max 45 mg/d)

Geriatric: **PO** Use lower doses

Renal or Hepatic Impairment

Use lower doses

ADMINISTRATION

Oral

- Give preferably prior to sleep to minimize injury potential.
- Begin drug no sooner than 14 d after discontinuation of an MAOI.
- Reduce dosage as warranted with severe renal or hepatic impairment and in older adults.
- Store at 20°–25° C (68°–77° F) in tight, light-resistant container.

ADVERSE EFFECTS (≥1%) **Body as a Whole:** Asthenia, flu syndrome, back pain, general and peripheral edema, malaise. **CNS:** *Somnolence,* dizziness, abnormal dreams, abnormal thinking, tremor, confusion, depression, agitation, vertigo, twitching. **CV:** Hypertension, vasodilation. **GI:** Nausea, vomiting, abdominal pain, *increased appetite/*weight gain, *dry mouth, constipation,* anorexia, cholecystitis, stomatitis, colitis, abnormal liver function tests. **Respiratory:** Dyspnea, cough, sinusitis. **Skin:** Pruritus, rash. **Urogenital:** Urinary frequency.

INTERACTIONS Drug: Additive cognitive and motor impairment with **alcohol** or BENZODIAZEPINES; increase risk of hypertensive crisis with MAOIS. **Herbal: Kava-kava, valerian** may potentiate sedative effects.

PHARMACOKINETICS Absorption: Rapidly absorbed from GI tract; 50% reaches systemic circulation. **Peak:** 2 h. **Distribution:** 85% protein bound. **Metabolism:** Metabolized in liver by cytochrome P-450 system (CYP2D6, CYP1A2, CYP3A). **Elimination:** 75% excreted in urine, 15% in feces. **Half-Life:** 20–40 h.

NURSING IMPLICATIONS

Assessment & Drug Effects

- Lab tests: Monitor WBC count with differential, lipid profile, and ALT/AST periodically.
- Assess for weight gain and excessive somnolence or dizziness.
- Monitor for orthostatic hypotension with a history of cardiovascular or cerebrovascular disease. Periodically monitor ECG especially in those with known cardiovascular disease.
- Monitor those with a history of increased intraocular pressure or urinary retention carefully for worsening or recurrence.
- Monitor those with history of seizures for lowering of the seizure threshold.

Client & Family Education

- Do not drive or engage in potentially hazardous activities until response to drug is known.
- Do not use alcohol while taking drug.
- Report immediately unexplained fever or S&S of infection, especially flu-like symptoms, to prescriber.
- Do not take other prescription or OTC drugs without consulting prescriber.
- Make position changes slowly, especially from lying or sitting to standing. Report dizziness, palpitations, and fainting.
- (Women) Notify prescriber immediately if you become pregnant.
- Monitor weight periodically and report significant weight gains.
- Do not breast feed while taking this drug without consulting prescriber.

ANTIDEPRESSANTS, TRICYCLIC

AMITRIPTYLINE HYDROCHLORIDE

(a-mee-trip'ti-leen)

Amitril, Apo-Amitriptyline ♣, Elavil, Emitrip, Endep, Enovil, Levate ♣, Meravil, Novotriptyn ♣, SK-Amitriptyline

Classifications: CENTRAL NERVOUS SYSTEM AGENT; PSYCHOTHERAPEUTIC; TRICYCLIC ANTIDEPRESSANT

Pregnancy Category: C

AVAILABILITY 10 mg, 25 mg, 50 mg, 75 mg, 100 mg, 150 mg tablets; 10 mg/mL injection

ACTIONS Among the most active of the tricyclic antidepressants (TCAs) in inhibition of serotonin uptake from synaptic gap; also inhibits norepinephrine reuptake to a moderate degree. Restoration of the levels of these neurotransmitters is a proposed mechanism of antidepressant action.

THERAPEUTIC EFFECTS Interference with the reuptake of serotonin and norepinephrine results in the antidepressant activity of amitriptyline.

USES Major depression.

UNLABELED USES Prophylaxis for cluster, migraine, and chronic tension headaches; intractable pain; peptic ulcer disease; to increase muscle strength in myotonic dystrophy; to treat pathologic weeping and laughing secondary to forebrain disease or

CVA; for eating disorders associated with depression (anorexia or bulimia); as sedative for nondepressed patients.

CONTRAINDICATIONS Acute recovery period after MI, history of seizure disorders, pregnancy (category C), lactation, children <12 y.

CAUTIOUS USE Prostatic hypertrophy, history of urinary retention or obstruction; angle-closure glaucoma; diabetes mellitus; hyperthyroidism; patient with cardiovascular, hepatic, or renal dysfunction; patient with suicidal tendency, electroconvulsive therapy (ECT); elective surgery; schizophrenia; respiratory disorders; older adults, adolescents.

ROUTE & DOSAGE

Antidepressant

Adult: **PO** 75–100 mg/d; may gradually increase to 150–300 mg/d (use lower doses in outpatients) **IM** 20–30 mg q.i.d. until patient can take PO
Geriatric: **PO** 10–25 mg h.s., may gradually increase to 25–150 mg/d
Adolescent: **PO** 25–50 mg/d in divided doses; may gradually increase to 100 mg/d (max 200 mg/d)

ADMINISTRATION

Oral

- Give with or immediately after food to reduce possibility of GI irritation. Tablet may be crushed if patient is unable to take it whole; administer with food or fluid.
- Give increased doses preferably in late afternoon or at bedtime due to sedative action that precedes antidepressant effect.
- Give as single dose at bedtime to promote sleep or for patients with dizziness or when daytime sedation interferes with work productivity.
- Note that dose is usually tapered over 2 wk at discontinuation to prevent withdrawal symptoms (headache, nausea, malaise, musculoskeletal pain, panic attack, weakness).

Intramuscular

- Reserve IM injections for patients unable or unwilling to take oral drug.
- Inject deep IM into a large muscle.
- Store drug at 15°–30° C (59°–86° F) and protect from light unless otherwise directed by manufacturer.

ADVERSE EFFECTS (≥1%) **CNS:** *Drowsiness, sedation, dizziness,* nervousness, restlessness, fatigue, headache, insomnia, abnormal movements (extrapyramidal symptoms), seizures. **CV:** *Orthostatic hypotension,* tachycardia, palpitation, ECG changes. **Special Senses:** Blurred vision, mydriasis. **GI:** *Dry mouth,* increased appetite especially for sweets, *constipation,* weight gain, sour or metallic taste, nausea, vomiting. **Urogenital:** *Urinary retention.* **Other:** (Rare) bone marrow depression.

INTERACTIONS Drug: ANTIHYPERTENSIVES may decrease some antihypertensive response; CNS DEPRESSANTS, **alcohol,** HYPNOTICS, BARBITURATES, SEDATIVES potentiate CNS depression; ORAL ANTICOAGULANTS may increase hypoprothombinemic effect; **ethchlorvynol,** transient delirium; **levodopa,** SYMPATHOMIMETICS (e.g., **epinephrine, norepinephrine**), possibility of sympathetic hyperactivity with hypertension and hyperpyrexia; MAOIS, possibility of severe reactions, toxic psychosis, cardiovascular instability; **methylphenidate** increases plasma TCA levels; THYROID DRUGS may increase possibility of arrhythmias; **cimetidine** may increase plasma TCA levels. **Herbal: Ginkgo** may decrease seizure threshold, **St. John's wort** may cause **serotonin** syndrome, **valerian** may enhance sedation.

PHARMACOKINETICS Absorption: Rapidly absorbed from GI and injection sites. **Peak:** 2–12 h. **Distribution:** Crosses placenta. **Metabolism:** Metabolized in liver to active metabolite. **Elimination:** Primarily excreted in urine; enters breast milk. **Half-Life:** 10–50 h.

NURSING IMPLICATIONS

Assessment & Drug Effects

- Monitor therapeutic effectiveness. It may take 1–6 wk to reduce attacks when used for migraine prophylaxis.
- Monitor for S&S of drowsiness and dizziness (initial stages of therapy); institute measures to prevent falling. Also monitor for overdose or suicide ideation in patients who use excessive amounts of alcohol.
- Lab tests: Baseline and periodic leukocyte and differential counts; renal and hepatic function tests; eye examinations (including glaucoma testing); recommended particularly for older adults, adolescents, and patients receiving high doses/prolonged therapy.
- Monitor BP and pulse rate in patients with preexisting cardiovascular disease. Assess for orthostatic hypotension especially

in older adults. Withhold drug if there is a rise or fall in systolic BP (by 10–20 mm Hg), or a sudden increase or a significant change in pulse rate or rhythm. Notify prescriber.
- Monitor I&O, including bowel elimination pattern.

Client & Family Education
- Monitor weight; drug may increase appetite or a craving for sweets.
- Understand that tolerance/adaptation to anticholinergic actions usually develops with maintenance regimen. Keep prescriber informed.
- Relieve dry mouth by taking frequent sips of water and increasing total fluid intake.
- Make position changes slowly and in stages to prevent dizziness.
- Do not drive or engage in potentially hazardous activities until response to drug is known.
- Do not use OTC drugs without consulting prescriber while on TCA therapy; many preparations contain sympathomimetic amines.
- Note: Amitriptyline may turn urine blue-green.
- Do not breast feed while taking this drug.

AMOXAPINE
(a-mox′a-peen)
Asendin
Classifications: CENTRAL NERVOUS SYSTEM AGENT; PSYCHOTHERAPEUTIC; TRICYCLIC ANTIDEPRESSANT
Pregnancy Category: C

AVAILABILITY 25 mg, 50 mg, 100 mg, 150 mg tablets

ACTIONS Tricyclic antidepressant (TCA) and secondary amine with mixed antidepressant and neuroleptic tranquilizing properties. Unlike some TCAs, not associated with severe cardiotoxicity, has mild sedative action, and causes slight orthostatic hypotension.
THERAPEUTIC EFFECTS Antidepressant activity is thought to be due to reduced reuptake of norepinephrine and serotonin. Also blocks response to dopamine by dopaminergic receptors.

USES Neurotic and endogenous depression accompanied by anxiety or agitation.

CONTRAINDICATIONS Hypersensitivity to other tricyclic compounds; acute recovery period after MI. Safety during pregnancy (category C), lactation, or children <16 y of age is not established.

CAUTIOUS USE History of convulsive disorders, schizophrenia, manic depression, electroshock therapy; alcohol abuse; history of urinary retention, benign prostatic hypertrophy; angle-closure glaucoma or increased intraocular pressure; cardiovascular disorders; impaired renal or hepatic function; elective surgery.

ROUTE & DOSAGE

Antidepressant

Adult: **PO** Start at 50 mg b.i.d. or t.i.d.; may increase on third day to 100 mg t.i.d. Maintenance doses ≤300 mg/d as single dose at bedtime
Geriatric: **PO** 25 mg h.s.; may increase q3–7d to 50–150 mg/d in divided doses (max 300 mg/d)

ADMINISTRATION

Oral

- Give with or after food to reduce GI irritation; tablet may be crushed and taken with fluid or mixed with food.
- Give maintenance dose as a single dose at bedtime to minimize daytime sedation and other annoying drug adverse effects.
- Do not abruptly discontinue drug. Doses should be tapered over 2 wk.
- Store at 15°–30° C (59°–86° F) in tightly closed container unless otherwise directed.

ADVERSE EFFECTS (≥1%) **CNS:** *Drowsiness,* dizziness, headache, fatigue, *sedation,* lethargy; extrapyramidal effects (acute dystonic reactions, panic attacks, parkinsonism, tardive dyskinesia), <u>seizures</u> (overdosage). **CV:** Orthostatic hypotension; arrhythmias **GI:** Constipation, diarrhea, flatulence, *dry mouth,* peculiar taste, nausea, heartburn. **Special Senses:** Blurred vision, dry eyes. **Urogenital:** Nephrotoxicity (overdosage).

INTERACTIONS Drug: May decrease response to ANTIHYPERTENSIVES; CNS DEPRESSANTS, **alcohol,** HYPNOTICS, BARBITURATES, SEDATIVES potentiate CNS depression; may increase hypoprothombinemic effect of ORAL ANTICOAGULANTS; **ethchlorvynol,** transient delirium; with **levodopa,** SYMPATHOMIMETICS (e.g., **epinephrine, norepinephrine**), possibility of sympathetic hyperactivity with hypertension and hyperpyrexia; with MAOIS, possibility of severe reactions: toxic psychosis, cardiovascular instability; **methylphenidate** increases plasma TCA levels; THYROID DRUGS may increase possibility of arrhythmias; **cimetidine** may increase plasma TCA levels. **Herbal: Ginkgo** may decrease seizure threshold, **St. John's wort** may cause **serotonin** syndrome.

PHARMACOKINETICS Absorption: Rapidly absorbed. **Peak:** 1–2 h. **Distribution:** Probably crosses placenta; distributed into breast milk. **Metabolism:** Metabolized active metabolite. **Elimination:** 60% excreted in urine in 6 d; 7–18% excreted in feces. **Half-Life:** parent drug 8 h; metabolite 30 h.

NURSING IMPLICATIONS

Assessment & Drug Effects

- Monitor therapeutic effectiveness. Initial antidepressant effect (mild euphoria, increased energy) may occur within 4–7 d; however, in most patients clinical response does not occur until after 2–3 wk of drug therapy.
- Supervise patient closely during therapy for suicidal ideation and potential serious adverse effects.
- Report immediately signs of neuroleptic malignant syndrome: fever, sweating, rigidity (catatonia), unstable BP, rapid, irregular pulse; changes in level of consciousness, coma. Although rare, it can be life threatening if drug is not stopped immediately. Death can result from acute respiratory, renal, or cardiovascular failure.
- Report immediately the onset of signs of tardive dyskinesia; careful observation/reporting may prevent irreversibility.
- Monitor I&O ratio and bowel elimination pattern. Report continuing constipation.

Client & Family Education

- Follow directions for taking this drug (see ADMINISTRATION).
- Do not abruptly discontinue drug. Dosage should be tapered over 2 wk. Maintain established dosage regimen. Do not skip, reduce, or double doses or change dose intervals.
- Minimize alcohol intake because it may potentiate drug effects, thus increasing the dangers of overdosage or suicidal ideation.
- Drink at least 2000 mL (approx 2 qt) fluid daily and eat foods with high fiber content (if allowed) to provide needed roughage.
- Monitor weight at least weekly and report significant weight gain.

- Do not drive or engage in potentially hazardous tasks until response to drug is known.
- Rinse mouth frequently with clear water, especially after eating, to relieve mouth dryness.
- Do not take any prescription or OTC drugs without consulting prescriber.
- Do not breast feed while taking this drug without consulting prescriber.

CLOMIPRAMINE HYDROCHLORIDE

(clo-mi′pra-meen)

Anafranil

Classifications: CENTRAL NERVOUS SYSTEM AGENT; PSYCHOTHERAPEUTIC; TRICYCLIC ANTIDEPRESSANT

Pregnancy Category: C

AVAILABILITY 25 mg, 50 mg, 75 mg capsules

ACTIONS Inhibits the reuptake of norepinephrine and serotonin at the presynaptic neuron. Elevates serum levels of these two amines.
THERAPEUTIC EFFECTS The basis of its antidepressant effects is thought to be due to the elevated serum levels of norepinephrine and serotonin. Exhibits anticholinergic, antihistaminic, hypotensive, sedative, mild analgesic, and peripheral vasodilator effects.

USES Obsessive-compulsive disorder (OCD).
UNLABELED USES Panic disorder, anxiety, agoraphobia.

CONTRAINDICATIONS Hypersensitivity to other tricyclic compounds; acute recovery period after MI, children <10 y, pregnancy (category C), lactation.
CAUTIOUS USE History of convulsive disorders, prostatic hypertrophy, urinary retention, cardiovascular, hepatic, GI, or blood disorders.

ROUTE & DOSAGE

Obsessive-Compulsive Disorder

Adult: **PO** 75–300 mg/d in divided doses
Child: **PO** *10–18 y,* 100–200 mg/d in divided doses, start at 50 mg/d

Depression

Adult: **PO** 50–150 mg/d in single or divided doses

ADMINISTRATION

Oral

- Give in divided doses with meals to reduce GI adverse effects.
- Following titration to the full dose, drug may be given as a single dose at bedtime to reduce daytime sedation.
- Store at 15°–30° C (59°–86° F).

ADVERSE EFFECTS (≥1%) **Body as a Whole:** Diaphoresis. **CV:** Hypotension, tachycardia. **GI:** Constipation, *dry mouth*. **Endocrine:** Galactorrhea, hyperprolactinemia, amenorrhea, *weight gain*. **Hematologic:** Leukopenia, <u>agranulocytosis</u>, thrombocytopenia, anemia. **CNS:** Mania, *tremor,* dizziness, hyperthermia, neuroleptic malignant syndrome, seizures (especially with abrupt withdrawal). **Urogenital:** Delayed ejaculation, anorgasmia.

DIAGNOSTIC TEST INTERFERENCE Clomipramine appears to elevate serum ***prolactin*** levels. ***Serum AST and ALT*** are elevated. Serum levels of ***triiodothyronine (T3) and free triiodothyronine (FT3)*** have been significantly reduced from baseline. ***Thyroxine-binding globulin (TBG)*** levels were increased from baseline, whereas ***thyroxine (T_4), free thyroxine (FT_4),*** and reverse ***T_3*** were unchanged.

INTERACTIONS Drug: MAOIS may precipitate hyperpyrexic crisis, tachycardia, or seizures; ANTIHYPERTENSIVE AGENTS potentiate orthostatic hypotension; CNS DEPRESSANTS, **alcohol** add to CNS depression; **norepinephrine** and other SYMPATHOMIMETICS may increase cardiac toxicity; **cimetidine** decreases hepatic metabolism, thus increasing imipramine levels; **methylphenidate** inhibits metabolism of **imipramine** and thus may increase its toxicity. **Herbal: Ginkgo** may decrease seizure threshold; **St. John's wort** may cause serotonin syndrome.

PHARMOCOKINETICS Absorption: Rapidly absorbed from GI tract; 20–78% reaches systemic circulation. **Onset:** Depression: approx. 2 wk; OCD: approx. 4–10 wk. **Peak:** 2–6 h. **Distribution:** Widely distributed including the CSF; crosses placenta. **Metabolism:** Extensive first-pass metabolism in the liver; active metabolite is desmethylclomipramine. **Elimination:** 50–60% excreted in urine, 24–32% in feces. **Half-Life:** 20–30 h.

NURSING IMPLICATIONS

Assessment & Drug Effects

- Monitor for seizures, especially in those with predisposing factors such as alcoholism, brain injury, or concurrent therapy with other drugs that lower seizure threshold.
- Lab tests: Periodic CBC with differential platelet count, and Hct and Hgb. Monitor liver functions, especially with long-term therapy.
- Monitor for and report signs of neuroleptic malignant syndrome.
- Monitor for sedation and vertigo, especially at the beginning of therapy and following dosage increases. Supervision of ambulation may be indicated.
- Notify prescriber of fever and complaints of sore throat; these may indicate need to rule out adverse hematologic changes.

Client & Family Education

- Do not take nonprescribed drugs or discontinue therapy without consulting prescriber. Abrupt discontinuation may cause nausea, headache, malaise, or seizures.
- Men should understand that the drug may cause impotence or ejaculation failure. Advise them to report this problem to prescriber.
- Report promptly a sore throat accompanied by fever.
- Use caution ambulating until response to drug is known.
- Avoid alcohol intake because it may potentiate adverse drug effects and is a depressant.
- Do not breast feed while taking this drug.

DESIPRAMINE HYDROCHLORIDE

(dess-ip′ra-meen)

Norpramin, Pertofrane

Classifications: CENTRAL NERVOUS SYSTEM AGENT; PSYCHOTHERAPEUTIC; TRICYCLIC ANTIDEPRESSANT

Pregnancy Category: C

AVAILABILITY 10 mg, 25 mg, 50 mg, 75 mg, 100 mg, 150 mg tablets

ACTIONS Dibenzoxazepine tricyclic antidepressant (TCA) and secondary amine. Desipramine is the active metabolite of

imipramine and has similar pharmacologic actions. Unlike imipramine, onset of action is more rapid, and it has lower potential for producing sedative and anticholinergic effects and orthostatic hypotension.
THERAPEUTIC EFFECTS In common with other TCAs, antidepressant activity appears to be related to inhibition of reuptake of norepinephrine and serotonin in the CNS. Restoration of the levels of these neurotransmitters is a proposed mechanism of antidepressant action.

USES Major depression and various depression syndromes.
UNLABELED USES Attention deficit disorder in children >6 y and adolescents; to prevent depression in cocaine withdrawal.

CONTRAINDICATIONS Hypersensitivity to tricyclic compounds; recent MI. Safe use during pregnancy (category C), lactation, or in children <12 y is not established.
CAUTIOUS USE Urinary retention, prostatic hypertrophy; narrow-angle glaucoma; epilepsy; alcoholism; adolescents, older adults; thyroid; cardiovascular, renal, and hepatic disease; suicidal tendency; ECT; elective surgery.

ROUTE & DOSAGE

Antidepressant

Adult: **PO** 75–100 mg/d at bedtime or in divided doses; may gradually increase to 150–300 mg/d (use lower doses in older adult patients)
Adolescent: **PO** 25–50 mg/d (max 100 mg/d) in divided doses
Child: **PO** *6–12 y,* 1–3 mg/kg/d in divided doses (max 5 mg/kg/d)

ADMINISTRATION

Oral

- Give drug with or immediately after food to reduce possibility of gastric irritation.
- Give maintenance dose at bedtime to minimize daytime sedation.
- Store drug in tightly closed container at 15°–30° C (59°–86° F) unless otherwise specified.

ADVERSE EFFECTS (≥1%) **Body as a Whole:** Hypersensitivity (rash, urticaria, photosensitivity). **CNS:** *Drowsiness,* dizziness, weakness, fatigue, headache, insomnia, confusional states, depressive reaction, paresthesias, ataxia. **CV:** *Postural hypotension,* hypotension, palpitation, tachycardia, ECG changes, flushing, heart block. **Special Senses:** Tinnitus, parotid swelling; blurred vision, disturbances in accommodation, mydriasis, increased IOP. **GI:** *Dry mouth, constipation,* bad taste, diarrhea, nausea. **Urogenital:** *Urinary retention,* frequency, delayed micturition, nocturia; impaired sexual function, galactorrhea. **Hematologic:** Bone marrow depression and agranulocytosis (rare). **Other:** Sweating, craving for sweets, weight gain or loss, SIADH secretion, hyperpyrexia, eosinophilic pneumonia.

INTERACTIONS Drug: May somewhat decrease response to ANTIHYPERTENSIVES; CNS DEPRESSANTS, **alcohol,** HYPNOTICS, BARBITURATES, SEDATIVES potentiate CNS depression; may increase hypoprothombinemic effect of ORAL ANTICOAGULANTS; **ethchlorvynol** may cause transient delirium; **levodopa,** SYMPATHOMIMETICS (e.g., **epinephrine, norepinephrine**) pose possibility of sympathetic hyperactivity with hypertension and hyperpyrexia; MAOIS pose possibility of severe reactions, toxic psychosis, cardiovascular instability; **methylphenidate** increases plasma TCA levels; THYROID AGENTS may increase possibility of arrhythmias; **cimetidine** may increase plasma TCA levels. **Herbal: Ginkgo** may decrease seizure threshold; **St. John's wort** may cause **serotonin** syndrome.

PHARMACOKINETICS Absorption: Rapidly absorbed from GI tract and injection sites. **Peak:** 4–6 h. **Distribution:** Crosses placenta. **Metabolism:** Metabolized in liver. **Elimination:** Primarily excreted in urine. **Half-Life:** 7–60 h.

NURSING IMPLICATIONS

Assessment & Drug Effects

- Monitor for therapeutic effectiveness: Usually not realized until after at least 2 wk of therapy.
- Monitor BP and pulse rate during early phase of therapy, particularly in older adult, debilitated, or cardiovascular patients. If BP rises or falls more than 20 mm Hg or if there is a sudden increase in pulse rate or change in rhythm, withhold drug and inform prescriber.
- Note: Drowsiness, dizziness, and orthostatic hypotension are signs of impending toxicity in patient on long-term, high-

dosage therapy. Prolonged QT or QRS intervals indicate possible toxicity. Report to prescriber.
- Observe patient with history of glaucoma. Report symptoms that may signal acute attack: Severe headache, eye pain, dilated pupils, halos of light, nausea, vomiting.
- Monitor bowel elimination pattern and I&O ratio. Severe constipation and urinary retention are potential problems of TCA therapy.
- Note: Norpramin tablets may contain tartrazine, which can cause allergic-type reactions, including bronchial asthma in susceptible individuals. Such individuals are frequently also sensitive to aspirin.

Client & Family Education
- Make all position changes slowly and in stages, particularly from recumbent to standing position.
- Do not drive or engage in other potentially hazardous activities until reaction to drug is known.
- Take medication exactly as prescribed; do not change dose or dose intervals.
- Note: Patients who receive high doses for prolonged periods may experience withdrawal symptoms including headache, nausea, musculoskeletal pain, and weakness if drug is discontinued abruptly.
- Do not take OTC drugs unless prescriber has approved their use.
- Stop, or at least limit, smoking because it may increase the metabolism of desipramine, thereby diminishing its therapeutic action.
- Do not breast feed while taking this drug without consulting prescriber.

DOXEPIN HYDROCHLORIDE

(dox′e-pin)

Adapin, Sinequan, Triadapin ♣, Zonalon

Classifications: CENTRAL NERVOUS SYSTEM AGENT; PSYCHOTHERAPEUTIC; TRICYCLIC ANTIDEPRESSANT

Pregnancy Category: C

AVAILABILITY 10 mg, 25 mg, 50 mg, 75 mg, 100 mg, 150 mg capsules; 10 mg/mL oral concentrate

ACTIONS Dibenzoxepin is a tricyclic antidepressant (TCA). One of the most sedating of the TCAs. Inhibits serotonin reuptake

from the synaptic gap; also inhibits norepinephrine reuptake to a moderate degree.
THERAPEUTIC EFFECTS Restores the level of the serotonin and norepinephrine neurotransmitters as the proposed mechanism of antidepressant action.

USES Anxiety or depressive reactions; mixed symptoms of anxiety and depression; anxiety or depression associated with alcoholism; organic disease; psychotic depressive disorders; topical for treatment of pruritus.
UNLABELED USES Peptic ulcer disease, neuralgia.

CONTRAINDICATIONS Prior sensitivity to any TCA; during acute recovery phase following MI; glaucoma; prostatic hypertrophy; tendency for urinary retention; concurrent use of MAOIS. Safe use during pregnancy (category C), lactation, or in children <12 y is not established.
CAUTIOUS USE Patients receiving electroconvulsive therapy (ECT), patients with suicidal tendency; renal, cardiovascular or hepatic dysfunction.

ROUTE & DOSAGE

Antidepressant

Adult: **PO** 30–150 mg/d h.s. or in divided doses; may gradually increase to 300 mg/d (use lower doses in older adult patients)
Geriatric: **PO** 10–25 mg h.s.; may gradually increase to 75 mg/d
Child: **PO** 1–3 mg/kg/d in single or divided doses

Pruritus

Adult: **Topical** Apply a thin film q.i.d. with at least 3–4 h between applications; may use up to 8 d

ADMINISTRATION

Oral

- Give oral concentrate diluted with approximately 120 mL water, milk, or fruit juice.
- Empty capsule and swallow contents with fluid or mix with food as necessary if it cannot be swallowed whole.
- Inform prescriber if daytime sedation is pronounced. Entire daily dose (up to 150 mg) may be prescribed for bedtime administration.

Topical

- Apply a thin film to affected areas; allow 3–4 h between applications.
- Store all forms at 15°–30° C (59°–86° F) in tightly closed, light-resistant container.

ADVERSE EFFECTS (≥1%) **Body as a Whole:** Anticholinergic. **CNS:** *Drowsiness,* dizziness, weakness, fatigue, headache, hypomania, confusion, tremors, paresthesias. **CV:** *Orthostatic hypotension,* palpitation, hypertension, tachycardia, ECG changes. **Special Senses:** Mydriasis, blurred vision, photophobia. **GI:** *Dry mouth,* sour or metallic taste, epigastric distress, constipation. **Urogenital:** Urinary retention, delayed micturition, urinary frequency. **Other:** Increased perspiration, tinnitus, weight gain, photosensitivity reaction, skin rash, agranulocytosis, *burning or stinging at application site,* edema.

INTERACTIONS Drug: May decrease some antihypertensive response to ANTIHYPERTENSIVES; CNS DEPRESSANTS, **alcohol,** HYPNOTICS, BARBITURATES, SEDATIVES potentiate CNS depression; may increase hypoprothombinemic effect of ORAL ANTICOAGULANTS; **ethchlorvynol** may cause transient delirium; **levodopa,** SYMPATHOMIMETICS (e.g., **epinephrine, norepinephrine**) introduce possibility of sympathetic hyperactivity with hypertension and hyperpyrexia; MAOIS introduce possibility of severe reactions, toxic psychosis, cardiovascular instability; **methylphenidate** increases plasma TCA levels; THYROID AGENTS may increase possibility of arrhythmias; **cimetidine** may increase plasma TCA levels. **Herbal: Ginkgo** may decrease seizure threshold; **St. John's wort** may cause **serotonin** syndrome; **valerian** may deepen sedation effect.

PHARMACOKINETICS Absorption: Rapidly absorbed from GI sites through intact skin. **Peak:** 2 h. **Distribution:** Crosses placenta; distributed into breast milk. **Metabolism:** Metabolized in liver. **Elimination:** Primarily excreted in urine. **Half-Life:** 6–8 h.

NURSING IMPLICATIONS

Assessment & Drug Effects

- Monitor use of other CNS depressants, including alcohol. Danger of overdosage or suicide attempt is increased when patient uses excessive amounts of alcohol.

- Be alert to changes in voiding and evaluate patient for constipation and abdominal distention; drug has moderate to strong anticholinergic effects.
- Monitor cognitions, especially with elderly, because anticholinergic effects can predictably worsen cognitive functioning and memory, cause agitation and delirium, and may cause psychosis.

Client & Family Education

- Maintain established dosage regimen and avoid change of intervals, doubling, reducing, or skipping doses.
- Consult prescriber about safe amount of ETOH, if any, that can be taken. The actions of both alcohol and doxepin are potentiated when used together and for up to 2 wk after doxepin is discontinued.
- Do not drive or engage in other potentially hazardous activities until response to drug is known.
- Do not breast feed while taking this drug without consulting prescriber.

IMIPRAMINE HYDROCHLORIDE

(im-ip′ra-meen)

Impril ♣, Janimine, Novopramine ♣, Tofranil

IMIPRAMINE PAMOATE

Tofranil-PM

Classifications: CENTRAL NERVOUS SYSTEM AGENT; PSYCHOTHERAPEUTIC; TRICYCLIC ANTIDEPRESSANT

Pregnancy Category: C

AVAILABILITY 10 mg, 25 mg, 50 mg tablets; 75 mg, 100 mg, 125 mg, 150 mg capsules

ACTIONS Tricyclic antidepressant (TCA) and tertiary amine, structurally related to the phenothiazines. In contrast with phenothiazines, which act on dopamine receptors, TCAs potentiate both norepinephrine and serotonin in the CNS by blocking their reuptake by presynaptic neurons. Decreases number of awakenings from sleep, markedly reduces time in REM sleep and increases stage 4 sleep.

THERAPEUTIC EFFECTS As a TCA antidepressant, imipramine potentiates the effects of both norepinephrine and serotonin in the CNS by blocking their reuptake by the neurons. Relief of nocturnal enuresis is perhaps due to anticholinergic activity and to nervous system stimulation, resulting in earlier arousal to sensation of full bladder.

USES Endogenous depression and occasionally for reactive depression. Imipramine is the only TCA used as temporary adjunctive treatment of enuresis in children >6 y.
UNLABELED USES Certain syndromes that mimic or overlap diagnostically with depression: Alcoholism, cocaine withdrawal; attention deficit disorder with or without hyperactivity (children >6 y and adolescents); with amphetamines or methylphenidate for narcolepsy; phobic anxiety syndromes such as panic disorders and agoraphobia; obsessive-compulsive neurosis; chronic intractable pain.

CONTRAINDICATIONS Hypersensitivity to tricyclic drugs; acute recovery period after MI, defects in bundle-branch conduction; severe renal or hepatic impairment; use of imipramine HCl in children <12 y except to treat enuresis; use of pamoate in children of any age. Safe use during pregnancy (category D) or lactation is not established.
CAUTIOUS USE Children, adolescents, older adults; respiratory difficulties; cardiovascular, hepatic, or GI diseases; blood disorders; increased intraocular pressure, narrow-angle glaucoma; schizophrenia, hypomania or manic episodes, patient with suicidal tendency, seizure disorders; prostatic hypertrophy, urinary retention; alcoholism, hyperthyroidism; electroshock therapy.

ROUTE & DOSAGE

Depression

Adult: **PO** 75–100 mg/d (max 300 mg/d) in 1 or more divided doses **IM** 50–100 mg/d in divided doses
Child: **PO** 1.5 mg/kg/d; may increase by 1 mg/kg/d q3–4d (max 5 mg/kg/d)

Enuresis in Childhood

Child: **PO** 25 mg 1 h before bedtime; *<12 y,* may increase to 50 mg nightly (max 2.5 mg/kg); *>12 y,* may increase to 75 mg nightly (max 2.5 mg/kg)

ADMINISTRATION

Oral

- Do NOT make dosage adjustments more frequently than q4d.
- Give with or immediately after food.
- Note: Single doses can be given h.s. or q a.m., respectively, if drowsiness or insomnia results.

Intramuscular

- Use IM form only for those unable/unwilling to take oral form.
- Dissolve crystals by immersing intact ampule in warm water for about 1 min.

ADVERSE EFFECTS (≥1%) **Body as a Whole:** Hypersensitivity (skin rash, erythema, petechiae, urticaria, pruritus, photosensitivity, *angioedema* of face, tongue, or generalized; drug fever). **CNS:** *Sedation, drowsiness,* dizziness, headache, fatigue, numbness, tingling (paresthesias) of extremities; incoordination, ataxia, tremors, peripheral neuropathy, extrapyramidal symptoms (including parkinsonism effects and tardive dyskinesia); lowered seizure threshold, altered EEG patterns, delirium, disturbed concentration, confusion, hallucinations, anxiety, nervousness, insomnia, vivid dreams, restlessness, agitation, shift to hypomania, mania; exacerbation of psychoses; hyperpyrexia. **CV:** *Orthostatic hypotension,* mild sinus tachycardia; *arrhythmias,* hypertension or hypotension, palpitation, <u>MI</u>, CHF, *heart block,* ECG changes, stroke, flushing, cold cyanotic hands and feet (peripheral vasospasm). **Endocrine:** Testicular swelling, gynecomastia (men), galactorrhea and breast enlargement (women), increased or decreased libido, ejaculatory and erectile disturbances, delayed or absent orgasm (male and female); elevation or depression of blood glucose levels. **Special Senses:** Nasal congestion, tinnitus; *blurred vision,* disturbances of accommodation, *slight mydriasis,* nystagmus. **GI:** *Dry mouth,* constipation, heartburn, excessive appetite, weight gain, nausea, vomiting, diarrhea, slowed gastric emptying time, flatulence, abdominal cramps, esophageal reflux, anorexia, stomatitis, increased salivation, black tongue, peculiar taste, paralytic ileus. **Urogenital:** *Urinary retention,* delayed micturition, nocturia, paradoxic urinary frequency. **Hematologic:** Bone marrow depression; <u>agranulocytosis</u>, eosinophilia, thrombocytopenia. **Other:** Excessive perspiration, cholestatic jaundice, precipitation of acute intermittent porphyria; dyspnea, changes in heat and cold tolerance, hair loss, syndrome of inappropriate antidiuretic hormone secretion (SIADH).

DIAGNOSTIC TEST INTERFERENCE Imipramine elevates ***serum bilirubin, alkaline phosphatase*** and may increase or decrease ***blood glucose.*** It decreases ***urinary 5-HIAA*** and ***VMA*** excretion and may falsely increase excretion of ***urinary catecholamines.***

INTERACTIONS Drug: MAOIS may precipitate hyperpyrexic crisis, tachycardia, or seizures; ANTIHYPERTENSIVE AGENTS potentiate orthostatic hypotension; CNS DEPRESSANTS, **alcohol** add to CNS depression; **norepinephrine** and other SYMPATHOMIMETICS may increase cardiac toxicity; **cimetidine** decreases hepatic metabolism, thus increasing imipramine levels; **methylphenidate** inhibits metabolism of imipramine and thus may increase its toxicity. **Herbal: Ginkgo** may decrease seizure threshold; **St. John's wort** may cause **serotonin** syndrome.

PHARMACOKINETICS Absorption: Completely absorbed from GI tract. **Peak:** 1–2 h PO; 30 min IM. **Metabolism:** Metabolized to the active metabolite desipramine in liver. **Elimination:** Primarily excreted in urine, small amount in feces; crosses placenta; may be secreted in breast milk. **Half-Life:** 8–16 h.

NURSING IMPLICATIONS

Assessment & Drug Effects

- Monitor for therapeutic effectiveness: May not occur for 2 wk or more.
- Prevent serious adverse effects by accurate early reporting to prescriber about patient's response to drug.
- Note: Dose sensitivity and adverse effects are most likely to occur in adolescents and older adults; use a lower initial dose in these patients.
- Lab tests: Monitor hepatic and renal function, CBC with differential, and fluid and electrolyte balance periodically.
- Monitor HR and BP frequently. Orthostatic hypotension may be marked in pretreatment hypertensive or cardiac patients.
- Monitor for potential signs of toxicity: QRS prolongation (to 100 ms or greater), arrhythmias, hypotension, respiratory depression, altered level of consciousness, seizures. Overdose onset may be sudden.
- Note: During the first 2 wk of therapy, older adults may develop confusion, restlessness, disturbed sleep, forgetfulness. Symptoms last 3–20 d. Report to prescriber.

- Weigh patient under standard conditions biweekly: Report a gain of 0.5–1.0 kg (1.5–2 lb) within 2–3 d and frank edema.
- Monitor urinary and bowel elimination, at least until maintenance dosage is stabilized, to detect urinary retention or frequency, constipation, or paralytic ileus.
- Report promptly early signs of agranulocytosis.
- Report signs of cholestatic jaundice: flu-like symptoms, yellow skin or sclerae, dark urine, light-colored stools, pruritus.
- Notify prescriber of extrapyramidal symptoms (tremors, twitching, ataxia, incoordination, hyperreflexia, drooling) in patients receiving large doses and especially in older adults.
- Monitor diabetic patients for loss of glycemic control. Hyperglycemia or hypoglycemia occur in some patients.
- Inspect oral mucosa frequently, especially gingival surfaces under dentures.

Client & Family Education

- Change position slowly and in stages, especially from lying down to upright posture and dangle legs over bed for a few minutes before walking.
- Note: Effectiveness can decrease with continued drug administration in some patients. Inform prescriber if this occurs.
- Do NOT use OTC drugs while on a TCA without consulting prescriber.
- Do not drive or engage in other potentially hazardous activities until response to drug is known.
- Avoid exposure to strong sunlight because of potential photosensitivity. Use sunscreen with at least SPF of 12–15 if allowed.
- Do not breast feed while taking this drug without consulting prescriber.

NORTRIPTYLINE HYDROCHLORIDE

(nor-trip′ti-leen)

Aventyl, Pamelor

Classifications: CENTRAL NERVOUS SYSTEM AGENT; PSYCHOTHERAPEUTIC; TRICYCLIC ANTIDEPRESSANT

Pregnancy Category: D

AVAILABILITY 10 mg, 25 mg, 50 mg, 75 mg capsules; 10 mg/5 mL solution

ACTIONS Secondary amine derivative of amitriptyline. Action mechanism unclear. Tricyclic antidepressant (TCA) with less sedative and anticholinergic effects than imipramine.
THERAPEUTIC EFFECTS Mood elevation may be due to its inhibition of reuptake of norepinephrine at the presynaptic membrane.

USES Endogenous depression. Similar in actions, uses, limitations, and interactions to imipramine.
UNLABELED USES Nocturnal enuresis in children.

CONTRAINDICATIONS Acute recovery period after MI; during or within 14 d of MAO inhibitor therapy. Children <12 y, pregnancy (category D), lactation.
CAUTIOUS USE Narrow-angle glaucoma, hyperthyroidism, concurrent administration of thyroid medications, concurrent use with electroshock therapy.

ROUTE & DOSAGE

Antidepressant

Adult: **PO** 25 mg t.i.d. or q.i.d., gradually increased to 100–150 mg/d
Geriatric: **PO** Start with 10–25 mg h.s., increase by 25 mg q3d to 75 mg h.s. (max 150 mg/d)
Adolescent: **PO** 30–50 mg/d in divided doses
Child: **PO** *6–12 y,* 10–20 mg/d in 3–4 divided doses

Nocturnal Enuresis

Child: **PO** *6–7 y,* 10 mg/d; *8–11 y,* 10–20 mg/d; *>11 y,* 25–35 mg/d given 30 min before h.s.

ADMINISTRATION

Oral

- Give with food to decrease gastric distress.
- In older adults, total daily dose may be given once a day h.s. (preferred).
- Be aware that Aventyl is a 4% alcohol solution.
- Supervise drug ingestion to be sure patient swallows medication.
- Store at 15°–30° C (59°–86° F) in tightly closed container.

ADVERSE EFFECTS (≥1%) **Body as a Whole:** Tremors, hyperhydrosis. **CV:** *Orthostatic hypotension.* **GI:** Paralytic ileus, *dry* *mouth*. **Hematologic:** Agranulocytosis (rare). **CNS:** Drowsiness, confusional state (especially in older adults and with high dosage). **Skin:** Photosensitivity reaction. **Special Senses:** Blurred vision. **Urogenital:** *Urinary retention*.

INTERACTIONS Drug: May decrease some antihypertensive response to ANTIHYPERTENSIVES; CNS DEPRESSANTS, **alcohol,** HYPNOTICS, BARBITURATES, SEDATIVES potentiate CNS depression; may increase hypoprothrombinemic effect of ORAL ANTICOAGULANTS; **ethchlorvynol** may cause transient delirium; **levodopa,** SYMPATHOMIMETICS (e.g., **epinephrine, norepinephrine**) pose possibility of sympathetic hyperactivity with hypertension and hyperpyrexia; MAOIS pose possibility of severe reactions—toxic psychosis, cardiovascular instability; **methylphenidate** increases plasma TCA levels; THYROID DRUGS may increase possibility of arrhythmias; **cimetidine** may increase plasma TCA levels. **Herbal: Ginkgo** may decrease seizure threshold. **St. John's wort** may cause **serotonin** syndrome (headache, dizziness, sweating, agitation).

PHARMACOKINETICS Absorption: Rapidly absorbed from GI tract. **Peak:** 7–8.5 h. **Distribution:** Crosses placenta; distributed in breast milk. **Metabolism:** Metabolized in liver. **Elimination:** Primarily excreted in urine. **Half-Life:** 16–90 h.

NURSING IMPLICATIONS

Assessment & Drug Effects

- Be aware that nortriptyline has a narrow therapeutic plasma level range, or "therapeutic window." Drug levels above or below the therapeutic window are associated with decreased rate of response.
- Therapeutic response may not occur for 2 wk or more.
- Monitor BP and pulse rate during adjustment period of TCA therapy. If systolic BP falls more than 20 mm Hg or if there is a sudden increase in pulse rate, withhold medication and notify the prescriber.
- Notify prescriber if psychotic signs increase. Because of the small therapeutic window, a substitute TCA may be prescribed rather than an increase in dosage.
- Inspect oral membranes daily if patient is on high doses of TCA. Urge outpatient to report stomatitis or dry mouth. Sore mouth can be a major cause of poor nutrition and noncompliance.

Consult prescriber about use of a saliva substitute (e.g., VA-Oralube, Moi-Stir).
- Monitor bowel elimination pattern and I&O ratio. Urinary retention and severe constipation are potential problems, especially in older adults. Advise increased fluid intake; consult prescriber about stool softener.
- Observe patient with history of glaucoma. Symptoms that may signal acute attack (severe headache, eye pain, dilated pupils, halos of light, nausea, vomiting) should be reported promptly.
- Report reduction or alleviation of fine tremors.
- Be aware that alcohol potentiation may increase the danger of overdosage or suicide attempt.

Client & Family Education
- Be aware that your ability to perform tasks requiring alertness and skill may be impaired.
- Do not use OTC drugs unless prescriber approves.
- Consult prescriber about safe amount of alcohol, if any, that can be ingested. Alcohol and nortriptyline both have increased effects when used together and for up to 2 wk after the TCA is discontinued.
- Nortriptyline enhances the effects of barbiturates and other CNS depressants are enhanced.
- Do not breast feed while taking this drug.

PROTRIPTYLINE HYDROCHLORIDE

(proe-trip′te-leen)

Triptil ♣, Vivactil

Classifications: CENTRAL NERVOUS SYSTEM AGENT; PSYCHOTHERAPEUTIC; TRICYCLIC ANTIDEPRESSANT

Pregnancy Category: C

AVAILABILITY 5 mg, 10 mg tablets

ACTIONS Tricyclic antidepressant (TCA) with more rapid onset of action than imipramine. Has little if any sedative properties characteristic of most other TCAs, but causes tachycardia, CNS stimulation, and strong anticholinergic activity. Orthostatic hypotension occurs frequently with usage.

THERAPEUTIC EFFECTS TCAs potentiate both norepinephrine and serotonin in CNS by blocking their reuptake by presynaptic neurons. Effective in the treatment of mentally depressed individuals, particularly those who are withdrawn.

USES Symptomatic treatment of endogenous depression in patients under close medical supervision. Particularly effective for depression manifested by psychomotor retardation, apathy, and fatigue.

CONTRAINDICATIONS Use in children; concurrent use of MAOIS; during acute recovery phase following MI; pregnancy (category C).
CAUTIOUS USE Hepatic, cardiovascular, or kidney dysfunction; diabetes mellitus; hyperthyroidism; patients with insomnia; lactation.

ROUTE & DOSAGE

Antidepressant
Adult: **PO** 15–40 mg/d in 3–4 divided doses (max 60 mg/d)
Adolescent: **PO** 15 mg/d in divided doses

ADMINISTRATION

Oral
- Give whole or crush and mix with fluid or food.
- Give dosage increases in the morning dose to prevent sleep interference and because this TCA has psychic energizing action.
- Give last dose of day no later than midafternoon; insomnia rather than drowsiness is a frequent adverse effect.
- Store at 15°–30° C (59°–86° F) in tightly closed container.

ADVERSE EFFECTS (≥1%) **Body as a Whole:** Photosensitivity, edema (general or of face and tongue). **GI:** *Xerostomia, constipation,* paralytic ileus. **Special Senses:** Blurred vision. **Urogenital:** *Urinary retention.* **CNS:** Insomnia, headache, confusion. **CV:** Change in heat or cold tolerance; *orthostatic hypotension, tachycardia.*

INTERACTIONS Drug: May decrease some response to ANTIHYPERTENSIVES; CNS DEPRESSANTS, **alcohol,** HYPNOTICS, BARBITURATES, SEDATIVES potentiate CNS depression; ORAL ANTICOAGULANTS may increase hypoprothrombinemic effects; **ethchlorvynol** causes transient delirium; **levodopa,** SYMPATHOMIMETICS (e.g., **epinephrine, norepinephrine**) increases possibility of sympathetic hyperactivity with hypertension and hyperpyrexia; MAOIS present possibility of severe reactions—toxic psychosis, cardiovascular instability; **methylphenidate** increases plasma TCA levels; THYROID DRUGS may increase possibility of arrhythmias; **cimetidine** may increase plasma TCA levels. **Herbal: Ginkgo** may decrease seizure threshold; **St. John's wort** may cause **serotonin** syndrome (headache, dizziness, sweating, agitation).

PHARMACOKINETICS Absorption: Rapidly absorbed from GI tract. **Peak:** 24–30 h. **Distribution:** Crosses placenta; distributed into breast milk. **Metabolism:** Metabolized in liver. **Elimination:** Primarily excreted in urine. **Half-Life:** 54–98 h.

NURSING IMPLICATIONS

Assessment & Drug Effects

- Monitor therapeutic effectiveness. Onset of initial effect characterized by increased activity and energy is fairly rapid, usually within 1 wk after therapy is initiated. Maximum effect may not occur for 2 wk or more.
- Monitor vital signs closely and CV system responses during early therapy, particularly in patients with cardiovascular disorders and older adults receiving daily doses in excess of 20 mg. Withhold drug and inform prescriber if BP falls more than 20 mm Hg or if there is a sudden increase in pulse rate.
- Lab tests: Obtain periodic liver function and blood cell counts in patients receiving large doses for prolonged periods or in combination with other drugs.
- Monitor I&O ratio and question patient about bowel regularity during early therapy and when patient is on large doses.
- Assess and advise prescriber as indicated for prominent anticholinergic effects (xerostomia, blurred vision, constipation, paralytic ileus, urinary retention, delayed micturition).
- Assess condition of oral membranes frequently; institute symptomatic treatment if necessary. Xerostomia can interfere with appetite, fluid intake, and integrity of tooth surfaces.
- Supervise patient closely during early treatment period. Suicide is an inherent risk with any depressed patient and may remain until there is significant improvement.
- Bear in mind that the potentiation of TCA effects may increase the danger of overdosage or suicide attempt (especially in patients who use excessive amounts of alcohol).

Client & Family Education

- Consult prescriber about safe amount of alcohol, if any, that can be taken. Actions of both alcohol and protriptyline are potentiated when used together for up to 2 wk after the TCA is discontinued.
- Stop or reduce smoking; smoking reduces TCAs' effectiveness. Apparent treatment failure may be due to the nicotine effect.
- Consult prescriber before taking any OTC medications.
- Be aware that effects of barbiturates and other CNS depressants are enhanced by TCAs.
- Avoid potentially hazardous activities requiring alertness and skill until response to drug is known.
- Avoid exposure to the sun without protecting skin with sunscreen lotion (SPF >12). Photosensitivity reactions may occur.
- Do not breast feed while taking this drug without consulting prescriber.

TRIMIPRAMINE MALEATE

(tri-mip′ra-meen)

Surmontil

Classifications: CENTRAL NERVOUS SYSTEM AGENT; PSYCHOTHERAPEUTIC; TRICYCLIC ANTIDEPRESSANT

Pregnancy Category: C

AVAILABILITY 25 mg, 50 mg, 100 mg capsules

ACTIONS Tricyclic antidepressant (TCA) pharmacologically similar to imipramine. Moderate anticholinergic and strong sedative effects; useful in depression associated with anxiety and sleep disturbances. Recent studies suggest strong, active H_2-receptor antagonism is a characteristic of TCAs.

THERAPEUTIC EFFECTS More effective in alleviation of endogenous depression than other depressive states.

USES Treatment of major depression.

UNLABELED USES Peptic ulcer disease.

CONTRAINDICATIONS Prostatic hypertrophy; during recovery period after MI. Safety during pregnancy (category C) or lactation is not established.

CAUTIOUS USE Schizophrenia, electroconvulsive therapy (ECT), suicidal tendency; cardiovascular, liver, thyroid, kidney disease.

ROUTE & DOSAGE

Depression

Adult: **PO** 75–100 mg/d in divided doses, may increase gradually up to 300 mg/d if needed. **PO Maintenance Dose** Usually 50–150 mg/d
Geriatric: **PO** 25 mg h.s.; may increase q3d (max 100 mg/d)

ADMINISTRATION

Oral

- Give with food to decrease gastric distress.
- Store in tightly closed container at 15°–30° C (59°–86° F) unless otherwise specified.

ADVERSE EFFECTS (≥1%) **CNS:** Seizures, tremor, confusion, *sedation*. **Special Senses:** Blurred vision. **CV:** Tachycardia, *orthostatic hypotension,* hypertension. **GI:** *Xerostomia, constipation,* paralytic ileus. **Urogenital:** *Urinary retention*. **Skin:** Photosensitivity, sweating.

INTERACTIONS Drug: May decrease some antihypertensive response to ANTIHYPERTENSIVES; CNS DEPRESSANTS, **alcohol,** HYPNOTICS, BARBITURATES, SEDATIVES potentiate CNS depression; may increase hypoprothrombinemic effect of ORAL ANTICOAGULANTS; **ethchlorvynol** may cause transient delirium; with **levodopa,** SYMPATHOMIMETICS (e.g., **epinephrine, norepinephrine**), possibility of sympathetic hyperactivity with hypertension and hyperpyrexia; with MAOIS, possibility of severe reactions, toxic psychosis, cardiovascular instability; **methylphenidate** increases plasma TCA levels; THYROID AGENTS may increase possibility of arrhythmias; **cimetidine** may increase plasma TCA levels. **Herbal: Ginkgo** may decrease seizure threshold; **St. John's wort** may cause **serotonin** syndrome.

PHARMACOKINETICS Absorption: Rapidly absorbed from GI tract. **Peak:** 2 h. **Metabolism:** Metabolized in liver. **Elimination:** Excreted in urine and feces. **Half-Life:** 9.1 h.

NURSING IMPLICATIONS

Assessment & Drug Effects

- Assess vital signs (BP and pulse rate) during adjustment period of tricyclic antidepressant (TCA) therapy. If BP falls more than

20 mm Hg or if there is a sudden increase in pulse rate, withhold medication and notify prescriber.

- Orthostatic hypotension may be sufficiently severe to require protective assistance when patient is ambulating. Instruct patient to change position from recumbency to standing slowly and in stages.
- Report signs of liver dysfunction: Yellow skin and sclerae, light-colored stools, pruritus, abdominal discomfort.
- Report fine tremors, a distressing extrapyramidal adverse effect, to prescriber.
- Monitor bowel elimination pattern and I&O ratio. Severe constipation and urinary retention are potential problems, especially in older adults. Advise increased fluid intake to at least 1500 mL/d (if allowed).
- Monitor patient carefully during initial drug therapy when therapeutic "lag period" may foster noncompliance.
- Inspect oral membranes daily with high-dose therapy. Urge outpatient to report symptoms of stomatitis or xerostomia.
- Regulate environmental temperature and patient's clothing carefully; drug may cause intolerance to heat or cold.
- Excessive alcohol may potentiate TCA effects and increase the danger of overdosage or suicide attempt.

Client & Family Education

- Be aware that your ability to perform tasks requiring alertness and skill may be impaired.
- Do not to use OTC drugs unless approved by prescriber.
- Understand that the actions of both alcohol and trimipramine are increased when used together during therapy and for up to 2 wk after the TCA is discontinued. Consult prescriber about safe amounts of alcohol, if any, that can be taken.
- Be aware that the effects of barbiturates and other CNS depressants may also be enhanced by trimipramine.
- Expect that therapeutic response will be delayed because TCAs have a "lag period" of 2–4 wk. Increased dosage does not shorten period but rather increases incidence of adverse reactions. Keep prescriber advised and do not interrupt therapy.
- Do not breast feed while taking this drug without consulting prescriber.

ANTIOBSESSIONAL AGENTS

CLOMIPRAMINE HYDROCHLORIDE

(clo-mi′ pra-meen)

Anafranil

Classifications: CENTRAL NERVOUS SYSTEM AGENT; PSYCHOTHERAPEUTIC; TRICYCLIC ANTIDEPRESSANT

Pregnancy Category: C

AVAILABILITY 25 mg, 50 mg, 75 mg capsules

ACTIONS Inhibits the reuptake of norepinephrine and serotonin at the presynaptic neuron. Elevates serum levels of these two amines.

THERAPEUTIC EFFECTS The basis of its antidepressant effects is thought to be due to the elevated serum levels of norepinephrine and serotonin. Exhibits anticholinergic, antihistaminic, hypotensive, sedative, mild analgesic, and peripheral vasodilator effects.

USES Obsessive-compulsive disorder (OCD).

UNLABELED USES Panic disorder, anxiety, agoraphobia.

CONTRAINDICATIONS Hypersensitivity to other tricyclic compounds; acute recovery period after MI, children <10 y, pregnancy (category C), lactation.

CAUTIOUS USE History of convulsive disorders, prostatic hypertrophy, urinary retention, cardiovascular, hepatic, GI, or blood disorders.

ROUTE & DOSAGE

Obsessive-Compulsive Disorder

Adult: **PO** 75–300 mg/d in divided doses

Child: **PO** *10–18 y,* 100–200 mg/d in divided doses, starting at 50 mg/d

Depression

Adult: **PO** 50–150 mg/d in single or divided doses

ADMINISTRATION

Oral

- Give in divided doses with meals to reduce GI adverse effects.

Common adverse effects in *italic;* life-threatening effects underlined; generic names in **bold;** drug classifications in SMALL CAPS; ♣Canadian drug name.

- Following titration to the full dose, drug may be given as a single dose at bedtime to reduce daytime sedation.
- Store at 15°–30° C (59°–86° F).

ADVERSE EFFECTS (≥1%) **Body as a Whole:** Diaphoresis. **CV:** Hypotension, tachycardia. **GI:** Constipation, *dry mouth*. **Endocrine:** Galactorrhea, hyperprolactinemia, amenorrhea, *weight gain*. **Hematologic:** Leukopenia, agranulocytosis, thrombocytopenia, anemia. **CNS:** Mania, *tremor*, dizziness, hyperthermia, neuroleptic malignant syndrome, seizures (especially with abrupt withdrawal). **Urogenital:** Delayed ejaculation, anorgasmia.

DIAGNOSTIC TEST INTERFERENCE Clomipramine appears to elevate serum ***prolactin*** levels. ***Serum AST and ALT*** are elevated. Serum levels of ***triiodothyronine*** (T_3) ***and free triiodothyronine*** (FT_3) have been significantly reduced from baseline. ***Thyroxine-binding globulin (TBG)*** levels were increased from baseline, whereas ***thyroxine*** (T_4), ***free thyroxine*** (FT_4), and reverse T_3 were unchanged.

INTERACTIONS Drug: MAOIS may precipitate hyperpyrexic crisis, tachycardia, or seizures; ANTIHYPERTENSIVE AGENTS potentiate orthostatic hypotension; CNS DEPRESSANTS, **alcohol** add to CNS depression; **norepinephrine** and other SYMPATHOMIMETICS may increase cardiac toxicity; **cimetidine** decreases hepatic metabolism, thus increasing imipramine levels; **methylphenidate** inhibits metabolism of **imipramine** and thus may increase its toxicity. **Herbal: Ginkgo** may decrease seizure threshold; **St. John's wort** may cause **serotonin** syndrome.

PHARMOCOKINETICS Absorption: Rapidly absorbed from GI tract; 20–78% reaches systemic circulation. **Onset:** OCD: approx 4–10 wk.; Depression: approx 2 wk. **Peak:** 2–6 h. **Distribution:** Widely distributed including the CSF; crosses placenta. **Metabolism:** Extensive first-pass metabolism in the liver; active metabolite is desmethylclomipramine. **Elimination:** 50–60% excreted in urine, 24–32% in feces. **Half-Life:** 20–30 h.

NURSING IMPLICATIONS

Assessment & Drug Effects

- Monitor for seizures, especially in those with predisposing factors such as alcoholism, brain injury, or concurrent therapy with other drugs that lower seizure threshold.

- Lab tests: Periodic CBC with differential, platelet count, and Hct and Hgb. Monitor liver functions, especially with long-term therapy.
- Monitor for and report signs of neuroleptic malignant syndrome.
- Monitor for sedation and vertigo, especially at the beginning of therapy and following dosage increases. Supervision of ambulation may be indicated.
- Notify prescriber of fever and complaints of sore throat; these may indicate need to rule out adverse hematologic changes.

Client & Family Education

- Do not take nonprescribed drugs or discontinue therapy without consent of prescriber. Abrupt discontinuation may cause nausea, headache, malaise, or seizures.
- Men should understand that the drug may cause impotence or ejaculation failure. Advise them to report this problem to prescriber.
- Report promptly a sore throat accompanied by fever.
- Use caution with ambulation until response to drug is known.
- Moderate alcohol intake because alcohol may potentiate adverse drug effects.
- Do not breast feed while taking this drug.

FLUVOXAMINE

(flu-vox'a-meen)

Luvox

Classifications: CENTRAL NERVOUS SYSTEM AGENT; PSYCHOTHERAPEUTIC; SELECTIVE SEROTONIN-REUPTAKE INHIBITOR (SSRI)

Pregnancy Category: B

AVAILABILITY 25 mg, 50 mg, 100 mg tablets; also available as a controlled-release (CR) formulation

ACTIONS Antidepressant with potent, selective, inhibitory activity on neuronal (5-HT) serotonin reuptake (SSRI); structurally unrelated to TCAs. Compared with TCAs, shows fewer anticholinergic effects and no severe cardiovascular effects.

THERAPEUTIC EFFECTS Effective for control of obsessive-compulsive disorders, as an antidepressant, and long-term treatment of social anxiety disorder.

USES Treatment of obsessive-compulsive disorder, depression.
UNLABELED USES Chronic tension-type headaches, panic attacks, and social anxiety disorder.

CONTRAINDICATIONS Hypersensitivity to fluvoxamine or fluoxetine.
CAUTIOUS USE Pregnancy (category B), lactation, liver disease, renal impairment, history of seizures.

ROUTE & DOSAGE

Obsessive-Compulsive Disorder, Depression
Adult: **PO** Start with 50 mg q.d.; may increase slowly up to 300 mg/d given q.h.s. or divided b.i.d.
Child: **PO** *8–11 y,* Start with 25 mg q.h.s.; may increase by 25 mg q4–7d (max 200 mg/d in divided doses)
CR Dosing: Once daily dose.

ADMINISTRATION

Oral
- Give starting doses at bedtime to improve tolerance to nausea and vomiting; both are common early in therapy.
- Assure time buffer between administration of a MAOI and fluvoxamine; do not coadminister a MAOI and fluvoxamine.
- Store at room temperature, 15°–30° C (59°–86° F), away from moisture and light.

ADVERSE EFFECTS (≥1%) **CNS:** *Somnolence, headache, agitation, insomnia, dizziness,* seizures. **CV:** Orthostatic hypotension, slight bradycardia. **GI:** *Nausea, vomiting, dry mouth, constipation, anorexia.* **Urogenital:** Sexual dysfunction. **Skin:** Stevens-Johnson syndrome, toxic epidermal necrolysis (rare).

DIAGNOSTIC TEST INTERFERENCE ***Gamma-glutamyl transferase*** increased by more than three-fold following 3 wk of therapy.

INTERACTIONS Drug: No coadministration of a MAOI and fluvoxamine. Fluvoxamine has been shown to significantly increase plasma levels of **amitriptyline, clomipramine,** and other TROCYCLIC ANTIDEPRESSANTS to mildly increase levels of their metabolites. May antagonize the blood pressure-lowering effects of **atenolol** and other BETA BLOCKERS. May increase levels and toxicity of **carbamazepine, mexiletine.** May increase **lithium** levels, causing neurotoxicity, **serotonin** syndrome, somnolence, and mania. One report of increased **theophylline** levels with toxicity. Increases prothrombin time in patients on **warfarin;** increased ergotamine toxicity with **dihydroergotamine, ergotamine. Herbal: Melatonin** may increase and prolong drowsiness; **St. John's wort** may cause **serotonin** syndrome.

PHARMACOKINETICS Absorption: Almost completely absorbed from GI tract. **Onset:** 4–7 d. **Distribution:** Approximately 77% bound to plasma proteins; excreted in human breast milk but in an amount that poses little risk to the nursing infant. CR has delayed, lower maximum concentration. **Metabolism:** Metabolized in liver. **Elimination:** Completely excreted in urine. **Half-Life:** 16–24 h.

NURSING IMPLICATIONS

Assessment & Drug Effects

- Monitor for significant nausea and vomiting, especially during initial therapy.
- Assess safety; drowsiness and dizziness are common adverse effects.
- Assess for use of OTC and complementary and alternative substances and assure MAOI (**St. John's wort**) is not ingested.
- Monitor PT and INR carefully with concurrent warfarin therapy; adjust warfarin as needed.

Client & Family Education

- Note: Nausea and vomiting are common in early therapy. Notify prescriber if these adverse effects last more than a few days.
- Use of some OTC and complementary and alternative substances containing a MAOI-like substance (such as **St. John's wort**) is not to be combined with this medication.
- Exercise caution with hazardous activity until response to the drug is known.
- Do not breast feed while taking this drug without consulting prescriber.

ANTIPARKINSONIAN AGENTS

AMANTADINE HYDROCHLORIDE

(a-man'ta-deen)

Symmetrel

Classifications: ANTI-INFECTIVE; ANTIVIRAL; AUTONOMIC NERVOUS SYSTEM AGENT; ANTICHOLINERGIC (PARASYMPATHOLYTIC); ANTIPARKINSONIAN AGENT

Pregnancy Category: C

AVAILABILITY 100 mg capsules; 50 mg/5 mL syrup

ACTIONS Because it does not suppress antibody formation, it can be administered for interim protection in combination with influenza A virus vaccine until antibody titer is adequate or to augment prophylaxis in a previously vaccinated individual. Mechanism of action in parkinsonism not understood, but may be related to release of dopamine and other catecholamines from neuronal storage sites.

THERAPEUTIC EFFECTS Active against several strains of influenza A virus; not effective against influenza B infections. Also provides anticholinergic effects.

USES In initial therapy or as adjunct with anticholinergic drugs or levodopa in treatment of all forms of parkinsonism (arteriosclerotic, idiopathic, postencephalitic) and for relief of drug-induced extrapyramidal reactions and symptomatic parkinsonism caused by carbon monoxide poisoning and psychotropics. Also used for prophylaxis and symptomatic treatment of influenza A infections.

UNLABELED USES Primary enuresis, pseudosclerosis, neuroleptic malignant syndrome (NMS), management of cocaine dependency and withdrawal.

CONTRAINDICATIONS Safety during pregnancy (category C), lactation, and in children <1 y is not established.

CAUTIOUS USE History of epilepsy or other types of seizures; CHF, peripheral edema, orthostatic hypotension; recurrent eczematoid dermatitis; psychoses, severe psychoneuroses; hepatic disease; renal impairment; older adults with cerebral arteriosclerosis.

ROUTE & DOSAGE

Influenza A

Adult: **PO** 200 mg once/d or 100 mg q12h
Child: **PO** *1–9 y,* 4.4–8.8 mg/kg in 2–3 equal doses (max 150 mg/d)

Parkinsonism

Adult: **PO** 100 mg 1–2 times/d, start with 100 mg/d if client is on other antiparkinsonian medications

Drug-Induced Extrapyramidal Symptoms

Adult: **PO** 100 mg b.i.d. (max 400 mg/d if needed)

Renal Impairment

Cl_{cr} 40–60 mL/min: 100 mg/d; 30–40 mL/min: 200 mg 2 times/wk; 10–20 mL/min: 100 mg 3 times/wk

ADMINISTRATION

Oral

- Give with water, milk, or food.
- Use supplied calibrated device for measuring syrup formulation.
- Influenza prophylaxis: Drug should be initiated when exposure is anticipated and continued for at least 10 d.
- Schedule medication in the morning or, with q12h dosing, schedule second dose several hours before bedtime. If insomnia is a problem, suggest client limit number of daytime naps.
- Store in tightly closed container preferably at 15°–30° C (59°– 86° F) unless otherwise directed by manufacturer. Avoid freezing.

ADVERSE EFFECTS (≥1%) **CNS:** *Dizziness, light-headedness,* headache, ataxia, irritability, anxiety, *nervousness, difficulty concentrating,* mood or other mental changes, confusion, visual and auditory hallucinations, *insomnia,* nightmares, convulsions. **CV:** Orthostatic hypotension, peripheral edema, dyspnea. **Special Senses:** Blurring or loss of vision. **GI:** Anorexia, *nausea,* vomiting, dry mouth. **Hematologic:** Leukopenia.

INTERACTIONS Drug: Alcohol enhances CNS effects; may potentiate effects of ANTICHOLINERGICS.

PHARMACOKINETICS Absorption: Readily and almost completely absorbed from GI tract. **Onset:** Within 48 h. **Peak:** 1–4 h. **Distribution:** Distributed to saliva, nasal secretions, breast milk, placenta, CSF. **Metabolism:** Not metabolized. **Elimination:** 90% excreted unchanged in urine. **Half-Life:** 9–37 h (prolonged in renal insufficiency).

NURSING IMPLICATIONS

Assessment & Drug Effects

- Monitor effectiveness. Note that with parkinsonism, maximum response occurs within 2 wk–3 mo. Effectiveness may wane after 6–8 wk of treatment; report change to prescriber.
- Monitor and report: Mental status changes; nervousness, difficulty concentrating, or insomnia; loss of seizure control; S&S of toxicity especially with doses above 200 mg/d.
- Establish a baseline profile of the client's disabilities to accurately differentiate disease symptoms and drug-induced neuropsychiatric adverse reactions.
- Monitor vital signs for at least 3 or 4 d after increases in dosage; also monitor urinary output.
- Lab tests: pH and serum electrolytes.
- Monitor for and report reduced salivation, increased akinesia or rigidity, and psychological disturbances that may develop within 4–48 h after initiation of therapy and after dosage increases with parkinsonism.

Client & Family Education

- Make all position changes slowly, particularly from recumbent to upright position, in order to minimize dizziness.
- Report any of the following: Shortness of breath, peripheral edema, significant weight gain, dizziness or light-headedness, inability to concentrate, and other changes in mental status, difficulty urinating, and visual impairment to prescriber.
- Do not drive; exercise caution during potentially hazardous activities until response to drug is known.
- Note: People with Parkinson's disease should not discontinue therapy abruptly; doing so may precipitate a parkinsonian crisis with severe akinesia, rigidity, tremor, and psychic disturbances. Adhere to established dosage regimen.
- Do not breast feed while taking this drug without consulting prescriber.

BENZTROPINE MESYLATE

(benz′troe-peen)

Apo-Benzotropine ♣, Bensylate ♣, Cogentin, PMS Benzotropine

Classifications: AUTONOMIC NERVOUS SYSTEM AGENT; ANTICHOLINERGIC (PARASYMPATHOLYTIC); ANTIPARKINSONIAN AGENT

Pregnancy Category: C

AVAILABILITY 0.5 mg, 1 mg, 2 mg tablets; 1 mg/mL ampules

ACTIONS Synthetic centrally acting anticholinergic (antimuscarinic) agent. Acts by diminishing excess cholinergic effect associated with dopamine deficiency.

THERAPEUTIC EFFECTS Suppresses tremor and rigidity; does not alleviate tardive dyskinesia.

USES Symptomatic treatment of all forms of parkinsonism (arteriosclerotic, idiopathic, postencephalitic) and to relieve extrapyramidal symptoms associated with neuroleptic drugs, e.g., haloperidol (Haldol), phenothiazines, thiothixene (Navane). Commonly used as supplement with trihexyphenidyl, carbidopa, or levodopa therapy.

CONTRAINDICATIONS Narrow-angle glaucoma; myasthenia gravis; obstructive diseases of GU and GI tracts; tendency to tachycardia; tardive dyskinesia, children <3 y. Safety during pregnancy (category C) or lactation is not established.

CAUTIOUS USE Older children, older adults or debilitated clients, clients with poor mental outlook, mental disorders; enlarged prostate; hypertension; history of renal or hepatic disease.

ROUTE & DOSAGE

Parkinsonism

Adult: **PO** 0.5–1 mg/d, may gradually increase q5–6d as needed up to 6 mg/d

Extrapyramidal Reactions

Adult: **PO** 1–2 mg b.i.d. **IM/IV** 1–2 mg as needed
Child: **PO/IM/IV** *>3 y,* 0.02–0.05 mg/kg, 1–2 times/d

Common adverse effects in *italic;* life-threatening effects underlined; generic names in **bold;** drug classifications in SMALL CAPS; ♣ Canadian drug name.

ADMINISTRATION

Oral

- Give immediately after meals or with food to prevent gastric irritation.
- Tablet can be crushed and sprinkled on or mixed with food.
- Initiate and withdraw drug therapy gradually; effects are cumulative.
- Store in tightly covered, light-resistant container at 15°–30° C (59°–86° F) unless otherwise directed.

Intravenous

IV administration to infants and children. Verify correct IV concentration with prescriber.

PREPARE **Direct:** Give undiluted.

ADMINISTER **Direct:** Give 1 mg or a fraction thereof over 1 min.

ADVERSE EFFECTS (≥1%) **CNS:** *Sedation,* drowsiness, dizziness, paresthesias; agitation, irritability, restlessness, nervousness, insomnia, hallucinations, delirium, mental confusion, toxic psychosis, muscular weakness, ataxia, inability to move certain muscle groups. **CV:** Palpitation, tachycardia, flushing. **Special Senses:** Blurred near vision, mydriasis, dilated pupils, photophobia, decreased sweating, hyperthermia, heat stroke. **GI:** Nausea, vomiting, *constipation, dry mouth,* distention, paralytic ileus. **Urogenital:** Dysuria.

INTERACTIONS Drug: Alcohol, CNS DEPRESSANTS have additive sedation and depressant effects; **amantidine,** TRICYCLIC ANTIDEPRESSANTS, MAOIS, PHENOTHIAZINES, **procainamide, quinidine** have additive anticholinergic effects and cause confusion, hallucinations, paralytic ileus.

PHARMACOKINETICS Onset: 15 min IM/IV; 1 h PO. **Duration:** 6–10 h.

NURSING IMPLICATIONS

Assessment & Drug Effects

- Assess therapeutic effectiveness. Clinical improvement may not be evident for 2–3 d after oral drug is started.
- Some clients may experience euphoric feelings from this medication, so assure veracity of extrapyramidal side effects (EPSE) prior to administration.
- Monitor I&O ratio and pattern. Advise client to report difficulty in urination or infrequent voiding. Dosage reduction may be indicated.

- Closely monitor for appearance of S&S of onset of paralytic ileus, including intermittent constipation, abdominal pain, diminution of bowel sounds on auscultation, and distention.
- Monitor for and report muscle weakness or inability to move certain muscle groups. Dosage reduction may be needed.
- Supervise ambulation and use bed side rails as necessary.
- Report immediately S&S of CNS depression or stimulation. These usually require interruption of drug therapy.

Client & Family Education

- Do not drive or engage in potentially hazardous activities until response to drug is known. Seek help walking as necessary.
- Avoid alcohol and other CNS depressants because they may cause additive drowsiness. Do not take OTC cold, cough, or hay fever remedies unless approved by prescriber.
- Chewing sugarless gum, sucking on hard candy, and rinsing mouth with tepid water will help dry mouth.
- Avoid doing manual labor or strenuous exercise in hot weather; diminished sweating may require dose adjustments because of possibility of heat stroke. This condition is most apt to occur in older adults.
- Do not breast feed while taking this drug without consulting prescriber.

BIPERIDEN HYDROCHLORIDE

(bye-per′i-den)

Akineton

BIPERIDEN LACTATE

Akineton

Classifications: AUTONOMIC NERVOUS SYSTEM AGENT; ANTICHOLINERGIC (PARASYMPATHOLYTIC); ANTIPARKINSONIAN AGENT

Pregnancy Category: C

AVAILABILITY 2 mg tablets; 5 mg/mL injection

ACTIONS Synthetic tertiary amine, antimuscarinic. In common with other antiparkinsonian drugs has atropine-like (anticholinergic) action. Antiparkinsonian activity is thought to be caused by reducing central excitatory action of acetylcholine on cholinergic receptors in the extrapyramidal system.

THERAPEUTIC EFFECTS This action helps to establish some balance between cholinergic (excitatory) and dopaminergic (inhibitory) activity in the basal ganglia with the result of controlling the effect of extrapyramidal symptoms.

USES Adjunct in all forms of parkinsonism, particularly postencephalitic and idiopathic parkinsonism (appears to be less effective in arteriosclerotic type). Also used to control drug-induced parkinsonism (extrapyramidal symptoms) associated with reserpine and phenothiazine therapy.

CONTRAINDICATIONS Narrow-angle glaucoma; GI or GU obstruction, megacolon; tardive dyskinesia. Safety during pregnancy (category C), lactation, or in children is not established.
CAUTIOUS USE Older adults or debilitated clients; prostatic hypertrophy; glaucoma; cardiac arrhythmias; epilepsy.

ROUTE & DOSAGE

Parkinsonism

Adult: **PO** 2 mg 1–4 times/d **IM/IV** 2 mg injected slowly; may repeat q30min up to 8 mg/24 h
Geriatric: **PO** 2 mg 1–2 times/d
Child: **IM/IV** 0.04 mg/kg or 1.2 mg/m^2, may repeat q30min (max 8 mg/24 h)

ADMINISTRATION

Oral

- Give with or after meals to relieve GI disturbances.

Intramuscular

- Give slowly, deep IM into a large muscle.
- Monitor ambulation following IM because incoordination may occur.

Intravenous

PREPARE **Direct:** Give undiluted.
ADMINISTER **Direct:** Infuse slowly at a rate of 2 mg or a fraction thereof over 1 min.

- Keep client recumbent when receiving parenteral biperiden and for at least 15 min thereafter. Postural hypotension, disturbances of coordination, and temporary euphoria can occur following IV administration.
- Store in tightly closed, light-resistant containers at 15°–30° C (59°–86° F) unless otherwise directed.

ADVERSE EFFECTS (≥1%) **CNS:** Drowsiness, dizziness, muscle weakness, lack of coordination, disorientation, euphoria, agitation, confusion. **CV:** Mild, transient postural hypotension (following IM), tachycardia. **Special Senses:** *Blurred vision*, photophobia. **GI:** *Dry mouth*, nausea, vomiting, constipation.

INTERACTIONS Drug: Alcohol and other CNS DEPRESSANTS increase sedation; **haloperidol,** PHENOTHIAZINES, OPIATES, TRICYCLIC ANTIDEPRESSANTS, **quinidine** increase risk of anticholinergic side effects.

PHARMACOKINETICS Unknown.

NURSING IMPLICATIONS

Assessment & Drug Effects

- Monitor BP and pulse after IV administration. Advise client to make position changes slowly and in stages, particularly from recumbent to upright position.
- Monitor for and report immediately: Mental confusion, drowsiness, dizziness, agitation, hematuria, and decrease in urinary flow.
- Assess for and report blurred vision.
- Monitor I&O ratio and pattern.
- Note: Biperiden usually reduces muscle rigidity. In clients with severe parkinsonism, tremors may increase as spasticity is relieved.

Client & Family Education

- Do not drive or engage in potentially hazardous activities until response to drug is known.
- Note: Clients on prolonged therapy can develop tolerance; an increase in dosage may be required.
- Do not breast feed while taking this drug without consulting prescriber.

DIPHENHYDRAMINE HYDROCHLORIDE

(dye-fen-hye′dra-meen)

Allerdryl ♣, Banophen, Belix, Ben-Allergin, Bena-D, Benadryl, Benadryl Dye-Free, Benahist, Benoject, Benylin, Compoz, Diahist, Dihydrex, Diphen, Diphenacen-50, Fenylhist, Hyrexin, Insomnal, Nordryl, Nytol with DPH, Sleep-Eze 3, Sominex Formula 2, Tusstat, Twilite, Valdrene, Wehdryl

Classifications: ANTIHISTAMINE; H_1-RECEPTOR ANTAGONIST

Pregnancy Category: C

AVAILABILITY 25 mg, 50 mg capsules, tablets; 6.25 mg/5 mL, 12.5 mg/5 mL syrup; 50 mg/mL injection

ACTIONS H_1-receptor antagonist and antihistamine with significant anticholinergic activity. High incidence of drowsiness, but GI side effects are minor. Effects in parkinsonism and drug-induced extrapyramidal symptoms are apparently related to its ability to suppress central cholinergic activity and to prolong action of dopamine by inhibiting its reuptake and storage.
THERAPEUTIC EFFECTS Competes for H_1-receptor sites on effector cells, thus blocking histamine release.

USES Temporary symptomatic relief of various allergic conditions and to treat or prevent motion sickness, vertigo, and reactions to blood or plasma in susceptible clients. Also used in anaphylaxis as adjunct to epinephrine and other standard measures after acute symptoms have been controlled; in treatment of parkinsonism and drug-induced extrapyramidal reactions; as a nonnarcotic cough suppressant; as a sedative-hypnotic; and for treatment of intractable insomnia.

CONTRAINDICATIONS Hypersensitivity to antihistamines of similar structure; lower respiratory tract symptoms (including acute asthma); narrow-angle glaucoma; prostatic hypertrophy, bladder neck obstruction; GI obstruction or stenosis; pregnancy (category C), lactation, premature neonates, and neonates; use as nighttime sleep aid in children <12 y.
CAUTIOUS USE History of asthma; convulsive disorders; increased IOP; hyperthyroidism; hypertension, cardiovascular disease; diabetes mellitus; older adults, infants, and young children.

ROUTE & DOSAGE

Allergy Symptoms, Parkinsonism, Motion Sickness, Nighttime Sedation

Adult: **PO** 25–50 mg t.i.d. or q.i.d. (max 300 mg/d) **IV/IM** 10–50 mg q4–6h (max 400 mg/d)
Child: **PO/IV/IM** *2–6 y,* 6.25 mg q4–6h (max 300 mg/24 h); *6–12 y,* 12.5–25 mg q4–6h (max 300 mg/24 h)

Nonproductive Cough

Adult: **PO** 25 mg q4–6h (max 100 mg/d)
Child: **PO** *2–6 y,* 6.25 mg q4–6h (max 25 mg/24 h); *6–12 y,* 12.5 mg q4–6h (max 50 mg/24 h)

ADMINISTRATION

Oral

- Give with food or milk to lessen GI adverse effects.

Intramuscular

- Give IM injection deep into large muscle mass; alternate injection sites. Avoid perivascular or SC injections because of the drug's irritating effects.
- Note: Hypersensitivity reactions (including anaphylactic shock) are more likely to occur with parenteral than PO administration.

Intravenous

PREPARE **Direct:** Give undiluted.
ADMINISTER **Direct:** Give at a rate of 25 mg or a fraction thereof over 1 min.
INCOMPATIBILITY **Y-Site: Furosemide.**

- Store in tightly covered containers at 15°–30° C (59°–86° F) unless otherwise directed by manufacturer. Keep injection and elixir formulations in light-resistant containers.

ADVERSE EFFECTS (≥1%) **CNS:** *Drowsiness*, dizziness, headache, fatigue, disturbed coordination, tingling, heaviness and weakness of hands, tremors, euphoria, nervousness, restlessness, insomnia; confusion; (especially in children): excitement, fever. **CV:** Palpitation, *tachycardia*, mild hypotension or hypertension, cardiovascular collapse. **Special Senses:** Tinnitus, vertigo, dry nose, throat, nasal stuffiness; blurred vision, diplopia, photosensitivity, dry eyes. **GI:** *Dry mouth*, nausea, epigastric distress, anorexia, vomiting, constipation, or diarrhea. **Urogenital:** Urinary frequency or retention, dysuria. **Body as a Whole:** Hypersensitivity (skin rash, urticaria, photosensitivity, anaphylactic shock). **Respiratory:** Thickened bronchial secretions, wheezing, sensation of chest tightness.

DIAGNOSTIC TEST INTERFERENCE In common with other antihistamines, diphenhydramine should be discontinued 4 d prior to ***skin testing*** procedures for allergy because it may obscure otherwise positive reactions.

INTERACTIONS Drug: Alcohol and other CNS DEPRESSANTS, MAOIS, compound CNS depression.

PHARMACOKINETICS Absorption: Readily absorbed from GI tract but only 40–60% reaches systemic circulation. **Onset:** 15–30 min. **Peak:** 1–4 h. **Duration:** 4–7 h. **Distribution:** Crosses placenta; distributed into breast milk. **Metabolism:** Metabolized in liver; some degradation in lung and kidney. **Elimination:** Mostly excreted in urine within 24 h.

NURSING IMPLICATIONS

Assessment & Drug Effects

- Monitor cardiovascular status especially with preexisting cardiovascular disease.
- Monitor for adverse effects especially in children and the older adult.
- Supervise ambulation and use side rails as necessary. Drowsiness is most prominent during the first few days of therapy and often disappears with continued therapy. Older adults are especially likely to manifest dizziness, sedation, and hypotension.
- Monitor for paradoxical effects when used for sedation—patient may instead become agitated and uncomfortable.

Client & Family Education

- Do not use alcohol and other CNS depressants because of the possible additive CNS depressant effects with concurrent use.
- Do not drive or engage in other potentially hazardous activities until response to drug is known.
- Increase fluid intake, if not contraindicated; drug has an atropine-like drying effect (thickens bronchial secretions) that may make expectoration difficult.
- Do not breast feed while taking this drug.

PROCYCLIDINE HYDROCHLORIDE

(proe-sye′kli-deen)

Kemadrin, Procyclid ♣

Classifications: AUTONOMIC NERVOUS SYSTEM AGENT; ANTICHOLINERGIC (PARASYMPATHOLYTIC); ANTIMUSCARINIC; ANTISPASMODIC; ANTIPARKINSONISM AGENT

Pregnancy Category: C

AVAILABILITY 5 mg tablets

ACTIONS Centrally acting synthetic anticholinergic agent with actions similar to those of atropine. Selectively blocks muscarinic responses to acetylcholine (ACh), whether excitatory or inhibitory.

THERAPEUTIC EFFECTS Diminishes the characteristic tremor of parkinsonism.

USES To relieve symptoms of parkinsonism (postencephalitic, arteriosclerotic, and idiopathic) and drug-induced extrapyramidal symptoms.

CONTRAINDICATIONS Angle-closure glaucoma. Safety during pregnancy (category C), lactation, or in children is not established.
CAUTIOUS USE Hypotension; mental disorders; tachycardia; prostatic hypertrophy.

ROUTE & DOSAGE

Parkinsonism

Adult: **PO** 2.5 mg t.i.d.; may be gradually increased to 5 mg t.i.d. if tolerated with an additional 5 mg h.s. (max 45–60 mg/d)
Geriatric: **PO** Start with 2.5 mg 1–2 times/d

ADMINISTRATION

Oral

- Minimize adverse effects by administering drug during or after meals.
- Store at 15°–30° C (59°–86° F) in tightly closed containers unless otherwise directed.

ADVERSE EFFECTS (≥1%) **Body as a Whole:** Flushing of skin, decreased sweating, headache, light-headedness, dizziness, feeling of muscle weakness. **Special Senses:** Blurred vision, mydriasis, photophobia. **CV:** Palpitation, tachycardia, *hypotension*. **GI:** *Dry mouth*, nausea, vomiting, epigastric distress, constipation, paralytic ileus, acute suppurative parotitis. **Urogenital:** Urinary retention. **Skin:** Skin eruptions (occasionally). **CNS:** Mental confusion, psychotic-like symptoms.

INTERACTIONS Drug: Additive adverse effects with ANTICHOLINERGIC AGENTS.

PHARMACOKINETICS Onset: 35–40 min. **Duration:** 4–6 h.

NURSING IMPLICATIONS

Assessment & Drug Effects

- Monitor heart rate and rhythm and BP. Report palpitations, tachycardia, paradoxical bradycardia, or decreasing BP. Dosage adjustment or discontinuation of drug may be indicated.

- Monitor therapeutic effectiveness. Generally more effective in controlling rigidity than tremors. Tremors may temporarily appear to be exaggerated as rigidity is relieved, especially in clients with severe spasticity.
- Observe for and report to prescriber symptoms of mental confusion, disorientation, agitation, and psychotic-like symptoms, particularly in older adult clients who have low BP.
- Check for constipation and abdominal distention and provide information for preventing constipation.

Client & Family Education

- Void before taking drug if urinary hesitancy or retention is a problem.
- Avoid potentially hazardous activities until response to drug is known because drug may cause blurred vision and dizziness.
- Relieve dry mouth by rinsing frequently with water, chewing sugarless gum or sucking hard candy, or increasing noncaloric fluid intake. If these measures fail, a saliva substitute, available OTC, may help (e.g., Orex, Xero-Lube).
- Avoid alcohol and do not to take other CNS depressants unless otherwise advised by prescriber.
- Do not breast feed while taking this drug without consulting prescriber.

TRIHEXYPHENIDYL HYDROCHLORIDE

(trye-hex-ee-fen′i-dill)

Artane, Aparkane ♣, Apo-Trihex ♣, Novohexidyl ♣, Trihexy

Classifications: AUTONOMIC NERVOUS SYSTEM AGENT; ANTICHOLINERGIC (PARASYMPATHOLYTIC); ANTIPARKINSONIAN AGENT; ANTIMUSCARINIC; ANTISPASMODIC

Pregnancy Category: C

AVAILABILITY 2 mg, 5 mg tablets; 5 mg sustained-release capsules; 2 mg/5 mL elixir

ACTIONS Synthetic tertiary amine anticholinergic agent similar to atropine. Thought to act by blocking excess of acetylcholine at certain cerebral synaptic sites. Relaxes smooth muscle by direct effect and by atropine-like blocking action on the parasympathetic nervous system.

THERAPEUTIC EFFECTS Anticholinergic agent diminishes the characteristic tremor of Parkinson's disease. Antispasmodic action appears to be one-half that of atropine.

USES Symptomatic treatment of all forms of parkinsonism (arteriosclerotic, idiopathic, postencephalitic). Also to prevent or control drug-induced extrapyramidal disorders.
UNLABELED USES Huntington's chorea, spasmodic torticollis.

CONTRAINDICATIONS Narrow-angle glaucoma. Safety during pregnancy (category C), lactation, or in children is not established.
CAUTIOUS USE History of drug hypersensitivities; arteriosclerosis; hypertension; cardiac disease, kidney or liver disorders; obstructive diseases of GI or genitourinary tracts; older adults with prostatic hypertrophy.

ROUTE & DOSAGE

Parkinsonism

Adult: **PO** 1 mg day 1, 2 mg day 2, then increase by 2 mg q3–5d up to 6–10 mg/d in 3 or more divided doses (max 15 mg/d)

Extrapyramidal Effects

Adult: **PO** 5–15 mg/d in divided doses

ADMINISTRATION

Oral

- Give before or after meals, depending on how client reacts. Older adults and clients prone to excessive salivation (e.g., postencephalitic parkinsonism) may prefer to take drug after meals. If drug causes excessive mouth dryness, it may be better given before meals, unless it causes nausea.
- Once stabilized on conventional dosage forms, client may be switched to sustained-release capsules to permit once- or twice-a-day dosing.
- Do not crush, cut, or chew sustained-release capsules. These must be swallowed whole.
- Store at 15°–30° C (59°–86° F) in tight container unless otherwise directed.

ADVERSE EFFECTS (≥1%) **GI:** *Dry mouth, nausea,* constipation. **Special Senses:** *Blurred vision*, mydriasis, photophobia, angle-closure glaucoma. **Urogenital:** Urinary hesitancy or retention.

CNS: *Dizziness, nervousness,* insomnia, drowsiness, confusion, agitation, delirium, psychotic manifestations, euphoria. **CV:** Tachycardia, palpitations, hypotension, orthostatic hypotension. **Body as a Whole:** Hypersensitivity reactions.

INTERACTIONS Drug: Reduces therapeutic effects of **chlorpromazine, haloperidol,** PHENOTHIAZINES; increases bioavailability of **digoxin;** MAOIS potentiate actions of trihexyphenidyl.

PHARMACOKINETICS Absorption: Readily absorbed from GI tract. **Onset:** Within 1 h. **Peak:** 2–3 h. **Duration:** 6–12 h. **Elimination:** Excreted in urine.

NURSING IMPLICATIONS

Assessment & Drug Effects

- Be aware that incidence and severity of adverse effects are usually dose related and may be minimized by dosage reduction. Older adults appear more sensitive to usual adult doses.
- Some clients may experience euphoric feelings from this medication, so assure veracity of extrapyramidal side effects (EPSE) prior to administration.
- Monitor vital signs. Pulse is a particularly sensitive indicator of response to drug. Report tachycardia, palpitations, paradoxical bradycardia, or fall in BP.
- Assess for and report severe CNS stimulation (see ADVERSE EFFECTS) that occurs with high doses, and in clients with arteriosclerosis, or those with history of hypersensitivity to other drugs.
- In clients with severe rigidity, tremors may appear to be accentuated during therapy as rigidity diminishes.
- Monitor daily I&O if client develops urinary hesitancy or retention. Voiding before taking drug may relieve problem.
- Check for abdominal distention and bowel sounds if constipation is a problem.
- Monitor intraocular pressure at regular intervals.
- Provide close follow-up care. Tolerance may develop, necessitating dosage adjustment or use of combination therapy. Clients ≥60 y frequently develop sensitivity to drug action.

Client & Family Education

- Learn measures to relieve drug-induced dry mouth; rinse mouth frequently with water and suck ice chips or hard candy, chew sugarless gum. Maintain adequate total daily fluid intake.

- Avoid excessive heat because drug suppresses perspiration and, therefore, heat loss.
- Do not to engage in potentially hazardous activities requiring alertness and skill. Drug causes dizziness, drowsiness, and blurred vision. Help walking may be indicated.
- Do not breast feed while taking this drug without consulting prescriber.

ANTIPSYCHOTICS (NEUROLEPTICS)

ARIPIPRAZOLE

(ari-pip′ra-zole)

Abilify

Classifications: CENTRAL NERVOUS SYSTEM AGENT; PSYCHOTHERAPEUTIC; ANTIPSYCHOTIC; ATYPICAL

Pregnancy Category: C

AVAILABILITY 5 mg, 10 mg, 15 mg, 20 mg, 30 mg tablets

ACTIONS Exhibits high affinity for dopamine D_2 and D_3, serotonin 5-HT_{1A} and 5-HT_{2A} receptors, moderate affinity for dopamine D_4, serotonin 5-HT_{2C} and 5-HT_7, alpha$_1$-adrenergic and histamine H_1 receptors, and moderate affinity for the serotonin-reuptake site. Functions as a partial agonist at the dopamine D_2 and the serotonin 5-H_{1A} receptors, and as an antagonist at serotonin 5-HT_{2A} receptors.

THERAPEUTIC EFFECTS The mechanism of action is unknown. Efficacy of aripiprazole may be mediated through a combination of partial agonist activity at D_2 and 5-HT_{1A} receptors and antagonist activity at 5-HT_{2A} receptors. Actions at other receptors may explain some other clinical effects of aripiprazole (e.g., orthostatic hypotension).

USES Treatment of schizophrenia.

CONTRAINDICATIONS Hypersensitivity to aripiprazole; lactation; pregnancy (category C).

CAUTIOUS USE History of seizures or conditions that lower seizure threshold (e.g., Alzheimer's dementia); patients with known cardiovascular disease (history of MI or ischemic heart disease, heart failure, or conduction abnormalities), cerebrovascular disease, or conditions that predispose to hypotension (dehydration, hypovolemia, and treatment with antihypertensive medications).

ROUTE & DOSAGE

Schizophrenia

Adult: **PO** 10–15 mg q.d. May increase at 2 wk intervals to max of 30 mg/d if needed

ADMINISTRATION

Oral

- Note that carbamazepine decreases levels of aripiprazole, dose should be adjusted, and that each of **ketoconazole, quinidine, fluoxetine,** and **paroxetine** raise levels of aripiprazole as its clearance is inhibited.
- Store at 15°–30° C (59°–86° F).

ADVERSE EFFECTS (≥1%) **Body as a Whole:** *Headache,* asthenia, fever, flu-like symptoms, peripheral edema, chest pain, neck pain, neck rigidity. **CNS:** *Anxiety, insomnia, light-headedness, somnolence, akathisia,* tremor, extrapyramidal symptoms, depression, nervousness, increased salivation, hostility, suicidal thoughts, manic reaction, abnormal gait, confusion, cogwheel rigidity. **CV:** Hypertension, tachycardia, hypotension, bradycardia. **GI:** *Nausea, vomiting, constipation,* anorexia. **Hematologic:** Echymosis, anemia. **Metabolic:** Weight gain, weight loss, increased creatine kinase. **Musculoskeletal:** Muscle cramp. **Respiratory:** Rhinitis, cough. **Skin:** Rash. **Special Senses:** Blurred vision.

INTERACTIONS Drug: Carbamazepine will decrease aripiprazole levels (may need to double aripiprazole dose); **ketoconazole, quinidine, fluoxetine, paroxetine** may increase aripiprazole levels (reduce dose by 1/2); may enhance effects of ANTIHYPERTENSIVE AGENTS.

PHARMACOKINETICS Absorption: Well absorbed, 87% bioavailable. **Peak:** 3–5 h. **Metabolism:** Metabolized in liver by CYP3A4 and 2D6. Major metabolite, dehydroaripiprazole, has some activity. **Elimination:** 55% excreted in feces, 25% in urine. **Half-Life:** 75 h (94 h for metabolite).

NURSING IMPLICATIONS

Assessment & Drug Effects

- Monitor cardiovascular status. Assess for and report orthostatic hypotension. Take BP supine then in sitting position. Report systolic drop of >15–20 mm Hg. Patients at increased risk are those who are dehydrated, hypovolemic, or receiving concurrent antihypertensive therapy.
- Monitor body temperature in situations likely to elevate core temperature (e.g., exercising strenuously, exposure to extreme heat, receiving drugs with anticholinergic activity, or being subject to dehydration.)
- Monitor for and report signs of tardive dyskinesia.
- Monitor for and immediately report S&S of neuroleptic malignant syndrome (NMS), including hyperpyrexia, muscle rigidity, altered mental status, irregular pulse or blood pressure, tachycardia, diaphoresis, and cardiac dysrhythmia. Withhold drug if NMS is suspected.
- Lab tests: Monitor periodically Hct & Hgb. Monitor for elevated CPK and myoglobinuria if NMS is suspected.
- Monitor for diabetes, worsening of glucose control. Those with risk factors should undergo fasting glucose testing at baseline and periodically throughout treatment.

Client & Family Education

- Do not drive or engage in other potentially hazardous activities until reaction to drug is known.
- Avoid situations where you are likely to become overheated or dehydrated.
- Notify prescriber if you become pregnant or intend to become pregnant while taking this drug.
- Do not breast feed while taking this drug.

CHLORPROMAZINE

(klor-proe′ma-zeen)

CHLORPROMAZINE HYDROCHLORIDE

Chlorpromanyl ♣, Largactil ♣, Novochlorpromazine ♣, Ormazine, Promapar, Promaz, Sonazine, Thorazine, Thor-Prom

Classifications: CENTRAL NERVOUS SYSTEM AGENT; PSYCHOTHERAPEUTIC; ANTIPSYCHOTIC; PHENOTHIAZINE; ANTIEMETIC

Pregnancy Category: C

AVAILABILITY 10 mg, 25 mg, 50 mg, 100 mg, 200 mg tablets; 30 mg, 75 mg, 150 mg sustained-release capsules; 10 mg/5 mL syrup; 30 mg/mL, 100 mg/mL oral concentrate; 25 mg, 100 mg suppositories; 25 mg/mL injection

ACTIONS Phenothiazine derivative with actions at all levels of CNS with a mechanism that produces strong antipsychotic effects. Actions on hypothalamus and reticular formation produce strong sedation, hypotension, and depressed temperature regulation. Has strong alpha-adrenergic blocking action and weak anticholinergic effects. Directly depresses the heart; may increase coronary blood flow. Exerts quinidine-like antiarrhythmic action. Antiemetic effect due to suppression of the chemoreceptor trigger zone (CTZ). Inhibitory effect on dopamine reuptake may be the basis for moderate extrapyramidal symptoms. Antipsychotic drugs are sometimes called neuroleptics because they tend to reduce initiative and interest in the environment, decrease displays of emotions or affect, suppress spontaneous movements and complex behavior, and decrease psychotic symptoms. Spinal reflexes and unconditioned nociceptive-avoidance behaviors remain intact.

THERAPEUTIC EFFECTS Mechanism that produces strong antipsychotic effects is unclear, but thought to be related to blockade of postsynaptic dopamine receptors in the brain. Also has antiemetic effects due to its action on the CTZ.

USES To control manic phase of manic-depressive illness, for symptomatic management of psychotic disorders, including schizophrenia, in management of severe nausea and vomiting, to control excessive anxiety and agitation before surgery, and for treatment of severe behavior problems in children, e.g., attention deficit disorder. Also used for treatment of acute intermittent porphyria, intractable hiccups, and as adjunct in treatment of tetanus.

CONTRAINDICATIONS Hypersensitivity to phenothiazine derivatives; withdrawal states from alcohol; comatose states, brain damage, bone marrow depression, Reye's syndrome; children <6 mo; pregnancy (category C), lactation.

CAUTIOUS USE Agitated states accompanied by depression, seizure disorders, respiratory impairment due to infection or COPD; glaucoma, diabetes, hypertensive disease, peptic ulcer, prostatic hypertrophy; thyroid, cardiovascular, and hepatic disorders; patients exposed to extreme heat or organophosphate insecticides; previously detected breast cancer.

ROUTE & DOSAGE

Psychotic Disorders, Agitation

Adult: **PO** 25–100 mg t.i.d. or q.i.d.; may need up to 1000 mg/d **IM/IV** 25–50 mg up to 600 mg q4–6h
Child: **PO** *>6 mo,* 0.55 mg/kg q4–6h prn up to 500 mg/d **PR** *>6 mo,* 1.1 mg/kg q6–8h **IM/IV** *>6 mo,* 0.55 mg/kg q6–8h

Nausea and Vomiting

Adult: **PO** 10–25 mg q4–6h prn **PR** 50–100 mg q6–8h **IM/IV** 25–50 mg q3–4h prn
Child: **PO** *>6 mo,* 0.55 mg/kg q4–6h prn up to 500 mg/d **PR** *>6 mo,* 1.1 mg/kg q6–8h **IM/IV** *>6 mo,* 0.55 mg/kg q6–8h

Dementia

Geriatric: **PO** Initial 10–25 mg 1–2 times/d; may increase q4–7d by 10–25 mg/d (max 800 mg/d)

Intractable Hiccups

Adult: **PO/IM/IV** 25–50 mg t.i.d. or q.i.d.

ADMINISTRATION

Oral

- Give with food or a full glass of fluid to minimize GI distress.
- Ensure that oral drug is swallowed and not hoarded. Suicide attempt is a constant possibility in depressed patients, particularly when they are improving.
- Mix chlorpromazine concentrate just before administration in at least 1/2 glass juice, milk, water, coffee, tea, carbonated beverage, or with semisolid food.
- Ensure that sustained-release form of drug is not chewed or crushed. It must be swallowed whole.

Intramuscular/Intravenous

- Avoid parenteral drug contact with skin, eyes, and clothing because of its potential for causing contact dermatitis.
- Keep patient recumbent for at least 1/2 h after parenteral administration. Observe closely. Report hypotensive reactions.

Intramuscular

- Inject IM preparations slowly and deep into upper outer quadrant of buttock. Avoid SC injection, which can cause tissue irritation and nodule formation. If irritation is a problem, consult prescriber about diluting medication with normal saline or 2% procaine. Rotate injection sites.

Intravenous

PREPARE **Direct:** Dilute 25 mg with 24 mL of NS to yield 1 mg/mL. **Continuous:** May be further diluted in up to 1000 mL of NS.
ADMINISTER **Direct:** Administer 1 mg or fraction thereof over 1 min for adults and over 2 min for children. **Continuous:** Give slowly at a rate not to exceed 1 mg/min.
INCOMPATIBILITIES **Solution/Additive: Aminophylline, amphotericin B, ampicillin, chloramphenicol, chlorothiazide, cimetidine, dimenhydrinate, furosemide, heparin, methohexital, penicillin G, pentobarbital, phenobarbital, thiopental. Y-site: Allopurinol, amifostine, aminophylline, amphotericin B, aztreonam, cefepime, chloramphenicol, chlorothiazide, cholesteryl complex, etoposide, fludarabine, melphalan, methotrexate, paclitaxel, piperacillin/tazobactam, remifentanil, sargramostim.**

- Lemon-yellow color of parenteral preparation does not alter potency; if otherwise colored or markedly discolored, solution should be discarded.
- All forms are stored preferably between 15°–30° C (59°–86° F) protected from light, unless otherwise specified by the manufacturer. Avoid freezing.

ADVERSE EFFECTS (≥1%) **Body as a Whole:** Idiopathic edema, muscle necrosis (following IM), SLE-like syndrome, <u>sudden unexplained death</u>. **CV:** Orthostatic hypotension, palpitation, tachycardia, ECG changes (usually reversible): prolonged QT and PR intervals, blunting of T waves, ST depression. **GI:** Dry mouth; constipation, <u>adynamic ileus</u>, cholestatic jaundice, aggravation of peptic ulcer, dyspepsia, increased appetite. **Hematologic:** <u>Agranulocytosis</u>, thrombocytopenic purpura, <u>pancytopenia</u> (rare). **Metabolic:** Weight gain, hypoglycemia, hyperglycemia, glycosuria (high doses), enlargement of parotid glands. **CNS:** *Sedation, drowsiness,* dizziness, restlessness, <u>neuroleptic malignant syndrome</u>, tardive dyskinesias, tumor, syncope, headache, weakness, insomnia, reduced REM sleep, bizarre dreams, cerebral edema, convulsive seizures, <u>hypothermia</u>, inability to sweat, depressed cough reflex, *extrapyramidal symptoms,* EEG changes. **Respiratory:** Laryngospasm. **Skin:** Fixed-drug eruption, urticaria, reduced perspiration, contact dermatitis, exfoliative dermatitis, photosensitivity, eczema, anaphylactoid reactions, hypersensitivity vasculitis; hirsutism (long-term therapy). **Special Senses:** Blurred vision, lenticular opacities, mydriasis, photophobia. **Urogenital:** Anovulation, infertility, pseudopregnancy, menstrual irregularity, gynecomastia, galactorrhea, priapism, inhibition of ejaculation, reduced libido, urinary retention and frequency.

DIAGNOSTIC TEST INTERFERENCE Chlorpromazine (phenothiazines) may increase ***cephalin flocculation,*** and possibly other ***liver function tests;*** also may increase ***PBI.*** False-positive result may occur for ***amylase, 5-hydroxyindoleacetic acid, porphobilinogens, urobilinogen (Ehrlich's reagent),*** and ***urine bilirubin (Bili-Labstix).*** False-positive or false-negative ***pregnancy test*** results possibly caused by a metabolite of phenothiazines, which discolors urine depending on test used.

INTERACTIONS Drug: Alcohol, CNS DEPRESSANTS increase CNS depression; ANTACIDS, ANTIDIARRHEALS decrease absorption—space administration 2 h before or after administration of chlorpromazine; **phenobarbital** increases metabolism of phenothiazine; GENERAL ANESTHETICS increase excitation and hypotension; antagonizes antihypertensive action of **guanethidine; phenylpropanolamine** poses possibility of sudden death; TRICYCLIC ANTIDEPRESSANTS intensify hypotensive and anticholinergic effects; ANTICONVULSANTS decrease seizure threshold—may need to increase anticonvulsant dose. **Herbal: Kava-kava** increases risk and severity of dystonic reaction.

PHARMACOKINETICS Absorption: Rapid absorption with considerable first-pass metabolism in liver; rapid absorption after IM. **Onset:** 30–60 min. **Peak:** 2–4 h PO; 15–20 min IM. **Duration:** 4–6 h. **Distribution:** Widely distributed; accumulates in brain; crosses placenta. **Metabolism:** Metabolized in liver. **Elimination:** Excreted in urine as metabolites; excreted in breast milk. **Half-Life:** Biphasic 2 and 30 h.

NURSING IMPLICATIONS

Assessment & Drug Effects

- Establish baseline BP (in standing and recumbent positions), and pulse, before initiating treatment.
- Monitor BP frequently. Hypotensive reactions, dizziness, and sedation are common during early therapy, particularly in patients on high doses and in the older adult receiving parenteral doses. Patients usually develop tolerance to these adverse effects; however, lower doses or longer intervals between doses may be required.

- Lab tests: Periodic CBC with differential, liver function tests, urinalysis, and blood glucose.
- Monitor cardiac status with baseline ECG in patients with preexisting cardiovascular disease.
- Be alert for signs of neuroleptic malignant syndrome. Report immediately.
- Observe and record smoking since it increases metabolism of phenothiazines, resulting in shortened half-life and more rapid clearance of drug. Higher dosage in smokers may be required. Advise patient to stop or at least reduce smoking, if possible.
- Monitor I&O ratio and pattern: Urinary retention due to mental depression and compromised renal function may occur. If serum creatinine becomes elevated, therapy should be discontinued.
- Monitor for antiemetic effect of chlorpromazine, which may obscure signs of overdosage of other drugs or other causes of nausea and vomiting.
- Be alert to complaints of diminished visual acuity, reduced night vision, photophobia, and a perceived brownish discoloration of objects. Patient may be more comfortable with dark glasses.
- Monitor diabetics or prediabetics on long-term, high-dose therapy for reduced glucose tolerance and loss of diabetes control.
- Ocular examinations, and EEG (in patients >50 y) are recommended before and periodically during prolonged therapy.

Client & Family Education

- Take medication as prescribed and keep appointments for follow-up evaluation of dosage regimen. Improvement may not be experienced until 7 or 8 wk into therapy.
- Do not alter dosing regimen, and do not give the drug to another person.
- May cause pink to red-brown discoloration of urine.
- Wear protective clothing and sunscreen lotion with SPF at/above 15 when outdoors, even on dark days. Photosensitivity associated with chlorpromazine therapy is a phototoxic reaction. Severity of response depends on amount of exposure and drug dose. Exposed skin areas have appearance of an exaggerated sunburn. If reaction occurs, report to prescriber.
- Practice meticulous oral hygiene. Oral candidiasis occurs frequently in patients receiving phenothiazines.

- Report extrapyramidal symptoms that occur most often in patients on high dosage, the pediatric patient with severe dehydration and acute infection, the older adult, and women.
- Avoid driving a car or undertaking activities requiring precision and mental alertness until drug response is known.
- Do not abruptly stop this drug. Abrupt withdrawal of drug or deliberate dose skipping, especially after prolonged therapy with large doses, can cause onset of extrapyramidal symptoms and severe GI disturbances. When drug is to be discontinued, dosage must be tapered off gradually over a period of several weeks.
- Do not breast feed while taking this drug.

CLOZAPINE

(clo′za-pin)

Clozaril

Classifications: CENTRAL NERVOUS SYSTEM AGENT; PSYCHOTHERAPEUTIC; ANTIPSYCHOTIC; ATYPICAL

Pregnancy Category: B

AVAILABILITY 25 mg, 100 mg tablets

ACTIONS Mechanism is not defined. Interferes with binding of dopamine to D_1 and D_2 receptors in the limbic region of brain. It binds primarily to nondopaminergic sites (e.g., alpha-adrenergic, serotonergic, and cholinergic receptors).
THERAPEUTIC EFFECTS Utilized for treatment of schizophrenia uncontrolled by other agents.

USE Indicated only in the management of severely ill schizophrenic patients who have failed to respond to other neuroleptic agents.

CONTRAINDICATIONS Severe CNS depression, blood dyscrasia, history of bone marrow depression; patients with myeloproliferative disorders, uncontrolled epilepsy; clozapine-induced agranulocytosis, severe granulocytosis, concurrent administration of benzodiazepines or other psychotropic drugs; pregnancy (category B), lactation.
CAUTIOUS USE Arrhythmias, GI disorders, narrow-angle glaucoma, hepatic and renal impairment, prostatic hypertrophy, history of seizures; patients with cardiovascular and/or pulmonary disease; previous history of agranulocytosis. Safety and efficacy in children have not been established.

ROUTE & DOSAGE

Schizophrenia

Adult: **PO** > *16 y,* Initiate at 25–50 mg/d and titrate to a target dose of 350–450 mg/d in 3 divided doses at 2 wk intervals; further increases can be made if necessary (max 900 mg/d)

ADMINISTRATION

Oral

- Drug is usually withdrawn gradually over 1–2 wk if therapy must be discontinued.
- Store the drug away from heat or light.

ADVERSE EFFECTS (≥1%) **CV:** Orthostatic hypotension, *tachycardia,* ECG changes, increased risk of myocarditis especially during first month of therapy, pericarditis, pericardial effusion, cardiomyopathy, heart failures, MI, mitral insufficiency. **GI:** Nausea, dry mouth, constipation, hypersalivation. **Hematologic:** Agranulocytosis. **CNS:** Seizures, *transient fever,* sedation neuroleptic malignant syndrome (rare), dystonic reactions (rare). **Urogenital:** Urinary retention.

INTERACTIONS Drug: Alcohol and other CNS DEPRESSANTS compound depressant effects; ANTICHOLINERGIC AGENTS potentiate anticholinergic effects; ANTIHYPERTENSIVE AGENTS may potentiate hypotension.

PHARMACOKINETICS Absorption: Readily absorbed from GI tract. **Onset:** 2–4 wk. **Peak:** 2.5 h. **Distribution:** Possibly distributed into breast milk. **Metabolism:** Metabolized in liver. **Elimination:** 50% excreted in urine, 30% in feces. **Half-Life:** 8–12 h.

NURSING IMPLICATIONS

Assessment & Drug Effects

- Lab tests: Baseline WBC and differential count must be made before initial treatment, every week for first 6 mo, then every 2 wk for next 6 mo, and for 4 wk after the drug is discontinued.
- Monitor for seizure activity; seizure potential increases at the higher dose level.
- Closely monitor for recurrence of psychotic symptoms if the drug is being discontinued.
- Monitor cardiovascular status, especially during the first month of therapy. Report promptly S&S of CHF and other potential cardiac problems.

- Monitor for development of tachycardia or hypotension, which may pose a serious risk for patients with compromised cardiovascular function.
- Monitor daily temperature and report fever. Transient elevation above 38° C (100.4° F), with peak incidence during first 3 wk of drug therapy, may occur.
- Monitor for diabetes, worsening of glucose control, and those with risk factors should undergo fasting glucose testing at baseline and periodically throughout treatment.

Client & Family Education

- Do not engage in any hazardous activity until response to the drug is known. Drowsiness and sedation are common adverse effects.
- Due to the risk of agranulocytosis it is important to comply with blood test regimen. Report flu-like symptoms, fever, sore throat, difficulty urinating, lethargy, malaise, or other signs of infection.
- Rise slowly to avoid orthostatic hypotension.
- Report immediately any of the following: Unexplained fatigue, especially with activity; shortness of breath, sudden weight gain, or edema of the lower extremities.
- Take drug exactly as ordered.
- Do not use OTC drugs or alcohol without permission of prescriber.
- Do not breast feed while taking clozapine.

FLUPHENAZINE DECANOATE

(floo-fen′a-zeen)

Prolixin Decanoate, Modecate Decanoate ♣

FLUPHENAZINE ENANTHATE

Moditen Enanthate ♣, Prolixin Enanthate

FLUPHENAZINE HYDROCHLORIDE

Moditen HCl ♣, Permitil, Prolixin

Classifications: CENTRAL NERVOUS SYSTEM AGENT; PSYCHOTHERAPEUTIC; ANTIPSYCHOTIC; PHENOTHIAZINE

Pregnancy Category: C

AVAILABILITY 1 mg, 2.5 mg, 5 mg, 10 mg tablets; 2.5 mg/5 mL elixir; 5 mg/mL oral concentrate; 2.5 mg/mL, 25 mg/mL injection

ACTIONS Potent phenothiazine, antipsychotic agent. Blocks postsynaptic dopamine receptors in the brain. Similar to other phenothiazines with the following exceptions: More potent per weight, higher incidence of extrapyramidal complications, and lower frequency of sedative, hypotensive, and antiemetic effects.
THERAPEUTIC EFFECTS Effective for treatment of antipsychotic symptoms including schizophrenia.

USES Management of manifestations of psychotic disorders.
UNLABELED USES As antineuralgia adjunct.

CONTRAINDICATIONS Known hypersensitivity to phenothiazines; subcortical brain damage, comatose or severely depressed states, blood dyscrasias, renal or hepatic disease. Safety during pregnancy (category C) or lactation is not established. Parenteral form not recommended for children <12 y.
CAUTIOUS USE With anticholinergic agents, other CNS depressants; older adults, previously diagnosed breast cancer; cardiovascular diseases; pheochromocytoma; history of convulsive disorders; patients exposed to extreme heat or phosphorous insecticides; peptic ulcer; respiratory impairment.

ROUTE & DOSAGE

Psychosis

Adult: **PO** 0.5–10 mg/d in 1–4 divided doses (max 20 mg/d) **IM/SC HCl** 2.5–10 mg/d divided q6–8h (max 10 mg/d) **Decanoate** 12.5–25 mg q1–4wk **Enanthate** 25 mg q2wk

Dementia Behavior

Geriatric: **PO** 1–2.5 mg/d; may increase every 4–7d by 1–2.5 mg/d (max 20 mg/d in 2–3 divided doses)

ADMINISTRATION

Note: Fluphenazine hydrochloride (HCl) is given PO and IM. Fluphenazine enanthate and decanoate are given IM or SC.

Oral

- Give sustained-release tablets whole (need to be swallowed whole; not recommended for children).
- Dilute oral concentrate in fruit juice, water, carbonated beverage, milk, soup. Avoid caffeine-containing beverages (cola, coffee) as a diluent, also tannic acid (tea) or pectinates (apple juice).
- Be careful not to contact skin or clothing with drug when preparing oral concentrate or liquid preparations for injection.

Warn patient to avoid spilling drug. If drug contacts skin, rinse/flush skin promptly with warm water.
- Give oral preparations at least 1 h before or 2 h after an antacid. Antacids diminish absorption.
- Protect all preparations from light and freezing. Solutions may safely vary in color from almost colorless to light amber. Discard dark or otherwise discolored solutions.
- Store in tightly closed container at 15°–30° C (59°–86° F) unless otherwise specified by manufacturer. Protect all forms from light.

ADVERSE EFFECTS (≥1%) **CNS:** *Extrapyramidal symptoms* (resembling Parkinson's disease), tardive dyskinesia, sedation, drowsiness, dizziness, headache, mental depression, catatonic-like state, impaired thermoregulation, grand mal seizures. **CV:** Tachycardia, hypertension, hypotension. **GI:** Dry mouth, nausea, epigastric pain, constipation, fecal impaction, cholecystic jaundice. **Urogenital:** Urinary retention, polyuria, inhibition of ejaculation. **Hematologic:** Transient leukopenia, agranulocytosis. **Skin:** Contact dermatitis. **Body as a Whole:** Peripheral edema. **Special Senses:** Nasal congestion, blurred vision, increased intraocular pressure, *photosensitivity*. **Endocrine:** Hyperprolactinemia.

INTERACTIONS Drug: Alcohol and other CNS DEPRESSANTS may potentiate depressive effects; decreases seizure threshold, may need to adjust dosage of ANTICONVULSANTS. **Herbal: Kava-kava** may increase risk and severity of dystonic reactions.

PHARMACOKINETICS Absorption: HCl is readily absorbed PO and IM; decanoate, enanthate have delayed IM absorption. **Onset:** 1 h HCl; 24–72 h decanoate, enanthate. **Peak:** 0.5 h PO; 1.5–2 h IM HCl. **Duration:** 6–8 h HCl; 1–6 wk decanoate; 2–4 wk enanthate. **Distribution:** Crosses blood–brain barrier and placenta. **Metabolism:** Metabolized in liver. **Half-Life:** 15 h HCl; 3.6 d enanthate; 7–10 d decanoate.

NURSING IMPLICATIONS

Assessment & Drug Effects

- Report immediately onset of mental depression and extrapyramidal symptoms. Both occur frequently, particularly with long-acting forms (decanoate and enanthate).
- Be alert for appearance of acute dystonia. Symptoms can be controlled by reducing dosage or by adding an antiparkinsonian drug such as benztropine.

- Be alert for red, dry, hot skin; full, bounding pulse, dilated pupils, dyspnea, mental confusion, elevated BP, temperature over 40.6° C (105° F). Inform prescriber and institute measures to reduce body temperature rapidly. Extended exposure to high environmental temperature, to sun's rays, or to a high fever places the patient taking this drug at risk for heat stroke.
- Lab tests: Monitor kidney function in patients on long-term treatment. Withhold drug and notify prescriber if BUN is elevated (normal BUN: 10–20 mg/dL). Also periodically perform WBC with differential, liver function tests.
- Monitor BP during early therapy. If systolic drop is more than 20 mm Hg, inform prescriber.
- Monitor I&O ratio and bowel elimination pattern. Check for abdominal distention and pain. Monitor for xerostomia and constipation.
- Note: Patients on large doses who undergo surgery and those with cerebrovascular, cardiac, or renal insufficiency are especially prone to hypotensive effects.

Client & Family Education

- Do not drive or engage in potentially hazardous activities until response to drug is known.
- Do not alter dosage regimen or stop taking drug abruptly. Do not give drug to anyone else.
- Seek and obtain prescriber approval before taking any OTC drugs.
- Be alert for adverse effects. Early detection is critical because both decanoate and enanthate have a long duration of action. Inform prescriber promptly if following symptoms appear: Light-colored stools, changes in vision, sore throat, fever, cellulitis, rash, any interference with your willful (volitional) movements.
- Make sure to eat and drink adequately in order to prevent constipation and dry mouth.
- Be aware that it may be difficult for you to adjust to extremes in temperature. Use caution because of this possible impaired thermoregulation.
- Avoid exposure to sun; wear protective clothing and cover exposed skin surfaces with sunscreen lotion (SPF above 12).
- Avoid alcohol while on fluphenazine therapy.
- Note: Fluphenazine may discolor urine pink to red or reddish brown.

- Do not breast feed while taking this drug without consulting prescriber.
- Periodic ophthalmologic exams are recommended.

HALOPERIDOL

(ha-loe-per′i-dole)

Haldol, Peridol ♣

HALOPERIDOL DECANOATE

Haldol LA

Classifications: CENTRAL NERVOUS SYSTEM AGENT; PSYCHOTHERAPEUTIC; ANTIPSYCHOTIC; BUTYROPHENONE

Pregnancy Category: C

AVAILABILITY 0.5 mg, 1 mg, 2 mg, 5 mg, 10 mg, 20 mg tablets; 2 mg/mL oral solution; 5 mg/mL, 50 mg/mL, 100 mg/mL injection

ACTIONS Potent, long-acting butyrophenone derivative with pharmacologic actions similar to those of piperazine phenothiazines but with higher incidence of extrapyramidal effects and less hypotensive and relatively low sedative activity.

THERAPEUTIC EFFECTS Decreases psychotic manifestations and exerts strong antiemetic effect.

USES Management of manifestations of psychotic disorders and for control of tics and vocal utterances of Gilles de la Tourette's syndrome; for treatment of agitated states in acute and chronic psychoses. Used for short-term treatment of hyperactive children and for severe behavior problems in children of combative, explosive hyperexcitability.

UNLABELED USES Cancer chemotherapy as an antiemetic in doses smaller than those required for antipsychotic effects; treatment of autism; alcohol dependence; chorea.

CONTRAINDICATIONS Parkinson's disease, parkinsonism, seizure disorders, coma; alcoholism; severe mental depression, CNS depression; thyrotoxicosis. Safe use during pregnancy (category C), lactation, or in children <3 y is not established.

CAUTIOUS USE Older adult or debilitated patients, urinary retention, glaucoma, severe cardiovascular disorders; patients receiving anticonvulsant, anticoagulant, or lithium therapy.

ROUTE & DOSAGE

Psychosis

Adult: **PO** 0.2–5 mg b.i.d. or t.i.d. **IM** 2–5 mg repeated q4h prn **Decanoate** 50–100 mg q4wk
Child: **PO** 0.5 mg/d in 2–3 divided doses; may be increased by 0.5 mg q5–7d to 0.05–0.15 mg/kg/d

Severe Psychosis

Adult: **PO** 3–5 mg b.i.d. or t.i.d.; may need up to 100 mg/d **IM** 2–5 mg; may repeat q.h. prn **Decanoate:** 50–100 mg q4wk
Child: **PO** 0.05–0.15 mg/kg/d in 2–3 divided doses

Dementia

Geriatric: **PO** 0.25–0.5 mg 1–2 times daily; may increase every 4–7 d (max 4 mg/d in 2–3 divided doses)

Tourette's Disorder

Adult: **PO** 0.2–5 mg b.i.d. or t.i.d.
Child: **PO** 0.05–0.075 mg/kg/d in 2–3 divided doses

ADMINISTRATION

Oral

- Give with a full glass (240 mL) of water or with food or milk.
- Taper dosing regimen when discontinuing therapy. Abrupt termination can initiate extrapyramidal symptoms.

Intramuscular

- Give by deep injection into a large muscle. Do not exceed 3 mL per injection site.
- Have patient recumbent at time of parenteral administration and for about 1 h after injection. Assess for orthostatic hypotension.
- Store in light-resistant container at 15°–30° C (59°–86° F), unless otherwise specified by manufacturer. Discard darkened solutions.

ADVERSE EFFECTS (≥1%) **CNS:** *Extrapyramidal reactions:* Parkinsonian symptoms, dystonia, akathisia, tardive dyskinesia (after long-term use); insomnia, restlessness, anxiety, euphoria, agitation, drowsiness, mental depression, lethargy, fatigue, weakness, tremor, ataxia, headache, confusion, vertigo; <u>neuroleptic malignant syndrome</u>, hyperthermia, grand mal seizures, exacerbation of psychotic symptoms. **CV:** Tachycardia,

ECG changes, hypotension, hypertension (with overdosage). **Endocrine:** Menstrual irregularities, galactorrhea, lactation, gynecomastia, impotence, increased libido, hyponatremia, hyperglycemia, hypoglycemia. **Special Senses:** Blurred vision. **Hematologic:** Mild transient leukopenia, agranulocytosis (rare). **GI:** Dry mouth, anorexia, nausea, vomiting, constipation, diarrhea, hypersalivation. **Urogenital:** Urinary retention, priapism. **Respiratory:** Laryngospasm, bronchospasm, increased depth of respiration, bronchopneumonia, respiratory depression. **Skin:** Diaphoresis, maculopapular and acneiform rash, photosensitivity. **Other:** Cholestatic jaundice, variations in liver function tests, decreased serum cholesterol.

INTERACTIONS Drug: CNS DEPRESSANTS, OPIATES, **alcohol** increase CNS depression; may antagonize activity of ORAL ANTICOAGULANTS; ANTICHOLINERGICS may increase intraocular pressure; **methyldopa** may precipitate dementia.

PHARMACOKINETICS Absorption: Well absorbed from GI tract; 60% reaches systemic circulation. **Onset:** 30–45 min IM. **Peak:** 2–6 h PO; 10–20 min IM; 6–7 d decanoate. **Distribution:** Distributes mainly to liver with lower concentration in brain, lung, kidney, spleen, heart. **Metabolism:** Metabolized in liver. **Elimination:** 40% excreted in urine within 5 d; 15% eliminated in feces; excreted in breast milk. **Half-Life:** 13–35 h.

NURSING IMPLICATIONS

Assessment & Drug Effects

- Monitor for therapeutic effectiveness. Because of long half-life, therapeutic effects are slow to develop in early therapy or when established dosing regimen is changed. "Therapeutic window" effect (point at which increased dose or concentration actually decreases therapeutic response) may occur after long period of high doses. Close observation is imperative when doses are changed.
- Target symptoms expected to decrease with successful haloperidol treatment include hallucinations, insomnia, hostility, agitation, and delusions.
- Monitor patient's mental status daily.
- Monitor for neuroleptic malignant syndrome (NMS), especially in those with hypertension or taking lithium. Symptoms of NMS can appear suddenly after initiation of therapy or after months

or years of taking neuroleptic (antipsychotic) medication. Immediately discontinue drug if NMS suspected.

- Monitor for parkinsonism and tardive dyskinesia. Risk of tardive dyskinesia appears to be greater in women receiving high doses and in older adults. It can occur after long-term therapy and even after therapy is discontinued.
- Monitor for extrapyramidal (neuromuscular) reactions that occur frequently during first few days of treatment. Symptoms are usually dose related and are controlled by dosage reduction or concomitant administration of antiparkinsonian drugs.
- Be alert for behavioral changes in patients who are concurrently receiving antiparkinsonian drugs.
- Monitor for exacerbation of seizure activity.
- Observe patients closely for rapid mood shift to depression when haloperidol is used to control mania or cyclic disorders. Depression may represent a drug adverse effect or reversion from a manic state.
- Lab tests: Monitor WBC count with differential and liver function in patients on prolonged therapy.

Client & Family Education

- Avoid use of alcohol during therapy.
- Do not drive or engage in other potentially hazardous activities until response to drug is known.
- Discuss oral hygiene with health care provider; dry mouth may promote dental problems. Drink adequate fluids.
- Avoid overexposure to sun or sunlamp and use a sunscreen; drug can cause a photosensitivity reaction.
- Do not breast feed while taking this drug without consulting prescriber.

LOXAPINE HYDROCHLORIDE

(lox′a-peen)

Loxitane C, Loxitane IM

LOXAPINE SUCCINATE

Loxitane, Loxapac ♣

Classifications: CENTRAL NERVOUS SYSTEM AGENT; PSYCHOTHERAPEUTIC; ANTIPSYCHOTIC

Pregnancy Category: C

AVAILABILITY 5 mg, 10 mg, 25 mg, 50 mg capsules; 25 mg/mL oral solution; 50 mg/mL injection

ACTIONS This dibenzoxazepine antipsychotic is chemically distinct from other antipsychotics. Its exact mode of action is not established. Sedative action is less than that produced by chlorpromazine, but anticholinergic effects are comparable and extrapyramidal effects may be more intense. Also has antiemetic activity; lowers seizure threshold in patients with history of convulsive disorders.
THERAPEUTIC EFFECTS Stabilizes emotional component of schizophrenia by acting on subcortical level of CNS.

USES Manifestations of psychotic disorders.
UNLABELED USES Anxiety associated with mental depression.

CONTRAINDICATIONS Severe drug-induced CNS depression; comatose states, children <16 y. Safe use during pregnancy (category C) or lactation is not established.
CAUTIOUS USE Glaucoma, prostatic hypertrophy, urinary retention, history of convulsive disorders, cardiovascular disease.

ROUTE & DOSAGE

Psychosis

Adult: **PO** Start with 10 mg b.i.d. and rapidly increase to maintenance levels of 60–100 mg/d in 2–4 divided doses (max 250 mg/d) **IM** 12.5–50 mg q4–6h

Dementia Behavior

Geriatric: **PO** 5–10 mg 1–2 times/d; may increase q4–7d (max 125 mg/d)

ADMINISTRATION

Oral

- Give with food, milk, or water to reduce possibility of stomach irritation.
- Dilute oral concentrate in about 2–3 oz (60–90 mL) water or orange or grapefruit juice shortly before administration. Measure concentrate with calibrated dropper dispensed with drug. Do not store diluted solution.

Intramuscular

- Use only with acute psychosis or when oral route not feasible.

- Reduce dosage gradually over period of several days when therapy is to be terminated.
- Protect from light and freezing. Intensification of straw color to light amber is acceptable. Discard if solution is noticeably discolored.

ADVERSE EFFECTS (≥1%) **CNS:** *Drowsiness,* sedation, dizziness, syncope, EEG changes, paresthesias, staggering gait, muscle weakness, *extrapyramidal effects,* akathisia, tardive dyskinesia, <u>neuroleptic malignant syndrome</u>. **CV:** *Orthostatic hypotension,* hypertension, tachycardia. **Special Senses:** Nasal congestion, tinnitus; blurred vision, ptosis. **GI:** Constipation, dry mouth. **Skin:** Dermatitis, facial edema, pruritus, photosensitivity. **Urogenital:** Urinary retention, menstrual irregularities. **Body as a Whole:** Polydipsia, weight gain or loss, hyperpyrexia, transient leukopenia.

INTERACTIONS Drug: Alcohol and other CNS DEPRESSANTS potentiate CNS depression; will inhibit vasopressor effects of **epinephrine.**

PHARMACOKINETICS Absorption: Readily absorbed from GI tract. **Onset:** 20–30 min. **Peak:** 1.5–3 h. **Duration** 12 h. **Distribution:** Widely distributed; crosses placenta; distributed into breast milk. **Metabolism:** Metabolized in liver. **Elimination:** 50% excreted in urine, 50% excreted in feces. **Half-Life:** 19 h.

NURSING IMPLICATIONS

Assessment & Drug Effects

- Monitor baseline BP pattern prior to and during therapy; both hypotension and hypertension have been reported as adverse reactions.
- Observe carefully for extrapyramidal effects such as acute dystonia during early therapy. Most symptoms disappear with dose adjustment or with antiparkinsonian drug therapy.
- Discontinue therapy and report promptly to prescriber the first signs of impending tardive dyskinesia (fine vermicular movements of the tongue) when patient is on long-term treatment.
- Monitor I&O and bowel elimination patterns and check for bladder distention. Depressed patients often fail to report urinary retention or constipation.
- Risk of seizures is increased in those with history of convulsive disorders.

Client & Family Education

- Do NOT change dosage regimen in any way without prescriber approval.
- Avoid self-dosing with OTC drugs unless approved by the prescriber.
- Drowsiness usually decreases with continued therapy. If it persists and interferes with daily activities, consult prescriber. A change in time of administration or dose may help.
- Avoid potentially hazardous activity until response to drug is known.
- Learn measures to relieve dry mouth; rinse mouth frequently with water, suck hard candy. Avoid commercial products that may contain alcohol, which enhances drying and irritation.
- Notify prescriber of blurred or colored vision.
- Do not take drug dose and notify prescriber of following: Light-colored stools, bruising, unexplained bleeding, prolonged constipation, tremor, restlessness and excitement, sore throat and fever, rash.
- Stay out of bright sun; cover exposed skin with sunscreen.
- Do not breast feed while taking this drug without consulting prescriber.

MESORIDAZINE BESYLATE

(mez-oh-rid'a-zeen)

Serentil

Classifications: CENTRAL NERVOUS SYSTEM AGENT; PSYCHOTHERAPEUTIC; PHENOTHIAZINE; ANTIPSYCHOTIC

Pregnancy Category: C

AVAILABILITY 10 mg, 25 mg, 50 mg, 100 mg tablets; 25 mg/mL oral solution; 25 mg/mL injection

ACTIONS Piperidine derivative of phenothiazine. Tranquilizer with stronger sedative action than produced by chlorpromazine, but has more antiemetic action and lower incidence of extrapyramidal adverse effects.

THERAPEUTIC EFFECTS Antipsychotic effect due to psychomotor slowing and reduction of emotional stress.

USES Second-line therapy for schizophrenia, behavioral problems in mental deficiency and chronic brain syndrome, acute and chronic alcoholism. Also to reduce symptoms of anxiety and tension associated with many neurotic disorders.

CONTRAINDICATIONS Known sensitivity to other phenothiazines; severely depressed (drug-induced) patient; comatose state; children <12 y. Safety during pregnancy (category C) or lactation is not established.

CAUTIOUS USE Previously detected cancer of breast; glaucoma; prostatic hypertrophy, urinary retention; history of cardiovascular disease (can prolong QTc interval).

ROUTE & DOSAGE

Psychotic Disorders

Adult: **PO** 10–50 mg b.i.d. or t.i.d.; may increase as needed up to 400 mg/d **IM** 25 mg; may repeat in 30–60 min if necessary

Dementia Behavior

Geriatric: **PO** 10 mg 1–2 times/d; may gradually increase q4–7d (max 250 mg/d)

Management of Hyperactivity

Adult: **PO** 25 mg t.i.d. up to 75–300 mg/d

Alcohol Dependence

Adult: **PO** 25 mg b.i.d. up to 50–200 mg/d

Anxiety & Tension

Adult: **PO** 10 mg b.i.d. up to 150 mg/d

ADMINISTRATION

Oral

- Measure drug with calibrated dispenser included in original package. Dilute oral concentrate in about 1/2 glass (120 mL) of fluid just before administration. Use fruit juices, water, soup, carbonated beverage.

Intramuscular

- Inject IM solution slowly and deeply into upper outer quadrant of buttock. Advise patient to lie still for 20–30 min after the injection to minimize possible dizziness.
- Slight yellowing of the solution will not change potency; however, darkened solution should be discarded.
- Store at 15°–30° C (59°–86° F); refrigeration is not necessary. Protect solution from light and freezing.

ADVERSE EFFECTS (≥1%) **CNS:** Dizziness, *sedation,* fainting, extrapyramidal effects, dystonic reactions, akathisia, tardive dyskinesia, neuroleptic malignant syndrome. **Special Senses:** Blurred vision, xerostomia, nasal congestion. **Urogenital:** Urinary retention or incontinence, ejaculation dysfunction, impotence, priapism. **GI:** Constipation. **Body as a Whole:** Decreased sweating. **Skin:** Rash, exfoliative dermatitis photosensitivity. **CV:** Tachycardia, *orthostatic hypotension,* arrhythmias (prolong QTc interval) heart block.

INTERACTIONS Drug: Amiodarone, amoxapine, astemizole, bepridil, cisapride, clarithromycin, daunorubicin, diltiazem, disopyramide, dofetilide, dolasetron, doxorubicin, encainide, erythromycin, flecainide, gatifloxacin, grepafloxacin, haloperidol, ibutilide, indapamide, LOCAL ANESTHETICS, **maprotiline, moxifloxacin, octreotide, pentamidine, pimozide, procainamide, probucol, quinidine, risperidone, sotalol, sparfloxacin, tocainide**, TRICYCLIC ANTIDEPRESSANTS, **verapamil,** and **ziprasidone** prolong the QTc interval and can cause arrhythmias; **amantadine, clozapine, cyclobenzaprine, diphenoxylate, olanzapine, orphenadrine,** SEDATING H_1-BLOCKERS may have additive anticholinergic effects; **entacapone, tolcapone, pramipexole, ropinirole,** ANTICONVULSANTS may cause additive drowsiness and CNS depressant effects. **Herbal: Kava-kava** may increase risk and severity of dystonic reactions.

PHARMACOKINETICS Absorption: Readily absorbed from GI tract. **Peak:** 2 h PO; 30 min IM. **Duration:** 4–6 h PO; 6–8 h IM. **Metabolism:** Metabolized in liver. **Elimination:** Excreted in urine and bile. **Half-Life:** 24–48 h.

NURSING IMPLICATIONS

Assessment & Drug Effects

- Monitor I&O and bowel elimination patterns and check bladder for distention. Depressed patients often fail to report urinary discomfort or constipation.
- Report to prescriber if patient complains of blurred vision. Periodic ophthalmic examinations are advisable with long-term therapy.
- Monitor BP with patient supine and standing.

Client & Family Education

- Avoid spilling drug on skin since it may cause contact dermatitis. Thoroughly rinse off with water if spilling occurs.

- Do not drive or engage in potentially hazardous activities until response to drug is known. Dizziness and drowsiness are possible during early period of therapy.
- Expect drowsiness to decrease with continued therapy. If it persists, consult prescriber. A change in time of administration or dose may help to prevent interference with normal physical activities.
- Dangle legs at bedside when rising because of possible orthostatic hypotension.
- Avoid alcohol during therapy.
- Relieve dry mouth by rinsing frequently with water, sucking hard candy.
- Do not breast feed while taking this drug without consulting prescriber.

MOLINDONE HYDROCHLORIDE

(moe-lin′done)

Moban

Classifications: CENTRAL NERVOUS SYSTEM AGENT; PSYCHOTHERAPEUTIC; ANTIPSYCHOTIC PHENOTHIAZINE

Pregnancy Category: C

AVAILABILITY 5 mg, 10 mg, 25 mg, 50 mg, 100 mg tablets; 20 mg/mL liquid

ACTIONS Tranquilizer structurally unrelated but pharmacologically similar to the piperazine phenothiazines; thought to block postsynaptic dopamine receptors in the brain. Has less sedative but comparable anticholinergic activity and greater incidence of extrapyramidal adverse effects than chlorpromazine. EEG studies suggest ascending reticular system is chief site of action.

THERAPEUTIC EFFECTS Reportedly lowers convulsive threshold and produces tranquilization without compromising alertness. Antipsychotic effect includes reduction in bizarre behavior, and control of aggressiveness.

USES Management of manifestations of psychotic disorders.

CONTRAINDICATIONS Known hypersensitivity to molindone or to phenothiazines; severe CNS depression; comatose states; children <12 y. Safety during pregnancy (category C) or lactation is not established.

CAUTIOUS USE Those harmed by increase in physical activity; prostatic hypertrophy; cardiovascular disease; previously detected cancer of breast.

ROUTE & DOSAGE

Psychotic Disorders

Adult: **PO** 50–75 mg/d in 3–4 divided doses; may be increased to 100 mg/d in 3–4 d or may be able to decrease to 15–60 mg/d in divided doses (max 225 mg/d)

ADMINISTRATION

Oral

- Be certain patient swallows the medication.
- Store medication in tightly capped, light-resistant bottles. Protect from heat and moisture.

ADVERSE EFFECTS (≥1%) **CNS:** *Transient drowsiness,* insomnia, *extrapyramidal symptoms* (dose related), euphoria, neuroleptic malignant syndrome. **GI:** Dry mouth, constipation, hepatotoxicity. **Special Senses:** Tinnitus, blurred vision, nasal congestion. **Urogenital:** Urinary retention. **Skin:** Mild photosensitivity. **CV:** Tachycardia. **Body as a Whole:** Change in weight. **Endocrine:** SLE-like syndrome, heavy menses, amenorrhea, galactorrhea, gynecomastia, increased libido, premature ejaculation.

INTERACTIONS Drug: May potentiate CNS depression with CNS DEPRESSANTS, **alcohol. Herbal: Kava-kava** may increase risk and severity of dystonic reactions.

PHARMACOKINETICS Absorption: Readily absorbed from GI tract. **Peak:** 1 h. **Duration:** 24–36 h. **Distribution:** Distributed into breast milk. **Metabolism:** Metabolized in liver. **Elimination:** Excreted in urine and feces. **Half-Life:** 1.5 h.

NURSING IMPLICATIONS

Assessment & Drug Effects

- Withhold dose and consult with prescriber if the following symptoms occur: Tremor, involuntary twitching, exaggerated restlessness, changes in vision, light-colored stools, sore throat, fever, rash.
- Monitor bowel pattern and urinary output. The depressed patient may not report constipation or urinary retention, both adverse effects of this medicine.

- Supervise ambulation and other ADL in the older adult or debilitated patient or those with impaired vision to prevent injury or falling because drug increases motor activity.
- Be alert early during treatment to onset of symptoms of parkinsonism (extrapyramidal side effects): Rigidity, immobility, reduction of voluntary movements, tremors, fine vermicular tongue movements. Withhold dose and report promptly to prescriber.

Client & Family Education

- Take drug as prescribed; do not alter dose regimen or stop medication without consulting prescriber.
- Dizziness during early therapy usually disappears as treatment continues.
- Do not drive or engage in potentially hazardous activities requiring mental or physical coordination until response to drug is known.
- Avoid alcohol and self-medication with other depressants during therapy. Get prescriber approval before using any OTC drug.
- Relieve dry mouth by rinsing frequently with warm water, increasing noncaloric fluid intake, sucking hard candy.
- Avoid overexertion (patient with angina) and report increase in frequency of precordial pain.
- Schedule periodic ophthalmic examinations when treatment is long term.
- Do not breast feed while taking this drug without consulting prescriber.

OLANZAPINE

(o-lan′za-peen)

Zyprexa, Zyprexa Zydis

Classifications: CENTRAL NERVOUS SYSTEM AGENT; PSYCHOTHERAPEUTIC; NEUROLEPTIC AGENT; ATYPICAL; SEROTONIN-REUPTAKE INHIBITOR; DOPAMINE-REUPTAKE INHIBITOR

Pregnancy Category: C

AVAILABILITY 2.5 mg, 5 mg, 7.5 mg, 10 mg, 15 mg tablets; 10 mg, 15 mg, 20 mg orally disintegrating tablets (Zydis)

ACTIONS Antipsychotic activity is thought to be due to antagonism for both serotonin 5-$HT_{2A/2C}$ and dopamine D_{1-4} receptors.

May inhibit the CNS presynaptic neuronal reuptake of serotonin and dopamine. Antagonism of alpha-adrenergic receptors results in the adverse effect of orthostatic hypotension.
THERAPEUTIC EFFECTS Produces antipsychotic and anticholinergic activity.

USE Management of psychotic disorders, short-term treatment of acute manic episodes in bipolar disorder.
UNLABELED USES Alzheimer's dementia.

CONTRAINDICATIONS Hypersensitivity to olanzapine; pregnancy (category C), lactation.
CAUTIOUS USE Known cardiovascular disease, cerebrovascular disease, Parkinson's disease, dementia, history of seizures, conditions that predispose to hypotension (i.e., dehydration, hypovolemia), history of syncopy, history of breast cancer, hepatic or renal impairment, concurrent use of hepatotoxic drugs, predisposition to aspiration pneumonia, history of or high risk for suicide. Safety and effectiveness in children <18 y are not established.

ROUTE & DOSAGE

Psychotic Disorders

Adult: **PO** Start with 5–10 mg once daily; may increase by 2.5–5 mg qwk until desired response (usual range of 10–15 mg/d; max 20 mg/d)
Geriatric: **PO** Start with 5 mg once daily

Bipolar Mania

Adult: **PO** Start with 10–15 mg once daily; may increase by 5 mg q24h if needed

ADMINISTRATION

Oral

- Do not push orally disintegrating tablet through blister foil. Peel foil back and remove tablet. Tablet will disintegrate with/without liquid.
- Disintegrating tablets have been shown to improve symptomatology and compliance.

ADVERSE EFFECTS (≥1%) **Body as a Whole:** *Weight gain,* fever, back and chest pain, peripheral and lower extremity edema, joint pain, twitching, premenstrual syndrome. **CNS:** *Somnolence, dizziness, headache, agitation, insomnia, nervousness, hostility,* anxiety, personality disorder, akathisia, hypertonia, tremor amnesia, euphoria, stuttering, extrapyramidal symptoms (dystonic events, *parkinsonism, akathisia*), tardive dyskinesia. **CV:** Postural hypotension, hypotension, tachycardia. **Special Senses:** Amblyopia, blepharitis. **GI:** Abdominal pain, constipation, dry mouth, increased appetite, increased salivation, nausea, vomiting, elevated liver function tests. **Urogenital:** Premenstrual syndrome, hematuria, urinary incontinence, metrorrhagia. **Respiratory:** Rhinitis, cough, pharyngitis, dyspnea. **Skin:** Rash.

INTERACTIONS Drug: May enhance hypotensive effects of ANTIHYPERTENSIVES. May enhance effects of other CNS ACTIVE DRUGS, **alcohol. Carbamazepine, omeprazole, rifampin** may increase metabolism and clearance of olanzapine. **Fluvoxamine** may inhibit metabolism and clearance of olanzapine. **Herbal: St. John's wort** may cause **serotonin** syndrome (headache, dizziness, sweating, agitation).

PHARMACOKINETICS Absorption: Rapidly absorbed from GI tract; 60% reaches systemic circulation. **Peak:** 6 h. **Distribution:** 93% protein bound, secreted into breast milk of animals (human secretion unknown). **Metabolism:** Metabolized in liver, primarily by cytochrome P-450 1A2 (CYP1A2). **Elimination:** Approximately 57% excreted in urine, 30% in feces. **Half-Life:** 21–54 h.

NURSING IMPLICATIONS

Assessment & Drug Effects

- Withhold drug and immediately report S&S of neuroleptic malignant syndrome; assess for and report S&S of tardive dyskinesia.
- Lab tests: Periodically monitor ALT, especially in those with hepatic dysfunction or being treated with other potentially hepatotoxic drugs.
- Monitor BP and HR periodically. Monitor temperature, especially under conditions such as strenuous exercise, extreme heat, or treatment with other anticholinergic drugs.
- Monitor for seizures, especially in older adults and cognitively impaired persons.
- Monitor for diabetes, worsening of glucose control; those with risk factors should undergo fasting glucose testing at baseline and periodically throughout treatment.

Client & Family Education

- Do not drive or engage in potentially hazardous activities until response to drug is known; drug increases risk of orthostatic hypotension and cognitive impairment.

- Learn common adverse effects and possible drug interactions.
- Avoid alcohol and do not take additional medications without informing prescriber.
- Do not become overheated; avoid conditions leading to dehydration.
- Do not breast feed while taking this drug.

PIMOZIDE

(pi′moe-zide)

Orap

Classifications: CENTRAL NERVOUS SYSTEM AGENT; PSYCHOTHERAPEUTIC; ANTIPSYCHOTIC; BUTYROPHENONE

Pregnancy Category: C

AVAILABILITY 2 mg tablet

ACTIONS Potent central dopamine antagonist that alters release and turnover of central dopamine stores; has no effect on turnover of norepinephrine.

THERAPEUTIC EFFECTS Blockade of CNS dopaminergic receptors results in suppression of the motor and phonic tics that characterize Tourette's disorder. Produces less sedation and fewer extrapyramidal reactions than haloperidol; lowers seizure threshold.

USES To suppress severe motor and phonic tics in patient with Tourette's disorder who has failed to respond satisfactorily to standard treatment (e.g., haloperidol).

CONTRAINDICATIONS Treatment of simple tics other than those associated with Tourette's disorder; drug-induced tics; history of cardiac dysrhythmias and conditions marked by prolonged QT syndrome, patient taking drugs that may prolong QT interval (e.g., quinidine); severe toxic CNS depression. Safety in children <12 y, during pregnancy (category C), or lactation is not established.

CAUTIOUS USE Kidney and liver dysfunction; patients receiving anticonvulsant therapy.

ROUTE & DOSAGE

Tourette's Disorder

Adult: **PO** 1–2 mg/d in divided doses; gradually increase dose q.o.d. up to 0.2 mg/kg/d or 7–16 mg/d in divided doses, whichever is less (max 0.2 mg/kg/d or 10 mg/d)

ADMINISTRATION

Oral

- Increase drug dose gradually, usually over 1–3 wk, until maintenance dose is reached.
- Follow regimen prescribed by prescriber for withdrawal: Usually slow, gradual changes over a period of days or weeks (drug has a long half-life). Sudden withdrawal may cause reemergence of original symptoms (motor and phonic tics) and of neuromuscular adverse effects of the drug.

ADVERSE EFFECTS (≥1%) **Body as a Whole:** *Akathisia,* speech disorder, *torticollis, tremor,* handwriting changes, *akinesia,* fainting, hyperpyrexia, tardive dyskinesia, *rigidity, oculogyric crisis,* hyperreflexia; seizures, neuroleptic malignant syndrome; *extrapyramidal dysfunction,* hyperthermia, autonomic dysfunction; diaphoresis, weight changes, asthenia, chest pain, periorbital edema. **CNS:** Headache, *sedation, drowsiness,* insomnia, seizures, stupor. **CV:** Prolongation of QT interval, inverted or flattened T wave, appearance of U wave, labile blood pressure. **Urogenital:** Loss of libido, impotence, nocturia, urinary frequency, amenorrhea, dysmenorrhea, mild glactorrhea, urinary retention, acute renal failure. **Respiratory:** Dyspnea, respiratory failure. **Skin:** Sweating, skin irritation. **Special Senses:** Visual disturbances, photosensitivity, decreased accommodation, blurred vision, cataracts. **GI:** Increased salivation, nausea, vomiting, diarrhea, anorexia, abdominal cramps, constipation.

INTERACTIONS Drug: Alcohol and other CNS DEPRESSANTS increase CNS depression; ANTICHOLINERGIC AGENTS (e.g., TRICYCLIC ANTIDEPRESSANTS, **atropine**) increase anticholinergic effects; PHENOTHIAZINES, TRICYCLIC ANTIDEPRESSANTS, ANTIARRHYTHMICS, MACROLIDE ANTIBIOTICS, AZOLE ANTIFUNGALS (**itraconazole, ketoconazole, fluconazole**), PROTEASE INHIBITORS, **nefazodone, zileuton, dofetilide, sotalol, quinidine**, **other Class Ia and III antiarrhythmics, mesoridazine, thioridazine, chlorpromazine, droperidol, sparfloxacin, gatifloxacin, moxifloxacin, halofantrine, mefloquine, pentamidine, arsenic trioxide, levomethadyl acetate, dolasetron mesylate, probucol, tacrolimus, ziprasidone,** or other drugs that have demonstrated QT prolongation as one of their pharmacodynamics because they increase risk of arrhythmias and heart block; pimozide antagonizes effects of ANTICONVULSANTS—there is loss of seizure control. **Food: Grapefruit juice** may inhibit metabolism of pimozide.

PHARMACOKINETICS Absorption: Slowly and variably absorbed from GI tract (40–50% absorbed). **Peak:** 6–8 h. **Metabolism:** Metabolized in liver to 2 major metabolites by CYP3A4. **Elimination:** 80–85% excreted in urine, 15–20% in feces. **Half-Life:** 55 h.

NURSING IMPLICATIONS

Note: See haloperidol for additional nursing implications.

Assessment & Drug Effects

- Obtain ECG baseline data at beginning of therapy and check periodically, especially during dosage adjustments.
- Notify prescriber immediately for widening or prolongation of the QT interval, which suggests developing cardiotoxicity [QT interval (QRS complex and T wave) representing both ventricular depolarization and repolarization].
- Risk of tardive dyskinesia appears to be greatest in women, older adults, and those on high-dose therapy.
- Be aware that extrapyramidal reactions often appear within the first few days of therapy, are dose related, and usually occur when dose is high.
- Be aware that anticholinergic effects (dry mouth, constipation) may increase as dose is increased.

Client & Family Education

- Adhere to established drug regimen (i.e., do not change dose or intervals and discontinue only with prescriber's guidance).
- Use measures to relieve dry mouth (rinse frequently with water, saliva substitute, increase fluid intake) and constipation (increase dietary fiber, drink 6–8 glasses of water daily).
- Do not drive or engage in potentially hazardous activities because drug-caused hand tremors, drowsiness, and blurred vision may impair alertness and abilities.
- Pseudoparkinsonian symptoms are usually mild and reversible with dose adjustment.
- Be alert to the earliest symptom of tardive dyskinesia ("fly-catching"—an involuntary movement of the tongue) and report promptly to the prescriber.
- Return to prescriber for periodic assessments of therapy benefit and cardiac status.
- Understand dangers of ingesting alcohol to prevent augmenting CNS depressant effects of pimozide.
- Do not breast feed while taking this drug without consulting prescriber.

PROCHLORPERAZINE

(proe-klor-per'a-zeen)

Compazine

PROCHLORPERAZINE EDISYLATE

Compazine

PROCHLORPERAZINE MALEATE

Compazine, Stemetil ♣

Classifications: PSYCHOTHERAPEUTIC; ANTIPSYCHOTIC PHENOTHIAZINE; GASTROINTESTINAL AGENT; ANTIEMETIC

Pregnancy Category: C

AVAILABILITY 5 mg, 10 mg, 25 mg tablets; 10 mg, 15 mg, 30 mg sustained-release capsules; 2.5 mg, 5 mg, 25 mg suppositories; 5 mg/mL injection **Edisylate** 5 mg/5 mL syrup, 5 mg/mL injection

ACTIONS Phenothiazine derivative similar to chlorpromazine. Mechanism that produces strong antipsychotic effects is unclear, but thought to be related to blockade of postsynaptic dopamine receptors in the brain. Action on the hypothalamus and reticular formation results in sedative effects. Antiemetic effect is produced by suppression of the chemoreceptor trigger zone (CTZ).

THERAPEUTIC EFFECTS Inhibits dopamine reuptake; may be basis for moderate extrapyramidal symptoms. Greater extrapyramidal effects and antiemetic potency but fewer sedative, hypotensive, and anticholinergic effects than chlorpromazine.

USES Management of manifestations of psychotic disorders, of excessive anxiety, tension, and agitation, and to control severe nausea and vomiting.

CONTRAINDICATIONS Hypersensitivity to phenothiazines; bone marrow depression; comatose or severely depressed states; children <9 kg (20 lb) or 2 y of age; pediatric surgery; short-term vomiting in children or vomiting of unknown etiology; Reye's syndrome or other encephalopathies; history of dyskinetic reactions or epilepsy; pregnancy (category C), lactation.

CAUTIOUS USE Patient with previously diagnosed breast cancer, children with acute illness or dehydration.

ROUTE & DOSAGE

Severe Nausea, Vomiting, Anxiety, Psychotic Disorders

Adult: **PO** 5–10 mg t.i.d. or q.i.d.; sustained release: 10–15 mg q12h **IM** 5–10 mg q3–4h up to 40 mg/d **IV** 2.5–10 mg q6–8h (max 40 mg/d) **PR** 25 mg b.i.d.
Child: **PO** 2.5 mg 1–3 times/d or 5 mg b.i.d. (max 15 mg/d) **IM** 0.13 mg/kg q3–4h **PR** 2.5 mg b.i.d. or t.i.d. up to 20–25 mg/d

ADMINISTRATION

Oral

- Dosages for older adults, emaciated patients, and children should be increased slowly.
- Ensure that sustained-release form is not chewed or crushed: Must be swallowed whole.
- Do not give oral concentrate to children.
- Avoid skin contact with oral concentrate or injection solution because of possibility of contact dermatitis.

Intramuscular

- Do not inject drug SC.
- Make injection deep into the upper outer quadrant of the buttock in adults. Follow agency policy regarding IM injection site for children.

Intravenous

PREPARE **Direct:** Dilute each 5 mg (1 mL) in 4 mL of NS or other compatible solution to yield 1 mg/mL.
IV Infusion: Dilute in 50–100 mL of D5W, NS, D5/0.45% NaCl, RL, or other compatible solution.
ADMINISTER **Direct:** Do not exceed 10 mg for a single dose. Do not give a bolus dose. Give at a maximum rate of 5 mg/min.
IV Infusion: Give over 15–30 min. Do not exceed direct IV rate.
INCOMPATIBILITIES **Solution/Additive: Aminophylline, amphotericin B, ampicillin, calcium gluceptate, calcium gluconate, cephalothin, chloramphenicol, chlorothiazide, dimenhydrinate, furosemide, hydrocortisone, hydromorphone, ketorolac, methohexital, midazolam, morphine, penicillin G sodium, pentobarbital, phenobarbital, sodium bicarbonate, thiopental. Y-Site: Aldesleukin, allopurinol, amifostine, amphotericin B cholesteryl complex, aztreonam, cefepime, etoposide, filgrastim, fludarabine, foscarnet, piperacillin-tazobactam.**

- Discard markedly discolored solutions; slight yellowing does not appear to alter potency.

ADVERSE EFFECTS (≥1%) **CNS:** *Drowsiness,* dizziness, *extrapyramidal reactions (akathisia, dystonia or parkinsonism),* persistent tardive dyskinesia, acute catatonia. **CV:** Hypotension. **GI:** Cholestatic jaundice. **Skin:** Contact dermatitis, photosensitivity. **Endocrine:** Galactorrhea, amenorrhea. **Special Senses:** Blurred vision. **Hematologic:** Leukopenia, agranulocytosis.

INTERACTIONS Drug: Alcohol, CNS DEPRESSANTS increase CNS depression; ANTACIDS, ANTIDIARRHEALS decrease absorption, therefore, administer 2 h apart; **phenobarbital** increases metabolism of prochlorperazine; GENERAL ANESTHETICS increase excitation and hypotension; antagonizes antihypertensive action of **guanethidine; phenylpropanolamine** poses possibility of sudden death; TRICYCLIC ANTIDEPRESSANTS intensify hypotensive and anticholinergic effects; decreases seizure threshold—ANTICONVULSANT dosage may need to be increased. **Herbal: Kava-kava** may increase risk and severity of dystonic reactions.

PHARMACOKINETICS Absorption: Readily absorbed from GI tract. **Onset:** 30–40 min PO; 60 min PR; 10–20 min IM. **Duration:** 3–4 h PO; 10–12 h sustained release PO; 3–4 h PR; up to 12 h IM. **Distribution:** Crosses placenta; distributed into breast milk. **Metabolism:** Metabolized in liver. **Elimination:** Excreted in urine.

NURSING IMPLICATIONS

Assessment & Drug Effects

- Position nauseated patients who have received prochlorperazine carefully to prevent aspiration of vomitus; may have depressed cough reflex.
- Most older adult and emaciated patients and children, especially those with dehydration or acute illness, appear to be particularly susceptible to extrapyramidal effects. Be alert to onset of symptoms: Early in therapy watch for pseudoparkinsonism and acute dyskinesia. After 1–2 mo, be alert to akathisia.
- Keep in mind that the antiemetic effect may mask toxicity of other drugs or make it difficult to diagnose conditions with a primary symptom of nausea, such as intestinal obstruction and increased intracranial pressure.
- Lab tests: Periodic CBC with differential in long-term therapy.

- Be alert to signs of high core temperature: Red, dry, hot skin; full bounding pulse; dilated pupils; dyspnea; confusion; temperature over 40.6° C (105° F); elevated BP.
- Exposure to high environmental temperature, to sun's rays, or to a high fever associated with serious illness places this patient at risk for heat stroke. Inform prescriber and institute measures to reduce body temperature rapidly.

Client & Family Education

- Take drug only as prescribed and do not alter dose or schedule. Consult prescriber before stopping the medication.
- Avoid hazardous activities such as driving a car until response to drug is known because drug may impair mental and physical abilities, especially during first few days of therapy.
- Be aware that drug may color urine reddish brown. It also may cause the sun-exposed skin to turn gray-blue.
- Protect skin from direct sun's rays and use a sunscreen lotion (SPF >12) to prevent photosensitivity reaction.
- Withhold dose and report to the prescriber if the following symptoms persist more than a few hours: Tremor, involuntary twitching, exaggerated restlessness. Other reportable symptoms include light-colored stools, changes in vision, sore throat, fever, rash.
- Do not breast feed while taking this drug.

PROMAZINE HYDROCHLORIDE

(proe′ma-zeen)

Prozine-50, Sparine

Classifications: CENTRAL NERVOUS SYSTEM AGENT; PSYCHOTHERAPEUTIC; ANTIPSYCHOTIC; PHENOTHIAZINE

Pregnancy Category: C

AVAILABILITY 25 mg, 50 mg tablets; 25 mg/mL, 50 mg/mL injection

ACTIONS Derivative of phenothiazine. Compared with chlorpromazine, has weak antipsychotic activity, and extrapyramidal effects occur less frequently. Thought to block the postsynaptic dopamine receptors in the brain, with a higher affinity for D_1 over D_2 dopamine receptors.

THERAPEUTIC EFFECTS Antipsychotic drugs are sometimes called neuroleptics (or tranquilizers) because they tend to reduce initiative and interest in the environment, decrease displays of emotions or affect, suppress spontaneous movements and complex behavior, and decrease psychotic symptoms.

USES Manifestations of psychotic disorders and for reducing agitation and paranoia associated with alcohol withdrawal.

CONTRAINDICATIONS Hypersensitivity to phenothiazines; myelosuppression; CNS depression; children <12 y of age, Reye's syndrome. Safety during pregnancy (category C) or lactation is not established.

CAUTIOUS USE Prostatic hypertrophy; cardiovascular or liver disease; paralytic ileus; xerostomia; angle-closure glaucoma; persons exposed to extremes in temperature or to organophosphorous insecticides; convulsive disorders.

ROUTE & DOSAGE

Psychotic Disorders

Adult: **PO/IM** 10–200 mg q4–6h up to 1000 mg/d
Adolescent: **PO/IM** >*12 y,* 10–25 mg q4–6h

Dementia Behavior

Geriatric: **PO/IM** Start with 25 mg 1–2 times/d; may increase q4–7d in divided doses (max 500 mg/d)

ADMINISTRATION

Oral

- Use oral route whenever possible. Reserve parenteral administration for acutely disturbed or uncooperative patients or those who cannot tolerate oral preparation.
- Give 1 h before or 2 h after antacid; absorption is inhibited by antacids.
- Dilute the concentrate immediately before administration with fruit juice, chocolate-flavored drinks, carbonated drinks, or soup (for best taste, 10 mL of diluent for each 25 mg of drug). Avoid coffee or tea ingestion at or near medication times. Explain dosage and dilution to patient if drug is to be self-administered.
- Avoid contact of liquid preparations with skin.

Intramuscular

- Make IM injection deep into upper outer quadrant of buttock. Carefully aspirate before injecting drug slowly. Tissue irritation can occur if given SC. Intra-arterial injection can cause arterial or arteriolar spasm and consequent impairment of local circulation. Rotate injection sites.

- Store at 15°–30° C (59°–86° F) in light-resistant container unless otherwise directed.

ADVERSE EFFECTS (≥1%) **Body as a Whole:** *Drowsiness, orthostatic hypotension,* syncope. **Special Senses:** Blurred vision, photosensitivity. **GI:** Constipation, xerostomia. **CNS:** Extrapyramidal effects, tardive dyskinesia, epileptic seizures in susceptible individuals, leukopenia, agranulocytosis (rare). **CV:** Hypotension, sinus tachycardia.

INTERACTIONS Drug: Alcohol, CNS DEPRESSANTS increases CNS depression; **phenobarbital** increases metabolism; GENERAL ANESTHETICS increase excitation and hypotension; antagonizes antihypertensive action of **guanethidine; phenylpropanolamine** poses possibility of sudden death; TRICYCLIC ANTIDEPRESSANTS intensify hypotensive and anticholinergic effects; ANTICONVULSANTS decrease seizure threshold—may need to increase anticonvulsant dose. **Herbal: Kava-kava** may increase risk and severity of dystonic reactions.

PHARMACOKINETICS Absorption: Variable, absorbed from GI tract. **Metabolism:** Metabolized in liver.

NURSING IMPLICATIONS

Assessment & Drug Effects

- Monitor BP and pulse before administration and between doses. Keep patient recumbent for about 1 h after IM dose is given because incidence of postural hypotension and drowsiness is particularly high after parenteral administration.
- Encourage adequate fluid intake as prophylaxis for constipation and xerostomia. The depressed patient may not seek help for either symptom or for urinary retention.
- Report symptoms suggesting agranulocytosis promptly.

Client & Family Education

- Make position changes slowly, particularly from lying down to upright positions. Dizziness or faintness may occur on arising.
- Avoid alcohol during therapy.
- Do not spill oral solutions on hands or clothing; wash exposed skin well with soap and water. Drug may cause contact dermatitis.
- Be aware that promazine may color urine pink to red to reddish brown.
- Do not take OTC drugs without prescriber approval.
- Do not breast feed while taking this drug without consulting prescriber.

QUETIAPINE FUMARATE

(ce-ti-a′peen)

Seroquel

Classifications: CENTRAL NERVOUS SYSTEM AGENT; PSYCHOTHERAPEUTIC; ATYPICAL; ANTIPSYCHOTIC

Pregnancy Category: C

AVAILABILITY 25 mg, 100 mg, 200 mg tablets

ACTIONS Antagonizes multiple neurotransmitter receptors in the brain, including serotonin ($5\text{-}HT_{1A}$ and $5\text{-}HT_2$) and dopamine D_1 and D_2 receptors. Mechanism of action is unknown, however, antipsychotic properties thought to be related to antagonized responses. Antagonizes histamine H_1 receptors, resulting in possible somnolence, and adrenergic $alpha_1$ and $alpha_2$ receptors, which may lead to orthostatic hypotension.

THERAPEUTIC EFFECTS Indicated by a reduction in psychotic behavior.

USES Management of psychotic disorders; monotherapy and adjunct therapy for treatment of mania associated with bipolar disorder.

UNLABELED USES Management of agitation and dementia.

CONTRAINDICATIONS Hypersensitivity to quetiapine; lactation; alcohol use.

CAUTIOUS USE Liver function impairment, older adults, pregnancy (category C); cardiovascular disease (history of MI or ischemic heart disease, heart failure, arrhythmias), CVA, hypotension, dehydration, treatment with antihypertensives; history of seizures, Alzheimer's, concurrent use of centrally acting drugs; patient at risk for aspiration pneumonia; debilitated patients.

ROUTE & DOSAGE

Psychosis

Adult: **PO** Initiate with 25 mg b.i.d.; may increase by 25–50 mg b.i.d. to t.i.d. on the second or third day as tolerated to a target dose of 300–400 mg/d divided b.i.d. to t.i.d.; may adjust dose by 25–50 mg b.i.d. qd as needed (max 800 mg/d)

Geriatric: **PO** Initiate with 25 mg b.i.d.; titrate more slowly than adult patients; target range 150–200 mg/day in divided doses. Reports of use in geriatrics up to 900 mg/d are showing safety and good tolerability.

Agitation, Dementia

Geriatric: **PO** Initiate with 25 mg b.i.d.; may increase by 25–50 mg b.i.d. q2–7d if needed (max 200 mg/d). Reports of use in geriatrics up to 900 mg/d are showing safety and good tolerability.

ADMINISTRATION

Oral

- Titrate dose over 4 d usually to a target range of 300–400 mg/d. Make further dose adjustments of 25–50 mg 2 times/d at intervals of at least 2 d.
- Retitrate to desired dose when patient has been off the drug for >1 wk.
- Follow recommended lower doses and slower titration for older adults, the debilitated, and those with hepatic impairment or a predisposition to hypotension.
- Store at 15°–30° C (59°–86° F).

ADVERSE EFFECTS (≥1%) **Body as a Whole:** Asthenia, fever, hypertonia, dysarthria, flu syndrome, weight gain, peripheral edema. **CNS:** *Dizziness, headache, somnolence.* **CV:** Postural hypotension, tachycardia, palpitations. **GI:** Dry mouth, dyspepsia, abdominal pain, constipation, anorexia. **Respiratory:** Rhinitis, pharyngitis, cough, dyspnea. **Skin:** Rash, sweating. **Hematologic:** Leukopenia.

INTERACTIONS Drug: BARBITURATES, **carbamazepine, phenytoin, rifampin, thioridazine** may increase clearance of quetiapine. Quetiapine may potentiate the cognitive and motor effects of **alcohol,** enhance the effects of ANTIHYPERTENSIVE AGENTS, antagonize the effects of **levodopa** and DOPAMINE AGONISTS. **Ketoconazole, itraconazole, fluconazole, erythromycin** may decrease clearance of quetiapine. **Herbal: St. John's wort** may cause **serotonin** syndrome (headache, dizziness, sweating, agitation).

PHARMACOKINETICS Absorption: Rapidly and completely absorbed from GI tract. **Peak:** 1.5 h. **Distribution:** 83% protein bound. **Metabolism:** Extensively metabolized in the liver by CYP3A4. **Elimination:** 73% excreted in urine, 20% in feces. **Half-Life:** 6 h.

Common adverse effects in *italic*; life-threatening effects underlined; generic names in **bold**; drug classifications in SMALL CAPS; ♣ Canadian drug name.

NURSING IMPLICATIONS

Assessment & Drug Effects

- Reassess need for continued treatment periodically.
- Withhold the drug and immediately report S&S of tardive dyskinesia or neuroleptic malignant syndrome.
- Lab tests: Periodically monitor liver function, lipid profile, thyroid function, blood glucose, CBC with differential.
- Monitor for diabetes, worsening of glucose control; those with risk factors should undergo fasting glucose testing at baseline and periodically throughout treatment.
- Monitor ECG periodically, especially in those with known cardiovascular disease.
- Preform baseline cataract exam when therapy is started and at 6-mo intervals thereafter.
- Monitor patients with a history of seizures for lowering of the seizure threshold.

Client & Family Education

- Exercise caution with potentially hazardous activities requiring alertness, especially during the first week of drug therapy or during dose increments.
- Make position changes slowly, especially when changing from lying or sitting to standing to avoid dizziness, palpitations, and fainting.
- Avoid alcohol consumption and activities that may cause overheating and dehydration.
- Inform prescriber immediately if you become pregnant.
- Do not breast feed while taking this drug.

RISPERIDONE

(ris-per′i-done)

Risperdal, Risperdal M-TAB

RISPERIDONE CONSTA

Consta

Classifications: CENTRAL NERVOUS SYSTEM AGENT; ANTIPSYCHOTIC; ATYPICAL

Pregnancy Category: C

AVAILABILITY 0.25 mg, 0.5 mg, 1 mg, 2 mg, 3 mg, 4 mg tablets; 1 mg/mL solution; long-acting injectable. **Consta** 25 mg, 37.5 mg, and 50 mg IM injection

ACTIONS Mechanism is not well understood. Interferes with binding of dopamine to D_2-interlimbic region of the brain, serotonin (5-HT_2) receptors, and alpha-adrenergic receptors in the occipital cortex. It has low to moderate affinity for the other serotonin (5-HT) receptors and no affinity to nondopaminergic sites (e.g., cholinergic, muscarinic, or beta-adrenergic receptors). **Consta** Active medication is encapsulated into polymer-based microspheres that are time released when the microspheres are broken down slowly, gradually releasing.

THERAPEUTIC EFFECTS Effective in controlling symptoms of schizophrenia as well as other psychotic symptoms. Seems to improve negative symptoms such as apathy, blunted affect, and emotional withdrawal.

USES Reduction or elimination of psychotic symptoms in schizophrenia and related psychoses. Seems to improve negative symptoms such as apathy, blunted affect, and emotional withdrawal. Short-term treatment of acute manic or mixed episodes associated with bipolar I disorder either alone or in combination with lithium or valproate.

UNLABELED USE Management of patients with dementia-related psychotic symptoms. Adjunctive treatment of behavioral disturbances in patients with mental retardation. **Consta** Bipolar disorder; adjunctive treatment of behavioral disturbances in patients with mental retardation.

CONTRAINDICATIONS Hypersensitivity to risperidone; lactation.

CAUTIOUS USE People with no previous history of taking risperidone should take oral risperidone first, for a few days, to make sure they can take it safely. This drug should be used with caution in people who have liver or kidney disease, heart disease, Parkinson's disease, or epilepsy. Arrhythmias, hypotension, history of seizures, breast cancer, blood dyscrasia, cardiac disorders, renal or hepatic impairment, pregnancy (category C). Safety and efficacy in children are not established.

ROUTE & DOSAGE

Psychosis

Adult: **PO** 1–3 mg b.i.d.; start with 1 mg b.i.d., increase by 1 mg b.i.d. daily to an initial target dose of 3 mg b.i.d. (max 8 mg/d) **IM** Deep gluteal IM every 2 wk. For people currently taking risperidone tablets of up to 4 mg daily, initially 25 mg every 2 wk; for people currently taking oral risperidone over

4 mg daily, initially 37.5 mg every 2 wk. The dose should then be adjusted at intervals of at least 4 wk, in steps of 12.5 mg, to a maximum of 50 mg (25 mg for those over 65 years), every 2 wk. Dosage adjustments will take at least 3 wk to have an effect. Oral risperidone or other antipsychotic agent must be continued for 3 wk following initial administration of long-acting injectable risperidone.
Geriatric: **PO** Start with 0.5 mg b.i.d. and increase by 0.5 mg b.i.d. daily to an initial target of 1.5 mg b.i.d. (max 4 mg/d)

Renal Impairment

Cl_{cr} <30 mL/min: Start with 0.5 mg b.i.d.; increase by 0.5 mg b.i.d. daily to an initial target of 1.5 mg b.i.d.; may increase by 0.5 mg b.i.d. at weekly intervals (max 6 mg/d)

Dementia-Related Psychotic Symptoms

Note: An increased risk of stroke and transient ischemic attack has been associated with the use of risperidone in elderly patients with dementia-related psychosis.
Geriatric: **PO** Start with 0.5 mg b.i.d.; increase by 0.5 mg b.i.d. daily to an initial target of 1 mg b.i.d. (max 2 mg/d)

ADMINISTRATION

Oral

- Do not exceed increases/decreases of 1 mg b.i.d. in normal populations or 0.5 mg b.i.d. in older adults or the debilitated during dosage adjustments.
- Make further increases at 1-wk or longer intervals after the target doses of 3 mg b.i.d. in normal populations and 1.5 mg b.i.d. in older adults or the debilitated are reached.
- Store at 15°–30° C (59°–86° F).

IM

- Supplied as a powder with a solvent to be reconstituted at time of injection.
- Use the injection system components specifically designed for risperidone consta. The components cannot be replaced with standard syringes or needles.
- Do not make upward dosage adjustments more frequently than every 4 wk (max 50 mg every 2 wk).
- Oral risperidone or other antipsychotic agent must be continued for 3 wk following initial administration of long-acting injectable risperidone.

- Store at or below 25° C (77° F). May be out of refrigerator for a total of 7 days.
- Follow directions for reconstituting medication. Vigorously shake for at least 10 sec to reconstitute. If 2 min or more have elapsed following reconstitution and prior to injection, shake syringe vigorously for at least 10 sec.
- Once reconstituted, Consta must be injected within 6 h or disposed of.
- Injection is not uncomfortable because it is not an oil-based solution.

ADVERSE EFFECTS (≥1%) **Body as a Whole:** Orthostatic hypotension with initial doses, weight gain, sweating, weakness, fatigue. **CNS:** *Sedation, drowsiness, headache,* transient blurred vision, *insomnia,* disinhibition, *agitation,* anxiety, increased dream activity, dizziness, catatonia, *extrapyramidal symptoms* (akathisia, dystonia, pseudoparkinsonism) especially with doses >10 mg/d (Consta 50 mg dose); <u>neuroleptic malignant syndrome</u> (rare). **CV:** Prolonged QTc interval, tachycardia. **GI:** Dry mouth, dyspepsia, nausea, vomiting, diarrhea, constipation, abdominal pain, elevated liver function tests (AST, ALT). **Endocrine:** Galactorrhea. **Respiratory:** Rhinitis, cough, dyspnea. **Skin:** Photosensitivity. **Urogenital:** Urinary retention, menorrhagia, decreased sexual desire, erectile dysfunction, sexual dysfunction male and female.

DIAGNOSTIC TEST INTERFERENCE ***Liver function tests (AST, ALT)*** are elevated.

INTERACTIONS Drug: Risperidone may enhance the effects of certain ANTIHYPERTENSIVE AGENTS. May antagonize the antiparkinsonian effects of **bromocriptine, cabergoline, levodopa, pergolide, pramipexole, ropinirole. Carbamazepine** may decrease risperidone levels. **Clozapine** may increase risperidone levels. **Cisapride** may cause dysrhythmias.

PHARMACOKINETICS Absorption: Rapidly absorbed; not affected by food. **Onset:** Therapeutic effect 1–2 wk. **Peak:** 1–2 h. **Distribution:** 0.7 L/kg; in animal studies, risperidone has been found in breast milk. **Metabolism:** Metabolized primarily in liver by cytochrome P-450 with an active metabolite, 9-hydroxyrisperidone. **Elimination:** 70% excreted in urine, 14% in feces. **Half-Life:** 20 h for slow metabolizers, 30 h for fast metabolizers.

NURSING IMPLICATIONS

Assessment & Drug Effects

- Reassess patients periodically and maintain on the lowest effective drug dose.
- Monitor cardiovascular status closely; assess for orthostatic hypotension, especially during initial dosage titration.
- Monitor those at risk for seizures carefully.
- Assess degree of cognitive and motor impairment, and assess for environmental hazards.
- Lab tests: Monitor periodically serum electrolytes, liver function, and complete blood counts.
- Monitor for diabetes, worsening of glucose control; those with risk factors should undergo fasting glucose testing at baseline and periodically throughout treatment.

Client & Family Education

- Do not engage in potentially hazardous activities until the response to drug is known.
- Be aware of the risk of orthostatic hypotension.
- Learn adverse effects and report those that are bothersome to prescriber.
- Wear sunscreen and protective clothing to avoid photosensitivity.
- Notify prescriber if you intend to or become pregnant.
- Risperidone is excreted in breast milk, so women who are taking risperidone should not breast feed.

TRIFLUOPERAZINE HYDROCHLORIDE

(trye-floo-oh-per'a-zeen)

Novoflurazine ♣, Solazine ♣, Stelazine, Terfluzine ♣

Classifications: CENTRAL NERVOUS SYSTEM AGENT; PSYCHOTHERAPEUTIC; ANTIPSYCHOTIC PHENOTHIAZINE

Pregnancy Category: C

AVAILABILITY 1 mg, 2 mg, 5 mg, 10 mg tablets; 10 mg/mL liquid; 2 mg/mL injection

ACTIONS Phenothiazine similar to chlorpromazine. Produces fewer sedative, cardiovascular, and anticholinergic effects and more prominent antiemetic and extrapyramidal effects than other phenothiazines. Antipsychotic effects thought related to blockade of postsynaptic dopamine receptors in the brain.

THERAPEUTIC EFFECTS Indicated by increase in mental and physical activity. Strong antipsychotic drug with more prolonged pharmacologic effects than that of chlorpromazine.

USES Management of manifestations of psychotic disorders; "possibly effective" control of excessive anxiety and tension associated with neuroses or somatic conditions.

CONTRAINDICATIONS Hypersensitivity to phenothiazines; comatose states; CNS depression; blood dyscrasias; children <6 y; bone marrow depression; preexisting liver disease; pregnancy (category C), lactation.
CAUTIOUS USE Previously detected breast cancer; compromised respiratory function; seizure disorders.

ROUTE & DOSAGE

Psychotic Disorders

Adult: **PO** 1–2 mg b.i.d.; may increase up to 20 mg/d in hospitalized patients **IM** 1–2 mg q4–6h (max 10 mg/d)
Child: **PO** *6–12 y,* 1 mg 1–2 times/d; may increase up to 15 mg/d in hospitalized patients **IM** *6–12 y,* 1 mg 1–2 times/d; may increase up to 15 mg/d

Dementia Behavior

Geriatric: **PO** 0.5–1 mg 1–2 times/d; may increase q4–7d (max 40 mg in divided doses) **IM** 1 mg q4–6h (max 6 mg/d)

ADMINISTRATION

Oral

- Separate antacid and phenothiazine doses by at least 2 h.
- Dilute oral concentrate just before administration with about 60–120 mL suitable diluent (e.g., water, fruit juices, carbonated beverage, milk, soups, puddings). Avoid coffee or tea near time of taking oral preparation. Explain dosage and dilution to patient if drug is to be self-administered.
- Crush tablet and give with fluid or mix with food if patient will not or cannot swallow pill.
- Monitor ingestion of tablet to ensure that patient does not hoard medication.

Intramuscular

- Give IM injection deep into upper outer quadrant of buttock.
- Note: Slight yellow discoloration of injectable drug reportedly

does not alter potency. If color is markedly changed, discard solution.

- Wash hands if undiluted concentrate is spilled on skin to prevent contact dermatosis.
- Store in light-resistant container at 15°–30° C (59°–86° F) unless otherwise directed.

ADVERSE EFFECTS (≥1%) **CNS:** *Drowsiness,* insomnia, dizziness, agitation, *extrapyramidal effects,* neuroleptic malignant syndrome. **Special Senses:** Nasal congestion, *dry mouth,* blurred vision, pigmentary retinopathy. **Hematologic:** Agranulocytosis. **Skin:** Photosensitivity, skin rash, sweating. **GI:** Constipation. **CV:** Tachycardia, *hypotension*. **Respiratory:** Depressed cough reflex. **Endocrine:** Gynecomastia, galactorrhea.

INTERACTIONS Drug: Alcohol and other CNS DEPRESSANTS add to CNS depression. **Herbal: Kava-kava** may increase risk and severity of dystonic reactions.

PHARMACOKINETICS Absorption: Well absorbed from GI tract. **Onset:** Rapid onset. **Peak:** 2–3 h. **Duration:** Up to 12 h. **Metabolism:** Metabolized in liver. **Elimination:** Excreted in bile and feces.

NURSING IMPLICATIONS

Assessment & Drug Effects

- Monitor HR and BP. Hypotension is a common adverse effect.
- Hypotension and extrapyramidal effects (especially akathisia and dystonia) are most likely to occur in patients receiving high doses or parenteral administration and in older adults. Withhold drug and notify prescriber if patient has dysphagia, neck muscle spasm, or if tongue protrusion occurs.
- Monitor I&O ratio and bowel elimination pattern. Check for abdominal distention and pain. Encourage adequate fluid intake as prophylaxis for constipation and xerostomia. The depressed patient may not seek help for either symptom or for urinary retention.
- Be aware that since trifluoperazine potentiates analgesics, its use may reduce amount of narcotic required in painful long-term illness such as cancer.
- Agitation, jitteriness, and sometimes insomnia may simulate original neurotic or psychotic symptoms. These adverse effects may disappear spontaneously.
- Expect maximum therapeutic response within 2–3 wk after initiation of therapy.

Client & Family Education

- Take drug as prescribed; do not alter dosing regimen or stop medication without consulting prescriber.
- Consult prescriber about use of any OTC drugs during therapy.
- Do not take alcohol and other depressants during therapy.
- Avoid potentially hazardous activities such as driving or operating machinery, until response to drug is known. Drowsiness and dizziness may be prominent during this time.
- Cover as much skin surface as possible with clothing when you must be in direct sunlight. Use a SPF >12 sunscreen on exposed skin.
- Urine may be discolored or reddish brown; this is harmless.
- Do not breast feed while taking this drug.

ZIPRASIDONE HYDROCHLORIDE

(zip-ra-si′done)

Geodon

Classifications: CENTRAL NERVOUS SYSTEM AGENT; PSYCHOTHERAPEUTIC; ANTIPSYCHOTIC; ATYPICAL

Pregnancy Category: C

AVAILABILITY 20 mg, 40 mg, 60 mg, 80 mg capsules; 20 mg/mL injection

ACTIONS Unrelated to phenothiazine or butrophenone antipsychotic agents. Exhibits high *in vitro* binding affinity for the following receptors: dopamine D_2 and D_3, serotonin 5-HT_{2A}, 5-HT_{2C}, 5-HT_{1A}, 5-HT_{1D}, and the $alpha_1$-adrenergic receptors, and moderate affinity for the histamine H_1 receptor. Antagonist at the D_2, 5-HT_{2A}, and 5-HT_{1D} receptors, and an agonist at the 5-HT_{1A} receptor. Additionally, inhibits synaptic reuptake of serotonin and norepinephrine. Antagonism at other receptors may explain some of the other therapeutic and adverse effects (e.g., orthostatic hypotension).

THERAPEUTIC EFFECTS Mechanism of action is unknown; probably related to inhibition of synaptic reuptake of serotonin and norepinephrine through antagonism of dopamine type 2 (D_2) and serotonin type 2 (5-HT_2) antagonism.

USES Treatment of schizophrenia.

UNLABELED USES Dementia-related problems, mood and behavioral disturbances, Tourette's syndrome.

CONTRAINDICATIONS Hypersensitivity to ziprasidone; history of QT prolongation including congenital long QT syndrome or with other drugs known to prolong the QT interval; recent MI or uncompensated heart failure; bradycardia; hypokalemia or hypomagnesemia; neuroleptic malignant syndrome and tardive dyskinesia; dehydration or hypovolemia; pregnancy (category C), lactation. Safety and efficacy in children are not established.

CAUTIOUS USE History of seizures, CVA, or Alzheimer's disease; known cardiovascular disease, conduction abnormalities, treatment with antihypertensive drugs; hepatic impairment; risk factors for elevated core body temperature; esophageal motility disorders and risk of aspiration pneumonia; suicide potential; seizure disorders.

ROUTE & DOSAGE

Schizophrenia

Adult: **PO** Start with 20 mg b.i.d. with food, may increase q2d up to 80 mg b.i.d. if needed. **IM** 10 mg q2h or 20 mg q4h up to max of 40 mg/d

ADMINISTRATION

Note CONTRAINDICATIONS for this drug. Do NOT administer to anyone with a history of cardiac arrhythmias or other cardiac disease, hypokalemia, hypomagnesemia, prolonged QT/QTc interval, or to anyone on other drugs known to prolong the QTc interval. Withhold drug and consult prescriber if any of the foregoing conditions are present.

Oral

- Give with food.
- Make dosage adjustments at intervals of ≥2 d.

Intramuscular

- Give deep IM into a large muscle.
- Store at 15°–30° C (59°–86° F).

ADVERSE EFFECTS (≥1%) **Body as a Whole:** Asthenia, myalgia, weight gain, flu-like syndrome, face edema, chills, hypothermia. **CNS:** *Somnolence,* akathisia, dizziness, extrapyramidal effects, dystonia, hypertonia, agitation, tremor, dyskinesias, hostility, paresthesia, confusion, vertigo, hypokinesia, hyperkinesias, abnormal gait, oculogyric crisis, hypesthesia, ataxia, amnesia, cogwheel rigidity, delirium, hypotonia, akinesia, dysarthria, withdrawal syndrome, buccoglossal syndrome, choreoathetosis, diplopia, incoordination, neuropathy. **CV:** Tachycardia, postural hypotension, prolonged QTc interval, hypertension. **GI:** *Nausea,* constipation, dyspepsia, diarrhea, dry mouth, anorexia, abdominal pain, vomiting. **Respiratory:** Rhinitis, increased cough, dyspnea. **Skin:** Rash, fungal dermatitis, photosensitivity. **Special Senses:** Abnormal vision.

INTERACTIONS Drug: Carbamazepine may decrease ziprasidone levels; **ketoconazole** may increase ziprasidone levels; may enhance hypotensive effects of ANTIHYPERTENSIVE AGENTS; may antagonize effects of **levodopa;** increased risk of arrhythmias and heart block due to prolonged QTc interval with ANTIARRHYTHMIC AGENTS, **quinidine, dofetilide, sotalol, amoxapine, arsenic trioxide, cisapride, chlorpromazine, clarithromycin, daunorubicin, diltiazem, dolasetron, doxorubicin, droperidol, erythromycin, halofantrine, indapamide, levomethadyl,** LOCAL ANESTHETICS, **maprotiline, mefloquine, mesoridazine, octreotide, pentamidine, pimozide, probucol, gatifloxacin, grepafloxacin, levofloxacin, moxifloxacin, sparfloxacin,** TRICYCLIC ANTIDEPRESSANTS, **tacrolimus, thioridazine, troleandomycin;** additive CNS depression with SEDATIVE-HYPNOTICS, ANXIOLYTICS, **ethanol,** OPIATE AGONISTS. Ziprasidone IM should not be given to patients already taking oral ziprasidone.

PHARMACOKINETICS Absorption: Well absorbed with 60% reaching systemic circulation. **Peak:** 6–8 h. **Metabolism:** Extensively metabolized in the liver. **Elimination:** 20% of metabolites excreted in urine, 66% of metabolites excreted in bile. **Half-Life:** 7 h.

NURSING IMPLICATIONS

Assessment & Drug Effects

- Lab tests: Baseline and periodic ECG, serum potassium and serum magnesium, especially with concomitant diuretic therapy.
- Monitor for S&S of torsade de pointes (e.g., dizziness, palpitations, syncope), tardive dyskinesia especially in older adult women and with prolonged therapy, and the appearance of an unexplained rash. Withhold drug and report to prescriber immediately if any of these develop.

- Monitor I&O ratio and pattern. Notify prescriber if diarrhea, vomiting or any other conditions develop that may cause electrolyte imbalance.
- Monitor for diabetes, worsening of glucose control; those with risk factors should undergo fasting glucose testing at baseline and periodically throughout treatment.
- Monitor BP lying, sitting, and standing. Report orthostatic hypotension to prescriber.
- Monitor cognitive status and take appropriate precautions.
- Monitor for loss of seizure control, especially with a history of seizures or dementia.

Client & Family Education

- Be aware that therapeutic effect may not be evident for several weeks.
- Report any of the following to a health care provider immediately: Palpitations, faintness or loss of consciousness, rash, abnormal muscle movements, vomiting, or diarrhea.
- Do not drive or engage in potentially hazardous activities until response to drug is known.
- Make position changes slowly and in stages to prevent dizziness upon arising.
- Avoid strenuous exercise, exposure to extreme heat, or other activities that may cause dehydration.
- Do not breast feed while taking this drug.

NONSTIMULANT TREATMENT FOR ADHD

ATOMOXETINE

(a-to-mox′e-teen)

Strattera

Classifications: CENTRAL NERVOUS SYSTEM AGENT; PSYCHOTHERAPEUTIC; NOREPINEPHRINE-REUPTAKE INHIBITOR

Pregnancy Category: C

AVAILABILITY 10 mg, 18 mg, 25 mg, 40 mg, 60 mg capsules

ACTIONS Exact mechanism of action is unknown, but is thought to be related to selective inhibition of the presynaptic norepinephrine transporter, resulting in norepinephrine-reuptake inhibition.

THERAPEUTIC EFFECTS Improved attentiveness, ability to follow through on tasks with less distraction and forgetfulness, diminished hyperactivity.

USES Treatment of attention deficit/hyperactivity disorder (ADHD) in adults and children.

CONTRAINDICATIONS Hypersensitivity to atomoxetine or any of its constituents; concomitant use or use within 2 wk of MAOIS; narrow-angle glaucoma; pregnancy (category C).
CAUTIOUS USE Hypertension, tachycardia, cardiovascular or cerebrovascular disease; any condition that predisposes to hypotension; urinary retention or urinary hesitancy; concomitant use of CYP2D6 inhibitors (e.g., paroxetine, fluoxetine, quinidine), albuterol or other $beta_2$-agonists, vasopressor drugs; safety and efficacy in children <6-y and older adults have not been established; lactation.

ROUTE & DOSAGE

ADHD

Adult: **PO** Start with 40 mg in morning. May increase after 3 days to target dose of 80 mg/d given either once in the morning or divided morning and late afternoon/early evening. May increase to max of 100 mg/d if needed
Child/Adolescent: **PO** *<70 kg,* Start with 0.5 mg/kg/d. May increase after 3 d to target dose of 1.2 mg/kg/d. Administer once daily in morning or divide dose and give morning and late afternoon/early evening. Max dose is 1.4 mg/kg or 100 mg, whichever is less. *>70 kg,* Max total daily dose is 100 mg

Hepatic Impairment

Child–Pugh Class B: Initial and target doses should be reduced to 50% of the normal dose
Child–Pugh Class C: Initial dose and target doses should be reduced to 25% of normal

ADMINISTRATION

Oral

- Note that total daily dose in children and adolescents is based on weight. Determine that ordered dose is appropriate for weight prior to administration of drug.

- Note manufacturer recommends dosage adjustments with concomitant administration of strong CYP2D6 inhibitors (e.g., paroxetine, fluoxetine, quinidine). Consult prescriber.
- Store at 15°–30° C (59°–86° F).

ADVERSE EFFECTS (≥1%) **Body as a Whole:** Flu-like syndrome, flushing, fatigue, fever, rigors. **CNS:** Dizziness, *headache,* somnolence, crying, tearfulness, irritability, mood swings, *insomnia,* depression, tremor, early morning awakenings, paresthesias, abnormal dreams, decreased libido, sleep disorder. **CV:** Increased blood pressure, sinus tachycardia, palpitations. **GI:** *Upper abdominal pain,* constipation, dyspepsia, *vomiting, decreased appetite,* anorexia, dry mouth, diarrhea, flatulence. **Endocrine:** Hot flushes. **Metabolic:** Weight loss. **Musculoskeletal:** Arthralgia, myalgia. **Respiratory:** *Cough,* rhinorrhea, nasal congestion, sinusitis. **Skin:** Dermatitis, pruritus, increased sweating. **Special Senses:** Mydriasis. **Urogenital:** Urinary hesitation/retention, dysmenorrhea, ejaculation dysfunction, impotence, delayed onset of menses, irregular menstruation, prostatitis.

INTERACTIONS Drug: Dosing adjustments necessary for coadministration with CYP2D6 inhibitors. **Albuterol** may potentiate cardiovascular effects of atomoxetine; **fluoxetine, paroxetine, quinidine** may increase atomoxetine levels and toxicity; MAOIS may precipitate a hypertensive crisis; may attenuate effects of ANTIHYPERTENSIVE AGENTS.

PHARMACOKINETICS Absorption: Well absorbed from GI tract. **Peak:** 1–2 h. **Metabolism:** Metabolized in liver by CYP2D6. **Elimination:** Primarily excreted in urine. **Half-Life:** 5.2 h.

NURSING IMPLICATIONS

Assessment & Drug Effects

- Requires dosage titration.
- Evaluate for continuing therapeutic effectiveness especially with long-term use.
- Monitor cardiovascular status especially with preexisting hypertension.
- Monitor HR and BP at baseline, following a dose increase, and periodically while on therapy.
- Report increased aggression and irritability because these responses may indicate a need to discontinue the drug.

Client & Family Education

- Report any of the following to prescriber: Chest pains or palpitations, urinary retention or difficulty initiating voiding of urine, appetite loss and weight loss, or insomnia.
- Make position changes slowly if you experience dizziness with arising from a lying or sitting position.
- Do not drive or engage in potentially hazardous activities until reaction to the drug is known.
- Do not breast feed while taking this drug without consulting prescriber.
- Is more costly than other ADHD treatments.
- Provides an alternative to those who fail or cannot tolerate conventional treatments.

OPIATE ANTAGONIST

NALTREXONE HYDROCHLORIDE

(nal-trex′one)

Depade, ReVia, Trexan

Classifications: CENTRAL NERVOUS SYSTEM AGENT; NARCOTIC (OPIATE) ANTAGONIST

Pregnancy Category: C

AVAILABILITY 50 mg tablets

ACTIONS Pure opioid antagonist with prolonged pharmacologic effect, structurally and pharmacologically similar to naloxone. Mechanism of action not clearly delineated, but it appears that its competitive binding at opioid receptor sites reduces euphoria and drug craving without supporting the addiction.

THERAPEUTIC EFFECTS Weakens or completely and reversibly blocks the subjective effects (the "high") of IV opioids and analgesics possessing both agonist and antagonist activity.

USES Adjunct to the maintenance of an opioid-free state in detoxified addicts who are and desire to remain narcotic free. Management of alcohol dependence as an adjunct to social and psychotherapeutic methods.

UNLABELED USES Obesity.

CONTRAINDICATIONS Patients receiving opioid analgesics or in acute opioid withdrawal; opioid-dependent patient; acute hepatitis, liver failure. Also contraindicated in any individual who (1) fails naloxone challenge, (2) has a positive urine screen for opioids, or (3) has a history of sensitivity to naltrexone. Safety during pregnancy (category C), lactation, or in children <18 y is not established.

ROUTE & DOSAGE

Treatment of Opiate Cessation

Adult: **PO** 25 mg followed by another 25 mg in 1 h if no withdrawal response; maintenance regimen is individualized (max 800 mg/d)

Alcohol Dependence

Adult: **PO** 50 mg once/d

ADMINISTRATION

Challenge Test

Give the naloxone challenge test (administered IV or SC) before starting the abstinence program with naltrexone.

- SC dose: The SC dose is followed by an observation period of 45 min for symptoms of withdrawal (see below).
- IV dose: A portion of the IV dose is injected and, with the needle left in place, the patient is observed for 30 sec for withdrawal symptoms. If none are observed, remainder of dose is injected and patient is observed for the next 20 min.
- Withdrawal symptoms: Stuffiness or runny nose; tearing; yawning; sweating; tremors; vomiting; gooseflesh; feeling of temperature change; bone, joint, and muscle pains; abdominal cramps.
- Interpretation: Evidence of withdrawal symptoms indicates that the patient is at potential risk and should not enter a naltrexone program.
- Do not give naltrexone until patient is opiate free for at least 7–10 d.

Oral

- Give without regard to food.

ADVERSE EFFECTS (≥1%) **GI:** Dry mouth, anorexia, *nausea, vomiting,* constipation, *abdominal cramps/pain,* <u>hepatotoxicity</u>. **Musculoskeletal:** *Muscle and joint pains.* **CNS:** *Difficulty sleeping, anxiety, headache, nervousness,* reduced or increased energy, irritability, dizziness, depression. **Skin:** Skin rash. **Body as a Whole:** Chills.

INTERACTIONS Drug: Increased somnolence and lethargy with PHENOTHIAZINES; reverses analgesic effects of NARCOTIC (OPIATE) AGONISTS and NARCOTIC (OPIATE) AGONIST-ANTAGONISTS.

PHARMACOKINETICS Absorption: Rapidly absorbed from GI tract; 20% reaches systemic circulation (first-pass effect). **Onset:** 15–30 min. **Peak:** 1 h. **Duration:** 24–72 h. **Metabolism:** Metabolized in liver to active metabolite. **Elimination:** Excreted in urine. **Half-Life:** 10–13 h.

NURSING IMPLICATIONS

Assessment & Drug Effects

- Lab tests: Check liver function before the treatment is started, at monthly intervals for 6 mo, and then periodically as indicated.

Client & Family Education

- Note: Naltrexone therapy may put you in danger of overdosing if you use opiates. Small doses even at frequent intervals will give no desired effects; however, a dose large enough to produce a high is dangerous and may be fatal.
- It may be possible to transfer from methadone to naltrexone. This can be done after gradual withdrawal and final discontinuation of methadone.
- Report promptly to prescriber onset of signs of hepatic toxicity. The drug will be discontinued.
- Do not self-dose with OTC drugs for treatment of cough, colds, diarrhea, or analgesia. Many available preparations contain small doses of an opioid. Consult prescriber for safe drugs if they are needed.
- Tell health care provider or dentist before treatment that you are using naltrexone.
- Wear identification jewelry indicating naltrexone use.
- Do not breast feed while taking this drug without consulting prescriber.

SEDATIVE-HYPNOTICS

AMOBARBITAL

(am-oh-bar′bi-tal)

Amytal, Isobec, Novamobarb

AMOBARBITAL SODIUM

Amytal Sodium

Classifications: CENTRAL NERVOUS SYSTEM AGENT; ANTICONVULSANT; BARBITURATE; SEDATIVE-HYPNOTIC

Pregnancy Category: D

Controlled Substance: Schedule II

AVAILABILITY 30 mg, 50 mg, 100 mg capsules; 250 mg, 500 mg vials

ACTIONS Intermediate-acting barbiturate similar to phenobarbital. CNS depressant action appears to be related to ability to interfere with ascending impulse transmission from reticular activating system (concerned with alertness) to cerebral cortex. Does not impair pain perception.

THERAPEUTIC EFFECTS Controls seizure activity by increasing the threshold for motor cortex stimuli.

USES Sedative, to relieve anxiety, and as short-term hypnotic to treat insomnia. Also used parenterally to control status epilepticus or acute convulsive episodes, agitated behavior, and for narcoanalysis and narcotherapy.

CONTRAINDICATIONS Hypersensitivity to barbiturates; history of addiction; family or client history of porphyria; severe respiratory, hepatic, or renal disease. Safety during pregnancy (category D), lactation, or in children <6 y is not established.

CAUTIOUS USE Hypotension, hypertension, cardiac disease; acute or chronic pain; older adults.

ROUTE & DOSAGE

Sedative

Adult: **PO** 30–50 mg b.i.d. or t.i.d.
Child: **PO** 2 mg/kg or 70 mg/m^2/d in 4 divided doses

Preoperative Sedation

Adult: **PO/IM** 200 mg 1 h before surgery

Labor

Adult: **PO** 200–400 mg repeated at 1–3 h intervals (max 1 g)

Hypnotic

Adult: **PO/IM** 65–200 mg (max 500 mg)
Child: **IM** 2–3 mg/kg

Anticonvulsant, Agitated Behavior, Hypnotic

Adult/Child: **IV** 65–500 mg, not to exceed 1 g

ADMINISTRATION

Oral

- Give on an empty stomach to increase rate of absorption.
- Give hypnotic dose 30–60 min before bedtime. Hypnotic use should be limited to 2 wk.

Intramuscular

- Give injection within 30 min after vial is opened.
- Inject deep IM in a large muscle mass (e.g., upper outer quadrant of gluteus maximus). Superficial injections are painful and can cause sterile abscess or sloughing.
- Do not inject more than 5 mL into any one site.

Intravenous

PREPARE **Direct:** Dilute each 125 mg with 1.25 mL of sterile water for injection.

- Add diluent slowly, rotate vial to dissolve but do not shake.
- Do not use if solution does not clear within 5 min or contains a precipitate.
- Consult manufacturer's package insert for reconstitution directions to prepare specific concentrations.

ADMINISTER **Direct:** Give at rate not to exceed 100 mg/min for adults or 60 mg/m²/min for children.

- Do not give >1 mL of a 10% solution/min.

INCOMPATIBILITIES **Solution/Additive: Codeine phosphate, dimenhydrinate, phenytoin, hydrocortisone, hydroxyzine, insulin, levophanol, meperidine, methadone, morphine, norepinephrine, pentazocine, procaine, streptomycin, tetracycline, vancomycin, penicillin G,** PHENOTHIAZINES, **cimetidine, pancuronium.**

- Store at 15°–30° C (59°–86° F) unless otherwise directed. Avoid freezing. Discard any vial that has been opened ≥30 min.

ADVERSE EFFECTS (≥1%) **CNS:** Drowsiness, dizziness, hangover, unsteadiness, lethargy, paradoxical excitement. **Hematologic:** Agranulocytosis and thrombocytopenia (rare). **Body as a Whole:** Rash, angioedema, pain at IM injection site. **Skin:** Stevens-Johnson syndrome. **CV:** Hypotension. **Respiratory:** Respiratory depression.

INTERACTIONS Drug: Antagonizes effects of **phenmetrazine;** CNS DEPRESSANTS, **alcohol,** SEDATIVES compound CNS depression; MAOIS cause excessive CNS depression; **methoxyflurane** presents risk of nephrotoxicity. **Herbal: Kava-kava, valerian** may potentiate sedation.

PHARMACOKINETICS Onset: 1 h PO; 5 min IV. **Duration:** 6–8 h PO; 3–6 h IV. **Distribution:** Crosses placenta; appears in breast milk. **Metabolism:** Metabolized primarily in liver. **Elimination:** 40–50% of dose excreted in urine. **Half-Life:** 20–25 h.

NURSING IMPLICATIONS

Assessment & Drug Effects

- Observe IV injection site during and after administration. Extravasation can cause thrombophlebitis and tissue necrosis.
- Monitor vital signs during IV infusion and for several hours after drug administration. Caution client not to get out of bed without assistance.
- Note: Personnel and equipment for management of respiratory depression and hypotension must be immediately available when IV drug is administered.
- Monitor for S&S of paradoxical restlessness, excitement, confusion, and depression in older adults and children. Dosage adjustments may be required.

Client & Family Education

- Do not take alcoholic beverages or other CNS depressants while taking this drug.
- Note: Excitement may occur with onset of pain while taking this drug. Report to your prescriber immediately.
- Do not drive or perform other potentially hazardous tasks until response to drug is known.
- Note: Prolonged use may lead to tolerance and dependence; take only as prescribed.
- Do not breast feed while taking this drug without consulting prescriber.

CHLORAL HYDRATE

(klor′al hye′drate)

Aquachloral Supprettes, Noctec, Novochlorhydrate ♣

Classifications: CENTRAL NERVOUS SYSTEM AGENT; ANXIOLYTIC, SEDATIVE-HYPNOTIC

Pregnancy Category: C

Controlled Substance: Schedule IV

AVAILABILITY 500 mg capsules; 250 mg/5 mL, 500 mg/5 mL syrup; 324 mg, 500 mg, 648 mg suppositories

ACTIONS Produces "physiologic sleep" by mild cerebral depression with little effect on respirations or BP and little or no hangover.
THERAPEUTIC EFFECTS Chloral hydrate is a sedative-hypnotic that does not affect sleep physiology (e.g., REM sleep) in low doses. Has little or no analgesic action.

USES Short-term management of insomnia, for general sedation (especially in the young and the older adult), for sedation before and after surgery, to reduce anxiety associated with drug withdrawal, and alone or with paraldehyde to prevent or suppress alcohol withdrawal symptoms.

CONTRAINDICATIONS Known hypersensitivity to chloral hydrate or chloral derivatives; severe hepatic, renal, or cardiac disease; rectal dosage form in clients with proctitis; oral use in clients with esophagitis, gastritis, gastric or duodenal ulcers; pregnancy (category C), lactation.
CAUTIOUS USE History of intermittent porphyria, asthma, history of or proneness to drug dependence, depression, suicidal tendencies.

ROUTE & DOSAGE

Sedative

Adult: **PO/PR** 250 mg t.i.d. p.c.
Child: **PO/PR** 25–50 mg/kg/d divided q6–8h (max 500 mg/dose)

Hypnotic

Adult: **PO/PR** 500 mg–1 g 15–30 min before h.s. or 30 min before surgery
Geriatric: **PO/PR** 250 mg h.s.
Child: **PO/PR** 50 mg/kg 15–30 min before h.s. or 30 min before surgery (max 1 g)

EEG Premedication

Child: **PO/PR** 20–25 mg/kg 30–60 min prior to procedure

ADMINISTRATION

Oral

- Dilute liquid preparations in chilled fluids to minimize unpleasant taste.
- Watch to see that drug is not cheeked and hoarded.

Rectal

- Moisten suppository with a water-based lubricant, such as K-Y jelly, prior to insertion.
- Solutions are preserved in tightly covered, light-resistant containers.

ADVERSE EFFECTS (≥1%) **Body as a Whole:** Angioedema, eosinophilia, breath odor, leukopenia, ketonuria, renal and hepatic damage, sudden death. **CV:** Arrhythmias, cardiac arrest. **GI:** *Nausea, vomiting, diarrhea,* severe gastritis. **CNS:** Dizziness, motor incoordination, headache. **Skin:** Purpura, urticaria, erythematous rash, eczema, erythema multiforme, fixed drug eruptions. **Special Senses:** Conjunctivitis.

DIAGNOSTIC TEST INTERFERENCE False-positive results for ***urine glucose*** with ***Benedict's solutions,*** and possibly with ***Clinitest*** but not with ***glucose oxidase methods*** (e.g., ***Clinistix, Diastix, TesTape***). Possible interference with fluorometric test for ***urine catecholamines*** (if chloral hydrate is administered within 48 h of test) and ***urinary 17-OHCS*** determinations (by modification of ***Reddy, Jenkins, Thorn procedure***).

INTERACTIONS Drug: Alcohol, BARBITURATES, **paraldehyde,** other CNS DEPRESSANTS potentiate CNS depression; tachycardia may also occur with **alcohol;** increases anticoagulant effect of ORAL ANTICOAGULANTS; ***furosemide IV*** can produce flushing, diaphoresis, BP changes.

PHARMACOKINETICS Absorption: Readily absorbed from oral or rectal administration. **Onset:** 30–60 min. **Peak:** 1–3 h. **Duration:** 4–8 h. **Distribution:** Well distributed to all tissues; 70–80% protein bound; crosses placenta. **Metabolism:** Metabolized in liver to the active metabolite trichloroethanol. **Elimination:** Excreted primarily by kidneys, with a small amount excreted in feces via bile. **Half-Life:** 8–11 h.

NURSING IMPLICATIONS

Assessment & Drug Effects

- Chloral hydrate is not intended for relief of pain. When used in the presence of pain, it may cause excitement and delirium.
- Do not discontinue abruptly following prolonged use. Sudden withdrawal from dependent clients may produce delirium, mania, or convulsions.
- Monitor for S&S of allergic skin reactions, which may occur within several hours or as long as 10 d after drug administration.
- Evaluate client's response to chloral hydrate and continued need for the drug.

Client & Family Education

- Do not ambulate without assistance until response to drug is known.
- Avoid concomitant use of alcoholic beverages.
- Avoid driving and other potentially hazardous activities while under the influence of chloral hydrate.
- Do not breast feed while taking this drug.

ESTAZOLAM

(es-ta-zo′lam)

Prosom

Classifications: CENTRAL NERVOUS SYSTEM AGENT; ANXIOLYTIC; SEDATIVE-HYPNOTIC; BENZODIAZEPINE

Pregnancy Category: X

Controlled Substance: Schedule IV

AVAILABILITY 1 mg, 2 mg tablets

ACTIONS Benzodiazepine whose effects (anxiolytic, sedative, hypnotic, skeletal muscle relaxant) are mediated by the inhibitory neurotransmitter gamma-aminobutyric acid (GABA).

GABA acts at the thalamic, hypothalamic, and limbic levels of CNS.

THERAPEUTIC EFFECTS Benzodiazepines generally decrease the number of awakenings from sleep. Stage 2 (unequivocal sleep) is increased with all benzodiazepines. Estazolam shortens stages 3 and 4 (slow-wave sleep), and REM sleep is shortened. The total sleep time, however, is increased with estazolam.

USES Short-term management of insomnia.

CONTRAINDICATIONS Known sensitivity to BENZODIAZEPINES; acute narrow-angle glaucoma, primary depressive disorders or psychosis; children <2 y old; coma, shock, acute alcohol intoxication; pregnancy (category X), lactation.

CAUTIOUS USE Renal and hepatic impairment, organic brain syndrome, myasthenia gravis, narrow-angle glaucoma, suicide tendency, GI disorders, older adult and debilitated clients, limited pulmonary reserve.

ROUTE & DOSAGE

Adult: **PO** 1 mg h.s. may increase up to 2 mg if necessary (some debilitated older adult clients should start with 0.5 mg h.s.)

ADMINISTRATION

Oral

- For older adult clients in good health, a 1-mg dose is indicated; reduce initial dose to 0.5 mg for debilitated or small older adult clients.
- Dosage reduction also may be needed in the presence of hepatic impairment.

ADVERSE EFFECTS (≥1%) **CNS:** Headache, dizziness, impaired coordination, headache, hypokinesia, *somnolence,* hangover. **CV:** Palpitations, arrhythmias, syncope (all rare). **Hematologic:** Leukopenia, agranulocytosis. **GI:** Constipation, xerostomia, anorexia, flatulence, vomiting. **Musculoskeletal:** Arthritis, arthralgia, myalgia, muscle spasm.

INTERACTIONS Drug: Cimetidine may decrease metabolism of estazolam and increase its effects; alcohol and other CNS DEPRESSANTS may increase drowsiness. **Herbal: Kava-kava, valerian** may potentiate sedation.

PHARMACOKINETICS Absorption: Rapidly absorbed from GI tract. **Onset:** 20–30 min. **Peak:** 2 h. **Distribution:** Crosses rapidly into brain; crosses placenta; distributed into breast milk. **Metabolism:** Extensively metabolized in liver. **Elimination:** Excreted in urine. **Half-Life:** 10–24 h.

NURSING IMPLICATIONS

Assessment & Drug Effects

- Monitor for improvement in S&S of insomnia.
- Assess for excess CNS depression or daytime sedation.
- Assess for safety, especially with older adult or debilitated clients, as dizziness and impaired coordination are known adverse effects.

Client & Family Education

- Learn adverse effects and report those experienced to the prescriber.
- Avoid using this drug in combination with other CNS depressant drugs or alcohol.
- Do not drive or engage in other potentially hazardous activities until response to drug is known.
- Do not breast feed while taking this drug.

ETHCHLORVYNOL

(eth-klor-vi′nole)

Placidyl

Classifications: CENTRAL NERVOUS SYSTEM AGENT; ANXIOLYTIC; SEDATIVE-HYPNOTIC; BARBITURATE

Pregnancy Category: C

Controlled Substance: Schedule IV

AVAILABILITY 200 mg, 500 mg, 750 mg capsules

ACTIONS CNS depressant effects similar to those of chloral hydrate and barbiturates. Mechanism of action not known. Also exhibits anticonvulsant and muscle relaxant activity. Has no analgesic properties. Effect on REM sleep not known. Not commonly used as a sedative because of its short duration of action.

THERAPEUTIC EFFECTS Hypnotic doses produce cerebral depression and quiet, deep sleep; sedative doses reduce anxiety and apprehension.

USES Short-term therapy of simple insomnia for periods up to 1 wk.

CONTRAINDICATIONS Porphyria; clients with uncontrolled pain; first and second trimesters of pregnancy (category C). Safety during lactation and in children is not established.
CAUTIOUS USE Third trimester of pregnancy; clients with mental depression or suicidal tendencies, addiction-prone individuals; impaired liver or kidney function; older adult or debilitated clients; clients who respond unpredictably to alcohol or barbiturates.

ROUTE & DOSAGE

Sedative

Adult: **PO** 200 mg b.i.d. or t.i.d.

Hypnotic

Adult: **PO** 500 mg–1 g h.s.; may give an additional 200 mg if client awakens early

ADMINISTRATION

Oral

- Minimize transient giddiness and ataxia by giving drug with milk or other food. Symptoms seen in clients who apparently absorb the drug rapidly.
- Store at 15°–30° C (59°–86° F) in tight, light-resistant containers (darkens on exposure to light; slight darkening does not affect potency).

ADVERSE EFFECTS (≥1%) **CNS:** Dizziness, facial numbness, headache, mild hangover, nightmares, coma, respiratory failure. **Special Senses:** Blurred vision. **GI:** Nausea, vomiting, aftertaste. **Body as a Whole:** Urticaria. **Musculoskeletal:** Muscle weakness, tremors.

DIAGNOSTIC TEST INTERFERENCE ***Phentolamine test:*** False-positive test results (ethchlorvynol should be withdrawn at least 24 h before the test).

INTERACTIONS Drug: Alcohol and other CNS DEPRESSANTS amplify CNS depression; decrease anticoagulation effect of ORAL ANTICOAGULANTS.

PHARMACOKINETICS Absorption: Readily absorbed from GI tract. **Onset:** 15–30 min. **Peak:** 1–2 h. **Duration:** 5 h. **Distribution:**

Localizes in adipose tissue, liver, kidney, spleen, brain, CSF, bile; crosses placenta; distribution into breast milk unknown. **Metabolism:** Metabolized in liver with enterohepatic cycling and possibly in kidney. **Elimination:** 10% excreted in urine within 24 h. **Half-Life:** 20–100 h.

NURSING IMPLICATIONS

Assessment & Drug Effects

- Report mental confusion, hallucinations, or drowsiness in clients receiving daytime sedation; decrease in dosage or drug discontinuation is indicated.
- Observe intensity and duration of drug action, particularly in older adults, who may not tolerate average adult doses.
- Do not discontinue abruptly; severe withdrawal symptoms may occur in clients taking regular doses.

Client & Family Education

- Caution client to avoid driving or engaging in other activities requiring mental alertness and physical coordination for at least 5 h after taking drug.
- Psychological and physical dependence is possible; therefore, prolonged administration is not recommended. Adhere to established drug regimen to minimize the chance of dependence.
- Do not breast feed while taking this drug without consulting prescriber.

FLURAZEPAM HYDROCHLORIDE

(flure-az′e-pam)

Apo-Flurazepam ♣, Dalmane, Durapam, Novoflupam ♣

Classifications: CENTRAL NERVOUS SYSTEM AGENT; ANXIOLYTIC; SEDATIVE-HYPNOTIC; BENZODIAZEPINE

Pregnancy Category: X

Controlled Substance: Schedule IV

AVAILABILITY 15 mg, 30 mg capsules

ACTIONS Benzodiazepine derivative, with hypnotic activity equal to or greater than that produced by barbiturates or chloral hydrate. Mode and site of action not known; appears to act at

limbic and subcortical levels of CNS to produce sedation, skeletal muscle relaxation, and anticonvulsant effects.
THERAPEUTIC EFFECTS Reduces sleep induction time; produces marked reduction of stage 4 sleep (deepest sleep stage) while at the same time increasing duration of total sleep time.

USES Hypnotic in management of all kinds of insomnia (e.g., difficulty in falling asleep, frequent nocturnal awakening or early morning awakening, or both). Also for treatment of poor sleeping habits.

CONTRAINDICATIONS Prolonged administration; sleep apnea; intermittent porphyria; acute narrow-angle glaucoma; children <15 y; pregnancy (category X), lactation.
CAUTIOUS USE Impaired renal or hepatic function; mental depression, psychoses, history of suicidal tendencies, addiction-prone individuals; older adult or debilitated clients; COPD.

ROUTE & DOSAGE

Sedative, Hypnotic
Adult: **PO** *≥15 y,* 15–30 mg h.s.
Geriatric: **PO** 15 mg h.s.

ADMINISTRATION

Oral
- Give once client is in bed and ready to fall asleep.
- Store in light-resistant container with childproof cap at 15°–30° C (59°–86° F) unless otherwise specified.

ADVERSE EFFECTS (≥1%) **CNS:** *Residual sedation, drowsiness,* light-headedness, dizziness, ataxia, headache, nervousness, apprehension, talkativeness, irritability, depression, hallucinations, nightmares, confusion, paradoxic reactions: Excitement, euphoria, hyperactivity, disorientation, <u>coma</u> (overdosage). **Special Senses:** Blurred vision, burning eyes. **GI:** Heartburn, nausea, vomiting, diarrhea, abdominal pain. **Body as a Whole:** Immediate allergic reaction, hypotension, granulocytopenia (rare), jaundice (rare).

DIAGNOSTIC TEST INTERFERENCE Flurazepam may increase serum levels of ***total and direct bilirubin, alkaline phosphatase, AST,*** and ***ALT.*** False-negative ***urine glucose*** reactions may occur with ***Clinistix*** and ***Diastix;*** no effect with ***TesTape.***

INTERACTIONS Drug: Alcohol, CNS DEPRESSANTS, ANTICONVULSANTS potentiate CNS depression; **cimetidine, disulfiram** may increase flurazepam levels, thus increasing its toxicity. **Herbal: Kava-kava, valerian** may potentiate sedation.

PHARMACOKINETICS Absorption: Readily absorbed from GI tract. **Onset:** 15–45 min. **Duration:** 7–8 h. **Distribution:** Crosses blood–brain barrier and placenta; distributed into breast milk. **Metabolism:** Metabolized in liver to active metabolites. **Elimination:** Excreted primarily in urine. **Half-Life:** 47–100 h.

NURSING IMPLICATIONS

Assessment & Drug Effects

- Monitor effectiveness. Hypnotic effect is apparent on second or third night of consecutive use and continues 1–2 nights after drug is stopped (drug has a long half-life).
- Supervise ambulation. Residual sedation and drowsiness are relatively common. Excessive drowsiness, ataxia, vertigo, and falling occur more frequently in older adults or debilitated clients.
- Monitor drug ingestion if client has a history of drug abuse. Prolonged use of large doses can result in psychic and physical dependence.
- Lab tests: Obtain blood counts and liver and kidney function with repeated use.
- Be aware that withdrawal symptoms have occurred 3 d after abrupt discontinuation after prolonged use and include worsening of insomnia, dizziness, blurred vision, anorexia, GI upset, nasal congestion, paresthesias.

Client & Family Education

- Avoid potentially hazardous activities until response to drug is known.
- Avoid alcohol. Concurrent ingestion with flurazepam intensifies CNS depressant effects; symptoms may occur even when alcohol is ingested as long as 10 h after last flurazepam dose.
- Be aware of the possible additive depressant effects when drug is combined with barbiturates, tranquilizers, or other CNS depressants.
- Do not change dose intervals or dosage. Do not take for a self-diagnosed problem.

- Ask prescriber about the desirability of discontinuing the drug if you become or intend to become pregnant during therapy.
- Note: Prolonged use of this hypnotic is inadvisable because insomnia is usually transient.
- Do not breast feed while taking this drug.

GLUTETHIMIDE

(gloo-teth'i-mide)

Doriglute

Classifications: CENTRAL NERVOUS SYSTEM AGENT; ANXIOLYTIC; SEDATIVE-HYPNOTIC

Pregnancy Category: C

Controlled Substance: Schedule III

AVAILABILITY 250 mg tablets

ACTIONS Pharmacologic actions similar to those of barbiturates. Can induce hypnosis without producing reliable analgesic, antitussive, or anticonvulsant action. Causes less respiratory depression but greater degree of hypotension than barbiturates. Addiction liability similar to that of barbiturates.

THERAPEUTIC EFFECTS Significantly suppresses REM sleep; but following drug withdrawal after chronic administration, REM rebound occurs, and client may experience markedly increased dreaming, nightmares, insomnia.

USES Short-term treatment of insomnia and for sedative effect preoperatively and during first stage of labor. Not indicated for routine sedation or persistent insomnia.

CONTRAINDICATIONS Uncontrolled pain; intermittent porphyria; severe hepatic and renal impairment; prolonged administration; lactation; children <12 y. Safe use during pregnancy [(category C) except with caution during first stage of labor] is not established.

CAUTIOUS USE Older adult or debilitated clients; prostatic hypertrophy, bladder neck obstruction; pyloroduodenal obstruction, stenosing peptic ulcer; narrow-angle glaucoma; hypotension, cardiac arrhythmias; mental depression (particularly in clients with suicidal tendencies), history of alcoholism or drug abuse.

ROUTE & DOSAGE

Insomnia

Adult: **PO** 250–500 mg h.s., may repeat prn but not <4 h before arising

Preoperative Sedation

Adult: **PO** 500 mg the night before surgery and 500 mg–1 g 1 h before anesthesia

ADMINISTRATION

Oral

- Give 4 h or more before the usual time of arising to avoid residual daytime effects when administered for insomnia.
- Withdraw drug gradually, using stepwise dose reduction over a period of several days or weeks. Abrupt withdrawal following regular use may produce nausea, vomiting, nervousness, tremors, abdominal cramps, nightmares, insomnia, tachycardia, chills, fever, numbness of extremities, dysphagia, delirium, hallucinations, or convulsions.

ADVERSE EFFECTS ($\geq$1%) **Body as a Whole:** Acute hypersensitivity reactions. **CNS:** CNS depression in fetus; paradoxic excitement, headache, vertigo. **GI:** Gastric irritation, nausea, drug "hangover," dry mouth. **Hematologic:** Blood dyscrasias. **Skin:** Generalized skin rash (occasionally, purpuric or urticarial), exfoliative dermatitis (rare). **Other:** Hiccups, blurred vision. **Acute Overdosage:** CNS depression (coma; depressed reflexes, including corneal reflex; dilated, fixed pupils; hypotension; hypothermia followed by hyperpyrexia; tachycardia; respiratory depression, cyanosis, sudden apnea; decreased intestinal motility, adynamic ileus; facial twitching; intermittent spasticity; flaccid paralysis; pulmonary and cerebral edema; renal tubular necrosis; severe infections). **Chronic Ingestion:** Toxic psychosis (slurred speech, impaired memory, inability to concentrate, mydriasis, dry mouth, nystagmus, ataxia, hyporeflexia, tremors, peripheral neuropathy).

INTERACTIONS Drug: Alcohol, BARBITURATES, other CNS DEPRESSANTS compound depressant effects; TRICYCLIC ANTIDEPRESSANTS add to anticholinergic effects; decreases anticoagulant effects of ORAL ANTICOAGULANTS.

PHARMACOKINETICS Absorption: Erratic absorption from GI tract. **Onset:** 30 min. **Duration:** 4–8 h. **Distribution:** Widely distributed; localizes in adipose tissue, liver, kidney, brain, and bile; crosses placenta; distributed into breast milk in small quantities. **Metabolism:** Metabolized in liver. **Elimination:** Metabolites excreted in urine. **Half-Life:** 10–12 h.

NURSING IMPLICATIONS

Assessment & Drug Effects

- Inform prescriber of client's response to drug. Smallest effective dosage should be used for the shortest period of time compatible with client's needs.
- Note: Overdosage of glutethimide is difficult to treat. Clients tend to go in and out of toxicity, possibly because of delayed absorption of the drug.

Client & Family Education

- Report onset of rash or any other unusual symptoms to prescriber. Discontinuation of drug is indicated if a rash occurs.
- Do not drive or engage in other potentially hazardous activities requiring mental alertness for 7–8 h after drug ingestion.
- Note: Possible adverse reactions are increased when glutethimide is combined with alcohol or other CNS depressants.
- Understand that prolonged use of moderate to high doses of glutethimide can produce tolerance and psychological and physical dependence.
- Follow prescriber's plan for discontinuing drug in a slow reduction because abruptly stopping drug is problematic.
- You may experience some difficulty sleeping for several days after you have stopped taking this medication. This is a temporary state but must be planned for.
- Do not breast feed while taking this drug.

PENTOBARBITAL

(pen-toe-bar'bi-tal)

Nembutal

PENTOBARBITAL SODIUM

Nembutal Sodium, Novopentobarb ♣

Classifications: CENTRAL NERVOUS SYSTEM AGENT; ANXIOLYTIC; SEDATIVE-HYPNOTIC; BARBITURATE

Pregnancy Category: D

Controlled Substance: Schedule II

AVAILABILITY 50 mg, 100 mg capsules; 20 mg/5 mL liquid; 30 mg, 60 mg, 120 mg, 200 mg suppositories; 50 mg/mL injection

ACTIONS Short-acting barbiturate. Potent respiratory depressant. Initially, barbiturates suppress REM sleep, but with chronic therapy REM sleep returns to normal. Has no analgesic properties, and small doses may increase reaction to painful stimuli.
THERAPEUTIC EFFECTS Effective as a sedative and hypnotic. CNS depression may range from mild sedation to coma, depending on dosage, route of administration, degree of nervous system excitability, and drug tolerance.

USES Sedative or hypnotic for preanesthetic medication, induction of general anesthesia, adjunct in manipulative or diagnostic procedures, and emergency control of acute convulsions.

CONTRAINDICATIONS Pregnancy (category D) or lactation. History of sensitivity to barbiturates; parturition, fetal immaturity, uncontrolled pain. Use of sterile injection containing polyethylene glycol vehicle in clients with renal insufficiency.
CAUTIOUS USE: Pregnant women with toxemia or history of bleeding.

ROUTE & DOSAGE

Sedative

Adult: **PO** 20–30 mg b.i.d. to q.i.d.
Child: **PO** 2–6 mg/kg/d in 3 divided doses (max 100 mg/d)

Preoperative Sedation

Adult: **PO** 150–200 mg in 2 divided doses **IM** 150–200 mg in 2 divided doses **IV** 100 mg; may increase to 500 mg if necessary

Hypnotic

Adult: **PO** 120–200 mg **IM** 150–200 mg
Child: **PO** 30–120 mg **IM** 2–6 mg/kg (max 100 mg)

ADMINISTRATION Note: Do not give within 14 d of starting/stopping a MAOI.

Intramuscular

- Do not use parenteral solutions that appear cloudy or in which a precipitate has formed.
- Make IM injections deep into large muscle mass, preferably upper outer quadrant of buttock. Aspirate needle carefully before

injecting it to prevent inadvertent entry into blood vessel. Inject no more than 5 mL (250 mg) in any one site because of possible tissue irritation.

Intravenous

- Use IV route ONLY when other routes are not feasible.

PREPARE **Direct:** Give undiluted or diluted (preferred) with sterile water, D5W, NS, or other compatible IV solutions.

ADMINISTER **Direct:** Give slowly. Do not exceed rate of 50 mg/min.

INCOMPATIBILITIES **Solution/Additive: Chlorpheniramine, codeine, ephedrine, hydrocortisone, hydroxyzine, inulin, levorphanol, methadone, norepinephrine,** TETRACYCLINES, **penicillin G, pentazocine, phenytoin, promazine, promethazine, sodium bicarbonate, streptomycin, succinylcholine, triflubromazine, vancomycin, cimetidine, benzquinamide, butorphanol, chlorpromazine, dimenhydrinate, diphenhydramine, droperidol, fentanyl, glycopyrrolate, meperidine, midazolam, morphine, nalbuphine, perphenazine, prochlorperazine, ranitidine. Y-Site: Cimetidine, butorphanol, glycopyrrolate, midazolam, nalbuphine, perphenazine, ranitidine.**

- Take extreme care to avoid extravasation. Necrosis may result because parenteral solution is highly alkaline.
- Do not use cloudy or precipitated solution.

ADVERSE EFFECTS (≥1%) **Body as a Whole:** Drowsiness, lethargy, hangover, paradoxical excitement in the older adult client. **CV:** Hypotension with rapid IV. **Respiratory:** With rapid IV (respiratory depression, laryngospasm, bronchospasm, apnea).

INTERACTIONS Drug: Phenmetrazine antagonizes effects of pentobarbital; CNS DEPRESSANTS, **alcohol,** SEDATIVES add to CNS depression; MAOIS cause excessive CNS depression; **methoxyflurane** creates risk of nephrotoxicity. **Herbal: Kava-kava, valerian** may potentiate sedation.

PHARMACOKINETICS Onset: 15–30 min PO; 10–15 min IM; 1 min IV. **Duration:** 1–4 h PO; 15 min IV. **Distribution:** Crosses placenta. **Metabolism:** Metabolized primarily in liver. **Elimination:** Excreted in urine. **Half-Life:** 4–50 h.

NURSING IMPLICATIONS

Assessment & Drug Effects

- Monitor BP, pulse, and respiration q3–5 min during IV administration. Observe client closely; maintain airway. Have equipment for artificial respiration immediately available.
- Observe client closely for adverse effects for at least 30 min after IM administration of hypnotic dose.

Client & Family Education

- There is potential for dependence on this compound. Use should be for as short a period of time as necessary to treat a serious problem.
- Exercise caution when driving or operating machinery for the remainder of day after taking drug.
- Avoid alcohol and other CNS depressants for 24 h after receiving this drug.

SECOBARBITAL SODIUM

(see-koe-bar′ bi-tal)

Seconal Sodium

Classifications: CENTRAL NERVOUS SYSTEM AGENT; SEDATIVE-HYPNOTIC; BARBITURATE; ANXIOLYTIC

Pregnancy Category: D

Controlled Substance: Schedule II

AVAILABILITY 100 mg capsules

ACTIONS Short-acting barbiturate with CNS depressant effects as well as mood alteration from excitation to mild sedation, hypnosis, and deep coma. Depresses the sensory cortex, decreases motor activity, alters cerebellar function, and produces drowsiness, sedation, and hypnosis.

THERAPEUTIC EFFECTS Alters cerebellar function and produces drowsiness, sedation and hypnosis.

USES Hypnotic for simple insomnia and preoperatively to provide basal hypnosis for general, spinal, or regional anesthesia.

CONTRAINDICATIONS History of sensitivity to barbiturates; porphyria; severe liver function; severe respiratory disease; nephritic syndrome; pregnancy (category D), parturition, fetal immaturity; uncontrolled pain. Use of sterile injection containing polyethylene glycol vehicle in clients with renal insufficiency.

CAUTIOUS USE Pregnant women with toxemia or history of bleeding; labor and delivery, lactation; liver or kidney function impairment, older adult, debilitated individuals; children.

ROUTE & DOSAGE

Sedative

Adult: **PO** 100–300 mg/d in 3 divided doses
Child: **PO** 4–6 mg/kg/d in 3 divided doses

Preoperative Sedative

Adult: **PO** 100–300 mg 1–2 h before surgery
Child: **PO** 50–100 mg 1–2 h before surgery

Hypnotic

Adult: **PO** 100–200 mg

ADMINISTRATION

Oral

- Give hypnotic dose only after client retires for the evening.
- Crush and mix with a fluid or with food if client cannot swallow pill.

ADVERSE EFFECTS (≥1%) **CNS:** Drowsiness, lethargy, hangover, paradoxical excitement in the older adult client. **Respiratory:** Respiratory depression, laryngospasm.

INTERACTIONS Drug: Phenmetrazine antagonizes effects of secobarbital; CNS DEPRESSANTS, **alcohol,** SEDATIVES compound CNS depression; MAOIS cause excessive CNS depression; **methoxyflurane** increases risk of nephrotoxicity. **Herbal: Kava-kava, valerian** may potentiate sedation.

PHARMACOKINETICS Absorption: 90% absorbed from GI tract. **Onset:** 15–30 min. **Duration:** 1–4 h. **Distribution:** Crosses placenta; distributed into breast milk. **Metabolism:** Metabolized in liver. **Elimination:** Excreted in urine. **Half-Life:** 30 h.

NURSING IMPLICATIONS

Assessment & Drug Effects

- Be alert to unexpected responses and report promptly. Older adult or debilitated clients and children sometimes have paradoxical response to barbiturate therapy (i.e., irritability, marked excitement as inappropriate tearfulness and aggression in children, depression, and confusion). Protect older adult clients from falling, irrational behavior, and effects of depression (anorexia, social withdrawal).

- Client may become irritable, and uncooperative after a subhypnotic dose of a short-acting barbiturate (uncommon response).
- Be aware that barbiturates do not have analgesic action and may produce restlessness when given to clients in pain.
- Long-term therapy may result in nutritional folate (B_9) and vitamin D deficiency.
- Lab tests: Obtain liver function and hematology tests, serum folate and vitamin D levels during prolonged therapy.
- Observe closely for changes in established drug regimen effectiveness whenever a barbiturate is added, at least during early phase of barbiturate use. Barbiturates increase the metabolism of many drugs, leading to decreased pharmacologic effects of those drugs.
- Be alert for acute toxicity (intoxication) characterized by profound CNS depression, respiratory depression that may progress to Cheyne-Stokes respirations, hypoventilation, cyanosis, cold clammy skin, hypothermia, constricted pupils (but may be dilated in severe intoxication), shock, oliguria, tachycardia, hypotension, respiration arrest, circulatory collapse, and death.

Client & Family Education

- Do not drive or engage in potentially hazardous activities until response to drug is established.
- There is potential for dependence on this compound. Use should be for as short a period of time as necessary to treat a serious problem.
- Store barbiturates in a safe place; not on the bedside table or other readily accessible places. It is possible to forget having taken the drug, and in half-wakened conditions take more and accidentally overdose.
- Barbiturates are reportedly teratogenic. Do not become pregnant. Use or add barrier contraception if using hormonal contraceptives.
- Report to prescriber onset of fever, sore throat or mouth, malaise, easy bruising or bleeding, petechiae, jaundice, rash during prolonged therapy.
- Do not consume alcohol in any amount when taking a barbiturate. It may severely impair judgment and abilities.
- Do not breast feed while taking this drug without consulting prescriber.

TEMAZEPAM

(te-maz′ e-pam)

Restoril

Classifications: CENTRAL NERVOUS SYSTEM AGENT; ANXIOLYTIC; SEDATIVE-HYPNOTIC; BENZODIAZEPINE

Pregnancy Category: X

Controlled Substance: Schedule IV

AVAILABILITY 7.5 mg, 15 mg, 30 mg capsules

ACTIONS Benzodiazepine derivative with hypnotic, anxiolytic, sedative effects. Principal effect is significant improvement in sleep parameters.

THERAPEUTIC EFFECTS Reduces night awakenings and early morning awakenings; increases total sleep times, absence of rebound effects. Minimal change in REM sleep.

USES To relieve insomnia associated with frequent nocturnal awakenings or early morning awakenings.

CONTRAINDICATIONS Pregnancy (category X); safety in children <8 y is not established; narrow-angle glaucoma; psychoses.

CAUTIOUS USE Severely depressed client or one with suicidal ideation; history of drug abuse or dependence, acute intoxication; liver or kidney dysfunction; older adult clients; sleep apnea; lactation.

ROUTE & DOSAGE

Insomnia

Adult: **PO** 7.5–30 mg h.s.

Geriatric: **PO** 7.5 mg h.s.

ADMINISTRATION

Oral

- Give 20–30 min before client retires.
- Store at 15°–30° C (59°–86° F) in tight container unless otherwise specified by manufacturer.

ADVERSE EFFECTS (≥1%) **CNS:** *Drowsiness,* dizziness, lethargy, confusion, headache, euphoria, relaxed feeling, weakness. **GI:** Anorexia, diarrhea. **CV:** Palpitations.

INTERACTIONS Drug: Alcohol, CNS DEPRESSANTS, ANTICONVULSANTS potentiate CNS depression; **cimetidine** increases temazepam plasma levels, thus increasing its toxicity; may decrease antiparkinsonian effects of **levodopa;** may increase **phenytoin** levels; smoking decreases sedative effects. **Herbal: Kava-kava, valerian** may potentiate sedation.

PHARMACOKINETICS Absorption: Readily absorbed from GI tract. **Onset:** 30–50 min. **Peak:** 2–3 h. **Duration:** 10–12 h. **Distribution:** Crosses placenta; distributed into breast milk. **Metabolism:** Metabolized in liver to oxazepam. **Elimination:** Excreted in urine. **Half-Life:** 8–24 h.

NURSING IMPLICATIONS

Assessment & Drug Effects

- Be alert to signs of paradoxical reaction (excitement, hyperactivity, and disorientation) in older adults. Psychoactive drugs are the most frequent cause of acute confusion in this age group.
- CNS adverse effects are more apt to occur in the client with hypoalbuminemia, liver disease, and in older adults. Report promptly incidence of bradycardia, drowsiness, dizziness, clumsiness, lack of coordination. Supervise ambulation, especially at night.
- Lab tests: Obtain liver and kidney function tests during long-term use.
- Be alert to S&S of overdose: Weakness, bradycardia, somnolence, confusion, slurred speech, ataxia, coma with reduced or absent reflexes, hypertension, and respiratory depression.

Client & Family Education

- Be aware that improvement in sleep will not occur until after 2–3 doses of drug.
- Notify prescriber if dreams or nightmares interfere with rest. An alternate drug or reduced dose may be prescribed.
- Be aware that difficulty getting to sleep may continue. Drug effect is evidenced by the increased amount of rest once asleep.
- Consult prescriber if insomnia continues in spite of medication.
- Do not smoke after medication is taken.
- Do not use OTC drugs (especially for insomnia) without advice of prescriber.
- Consult prescriber before discontinuing drug especially after long-term use. Gradual reduction of dose may be necessary to avoid withdrawal symptoms.

- Avoid use of alcohol and other CNS depressants.
- Do not drive or engage in other potentially hazardous activities until response to drug is known. This drug may depress psychomotor skills and causes sedation.
- Do not breast feed while taking this drug without consulting prescriber. Distribution in the breast milk may cause sedation and possibly feeding problems and weight loss in the infant.

ZALEPLON

(zal′ep-lon)

Sonata

Classifications: CENTRAL NERVOUS SYSTEM AGENT; ANXIOLYTIC; SEDATIVE-HYPNOTIC; NONBENZODIAZEPINE

Pregnancy Category: C

Controlled Substance: Schedule IV

AVAILABILITY 5 mg, 10 mg capsules

ACTIONS Short acting nonbenzodiazepine with sedative-hypnotic, muscle relaxant, and anticonvulsant activity.

THERAPEUTIC EFFECTS Effectiveness is indicated by less difficulty in initially falling asleep. Preserves deep sleep (stage 3 through stage 4) at hypnotic dose with minimal-to-absent rebound insomnia when discontinued.

USES Short-term treatment of insomnia.

CONTRAINDICATIONS Hypersensitivity to zaleplon.

CAUTIOUS USE Concurrent use of other CNS depressants (e.g., benzodiazepines, alcohol); history of drug abuse; hepatic or renal impairment; pulmonary disease; pregnancy (category C); lactation.

ROUTE & DOSAGE

Insomnia

Adult: **PO** 10 mg h.s. (max 20 mg h.s.)
Geriatric: **PO** 5 mg h.s. (max 10 mg h.s.)

ADMINISTRATION

Oral

- Give immediately before bedtime; not while client is still ambulating.

- Give lower dose of 5 mg to older adult or debilitated clients.
- Store at 20°–25° C (68°–77° F).

ADVERSE EFFECTS (≥1%) **Body as a Whole:** Asthenia, fever, *headache,* migraine, myalgia, back pain. **CNS:** Amnesia, dizziness, paresthesia, somnolence, tremor, vertigo, depression, hypertonia, nervousness, difficulty concentrating. **GI:** Abdominal pain, dyspepsia, nausea, constipation, dry mouth. **Respiratory:** Bronchitis. **Skin:** Pruritus, rash. **Special Senses:** Eye pain, hyperacusis, conjunctivitis. **Urogenital:** Dysmenorrhea.

INTERACTIONS Drug: Alcohol, imipramine, thioridazine may cause additive CNS impairment; **rifampin** increases metabolism of zaleplon; **cimetidine** increases serum levels of zaleplon. **Herbal: Valerian, melatonin** may produce additive sedative effects.

PHARMACOKINETICS Absorption: Rapidly and completely absorbed; 30% reaches systemic circulation. **Onset:** 15–20 min. **Peak:** 1 h. **Duration:** 3–4 h. **Distribution:** 60% protein bound. **Metabolism:** Extensively metabolized in liver to inactive metabolites. CYP3A4 is one of its metabolic pathways. **Elimination:** 70% excreted in urine, 17% in feces. **Half-Life:** 1 h.

NURSING IMPLICATIONS

Assessment & Drug Effects

- Monitor behavior and notify prescriber for significant changes. Use extra caution with preexisting clinical depression.
- Provide safe environment and monitor ambulation after drug is ingested.
- Monitor respiratory status with preexisting compromised pulmonary function.

Client & Family Education

- Take medication immediately before lying down to go to sleep.
- Do not take in combination with alcohol or any other sleep medication.
- Note: Exhibits altered effectiveness if taken with/immediately after high-fat meal.
- Exercise caution when walking; avoid all hazardous activities after taking zaleplon.
- Do not use longer than 2–3 wk.

- Expect possible mild/brief rebound insomnia after discontinuing regimen.
- Report use of OTC medications to prescriber (e.g., cimetidine).
- Report pregnancy to prescriber immediately.
- Do not breast feed while taking this drug.

ZOLPIDEM

(zol′ pi-dem)

Ambien

Classifications: CENTRAL NERVOUS SYSTEM AGENT; ANXIOLYTIC; SEDATIVE-HYPNOTIC; NONBENZODIAZEPINE

Pregnancy Category: B

Controlled Substance: Schedule IV

AVAILABILITY 5 mg, 10 mg tablets

ACTIONS Nonbenzodiazepine hypnotic. Does not have muscle relaxant or anticonvulsant effects.

THERAPEUTIC EFFECTS Preserves deep sleep (stages 3 and 4) at hypnotic doses.

USES Short-term treatment of insomnia.

CONTRAINDICATIONS Lactation.

CAUTIOUS USE Depressed clients, hepatic/renal impairment, older adults, pregnancy (category B), clients with compromised respiratory status. Safety and efficacy in children <18 y are not established.

ROUTE & DOSAGE

Short-Term Treatment of Insomnia

Adult: **PO** 5–10 mg h.s., limited to 7–10 d
Geriatric: **PO** start with 5 mg h.s., limited to 7–10 d

ADMINISTRATION

Oral

- Give immediately before bedtime; for more rapid sleep onset, do NOT give with or immediately after a meal.
- Use reduced dosage of 5 mg in older adult or debilitated clients.
- Store at room temperature, 15°–30° C (59°–86° F).

ADVERSE EFFECTS (≥1%) **CNS:** Headache on awakening, drowsiness or fatigue, lethargy, drugged feeling, depression, anxiety, irritability, dizziness, double vision. Confusion and falls reported in elderly. Doses >10 mg may be associated with anterograde amnesia or memory impairment. **GI:** Dyspepsia, nausea, vomiting. **Other:** Myalgia.

INTERACTIONS Drug: CNS DEPRESSANTS, **alcohol,** PHENOTHIAZINES by augmenting CNS depression. **Food:** Extent and rate of absorption of zolpidem is significantly decreased.

PHARMACOKINETICS Absorption: Readily absorbed from GI tract. 70% reaches systemic circulation. Food decreases rate and extent of absorption. **Onset:** 7–27 min. **Peak:** 0.5–2.3 h. **Duration:** 6–8 h. **Distribution:** Highly protein bound. Lowest concentrations in CNS, highest concentrations in glandular tissue and fat. Crosses placenta; very small amounts (<0.02%) distributed into breast milk. **Metabolism:** Metabolized in the liver to 3 inactive metabolites. **Elimination:** 79–96% of dose appears as metabolites in the bile, urine, and feces. **Half-Life:** 1.7–2.5 h.

NURSING IMPLICATIONS

Assessment & Drug Effects

- Assess respiratory function in clients with compromised respiratory status. Report immediately to prescriber significantly depressed respiratory rate (less than 12/min).
- Monitor clients for S&S of depression; zolpidem may increase level of depression.
- Monitor older adult or debilitated clients closely for impaired cognitive or motor function and unusual sensitivity to the drug's effects.

Client & Family Education

- Take medication immediately before lying down to go to sleep.
- Avoid taking alcohol or other CNS depressants while on zolpidem.
- Do not drive or engage in other potentially hazardous activities until response to drug is known.
- Report vision changes to prescriber.
- Note: Onset of drug is more rapid when taken on an empty stomach.
- Do not breast feed while taking this drug.

SIDE EFFECT MEDICATION

PROPRANOLOL HYDROCHLORIDE

(proe-pran'oh-lole)

Apo-Propranolol ♣, Detensol ♣, Inderal, Inderal LA, Novopranol ♣

Classifications: AUTONOMIC NERVOUS SYSTEM AGENT; BETA-ADRENERGIC ANTAGONIST (BLOCKING AGENT, SYMPATHOLYTIC); ANTIHYPERTENSIVE; ANTIARRHYTHMIC, CLASS II

Pregnancy Category: C

AVAILABILITY 10 mg, 20 mg, 40 mg, 60 mg, 80 mg, 90 mg tablets; 60 mg, 80 mg, 120 mg, 160 mg sustained-release capsules; 4 mg/mL, 8 mg/mL, 80 mg/mL solution; 1 mg/mL injection

ACTIONS Nonselective beta-blocker of both cardiac and bronchial adrenoreceptors that competes with epinephrine and norepinephrine for available beta-receptor sites. In higher doses, exerts direct quinidine-like effects, which depresses cardiac function including contractility and arrhythmias. Lowers both supine and standing blood pressures in hypertensive patients. Mechanism of antimigraine action unknown but thought to be related to inhibition of cerebral vasodilation and arteriolar spasms.

THERAPEUTIC EFFECTS Blocks cardiac effects of beta-adrenergic stimulation; as a result, reduces heart rate, myocardial irritability (Class II antiarrhythmic), and force of contraction, depresses automaticity of sinus node and ectopic pacemaker, and decreases AV and intraventricular conduction velocity. Hypotensive effect is associated with decreased cardiac output, suppressed renin activity, as well as beta blockade. Also decreases platelet aggregability.

USES Management of cardiac arrhythmias, myocardial infarction, tachyarrhythmias associated with digitalis intoxication, anesthesia, and thyrotoxicosis, hypertrophic subaortic stenosis, angina pectoris due to coronary atherosclerosis, pheochromocytoma, hereditary essential tremor; also treatment of hypertension alone, but generally with a thiazide or other antihypertensives.

UNLABELED USES Anxiety states, migraine prophylaxis, essential tremors, extrapyramidal side effects (low dose used for akathisia), tardive dyskinesia, shaking leg syndrome, acute panic symptoms (e.g., stage fright), recurrent GI bleeding in cirrhotic patients, treatment of aggression and rage.

CONTRAINDICATIONS Greater than first-degree heart block; CHF, right ventricular failure secondary to pulmonary hypertension; sinus bradycardia, cardiogenic shock, significant aortic or mitral valvular disease; bronchial asthma or bronchospasm, severe COPD, allergic rhinitis during pollen season; concurrent use with adrenergic augmenting psychotropic drugs or within 2 wk of MAO inhibition therapy. Safety during pregnancy (category C) or lactation is not established.

CAUTIOUS USE Peripheral arterial insufficiency; history of systemic insect sting reaction; patients prone to nonallergenic bronchospasm (e.g., chronic bronchitis, emphysema); major surgery; renal or hepatic impairment; diabetes mellitus; patients prone to hypoglycemia; myasthenia gravis; Wolff-Parkinson-White syndrome.

ROUTE & DOSAGE

Hypertension

Adult: **PO** 40 mg b.i.d.; usually need 160–480 mg/d in divided doses
Child: **PO** 1 mg/kg/d in 2 divided doses (1–5 mg/kg/d)
Neonate: **PO** 0.25 mg/kg q6–8h (max 5 mg/kg/d) **IV** 0.01 mg/kg slow IV push over 10 min q6–8h prn (max 0.15 mg/kg q6–8h)

Angina

Adult: **PO** 10–20 mg b.i.d. or t.i.d.; may need 160–320 mg/d in divided doses

Arrhythmias

Adult: **PO** 10–30 mg t.i.d. or q.i.d. **IV** 0.5–3 mg q4h prn
Child: **PO** 1–4 mg/kg/d in 4 divided doses (max 16 mg/kg/d) **IV** 10–20 mcg/kg/min over 10 min

Acute MI

Adult: **PO** 180–240 mg/d in divided doses

Migraine Prophylaxis

Adult: **PO** 80 mg/d in divided doses; may need 160–240 mg/d

ADMINISTRATION

- Do not give within 2 wk of a MAOI.
- Take apical pulse and BP before administering drug. Withhold drug if heart rate <60 bpm or systolic BP <90 mm Hg. Consult prescriber for parameters.
- Be consistent with regard to giving with food or on an empty stomach to minimize variations in absorption.
- Ensure that sustained-release form is not cut, chewed, or crushed. Must be swallowed whole.
- Reduce dosage gradually over a period of 1–2 wk and monitor patient closely when discontinued.

Intravenous

Note: Verify correct IV concentration and rate of infusion for neonates with prescriber.

PREPARE **Direct:** Give undiluted or dilute each 1 mg in 10 mL of D5W. **Intermittent:** Dilute a single dose in 50 mL of NS.

ADMINISTER **Direct:** Give each 1 mg over 1 min. **Intermittent:** Give each dose over 15–20 min.

INCOMPATIBILITIES **Y-Site: Amphotericin B cholesteryl complex, diazoxide.**

- Store at 15°–30° C (59°–86° F) in tightly closed, light-resistant containers.

ADVERSE EFFECTS (≥1%) **Body as a Whole:** Fever; pharyngitis; respiratory distress, weight gain, LE-like reaction, cold extremities, leg fatigue, arthralgia. **Urogenital:** Impotence or decreased libido. **Skin:** Erythematous, psoriasis-like eruptions; pruritus. Reversible alopecia, hyperkeratoses of scalp, palms, feet; nail changes, dry skin. **CNS:** Drug-induced psychosis, sleep disturbances, depression, *confusion,* agitation, giddiness, lightheadedness, *fatigue,* vertigo, syncope, weakness, *drowsiness,* insomnia, vivid dreams, visual hallucinations, delusions, reversible organic brain syndrome. **CV:** Palpitation, profound *bradycardia,* AV heart block, cardiac standstill, hypotension, angina pectoris, tachyarrhythmia, acute CHF, peripheral arterial insufficiency resembling Raynaud's disease, myotonia, *paresthesia of hands.* **Special Senses:** Dry eyes (gritty sensation), visual disturbances, conjunctivitis, tinnitus, hearing loss, nasal stuffiness. **GI:** Dry mouth, cheilostomatitis, nausea, vomiting, heartburn, diarrhea, constipation, flatulence, abdominal cramps, mesenteric arterial thrombosis, ischemic colitis, pancreatitis. **Hematologic:** Transient eosinophilia, thrombocytopenic or nonthrombocytopenic purpura, agranulocytosis. **Metabolic:** Hypoglycemia, hyperglycemia, hypocalcemia (patients with hyperthyroidism). **Respiratory:** Dyspnea, laryngospasm, bronchospasm.

DIAGNOSTIC TEST INTERFERENCE BETA-ADRENERGIC BLOCKERS may produce false-negative test results in exercise tolerance ECG tests, and elevations in ***serum potassium, peripheral platelet count, serum uric acid, serum transaminase, alkaline phosphatase, lactate dehydrogenase, serum creatinine, BUN,*** and an increase or decrease in ***blood glucose*** levels in diabetic patients.

INTERACTIONS Drug: PHENOTHIAZINES have additive hypotensive effects. BETA-ADRENERGIC AGONISTS (e.g., **albuterol**) antagonize effects. **Atropine** and TRICYCLIC ANTIDEPRESSANTS block bradycardia. DIURETICS and other HYPOTENSIVE AGENTS increase hypotension. High doses of **tubocurarine** may potentiate neuromuscular blockade. **Cimetidine** decreases clearance, increases effects. ANTACIDS may decrease absorption.

PHARMACOKINETICS Absorption: Completely absorbed from GI tract but undergoes extensive first-pass metabolism. **Peak:** 60–90 min immediate release; 6 h sustained release; 5 min IV. **Distribution:** Widely distributed including CNS, placenta, and breast milk. **Metabolism:** Almost completely metabolized in liver. **Elimination:** 90–95% excreted in urine as metabolites; 1–4% excreted in feces. **Half-Life:** 2.3 h.

NURSING IMPLICATIONS

Assessment & Drug Effects

- Obtain careful medical history to rule out allergies, asthma, and obstructive pulmonary disease. Propranolol can cause bronchiolar constriction even in normal subjects.
- Monitor apical pulse, respiration, BP, and circulation to extremities closely throughout period of dosage adjustment. Consult prescriber for acceptable parameters.
- Evaluate adequate control or dosage interval for patients being treated for hypertension by checking blood pressure near end of dosage interval or before administration of next dose.
- Be aware that adverse reactions occur most frequently following IV administration soon after therapy is initiated; however, incidence is also high following oral use in the older adult and in patients with impaired kidney function. Reactions may or may not be dose related.

- Lab tests: Obtain periodic hematologic, kidney, liver, and cardiac functions when propranolol is given for prolonged periods.
- Monitor I&O ratio and daily weight as significant indexes for detecting fluid retention and developing heart failure.
- Consult prescriber regarding allowable salt intake. Drug plasma volume may increase with consequent risk of CHF if dietary sodium is not restricted in patients not receiving concomitant diuretic therapy.
- Fasting for more than 12 h may induce hypoglycemic effects fostered by propranolol. This needs to be attended to if patient is religiously observant during fasting holidays.
- If patient complains of cold, painful, or tender feet or hands, examine carefully for evidence of impaired circulation. Peripheral pulses may still be present even though circulation is impaired. Caution patient to avoid prolonged exposure of extremities to cold.

Client & Family Education

- Learn usual pulse rate and take radial pulse before each dose. Report to prescriber if pulse is below the established parameter or becomes irregular.
- Be aware that propranolol suppresses clinical signs of hypoglycemia (e.g., BP changes, increased pulse rate) and may prolong hypoglycemia.
- Understand importance of compliance. Do not to alter established regimen (i.e., do not omit, increase, or decrease dosage or change dosage interval).
- Do not discontinue abruptly; can precipitate withdrawal syndrome (e.g., tremulousness, sweating, severe headache, malaise, palpitation, rebound hypertension, MI, and life-threatening arrhythmias in patients with angina pectoris).
- Be aware that drug may cause mild hypotension (experienced as dizziness or light-headedness) in patients with normal blood pressures on prolonged therapy. Make position changes slowly and avoid prolonged standing. Notify prescriber if symptoms persist.
- Do not drive or engage in potentially hazardous activities until response to drug is known.
- Notify prescriber if you have regular or intermittent fasting experiences.
- Consult prescriber before self-medicating with OTC drugs.
- Inform dentist, surgeon, or ophthalmologist that you are taking propranolol (drug lowers normal and elevated intraocular pressure).

- Do not breast feed while taking this drug without consulting prescriber.

STIMULANTS

CAFFEINE

(kaf-een′)

Caffedrine, Dexitac, NoDoz, Quick Pep, S-250, Tirend, Vivarin

CAFFEINE AND SODIUM BENZOATE CITRATED CAFFEINE

Cafcit

Classifications: CENTRAL NERVOUS SYSTEM AGENT; RESPIRATORY AND CEREBRAL STIMULANT; XANTHINE

Pregnancy Category: C

AVAILABILITY 100 mg, 150 mg, 200 mg tablets; 250 mg/mL solution; 20 mg/mL caffeine citrate injection

ACTIONS Chief action is thought to be related to inhibition of the enzyme phosphodiesterase, which results in higher concentrations of cyclic AMP. Releases epinephrine and norepinephrine from adrenal medulla, producing CNS stimulation. Small doses improve psychic and sensory awareness and reduce drowsiness and fatigue by stimulating cerebral cortex. Higher doses stimulate medullary, respiratory, vasomotor, and vagal centers. Produces smooth muscle relaxation (especially bronchi) and dilation of coronary, pulmonary, and systemic blood vessels by direct action on vascular musculature. Mild diuretic action may result from increase in renal blood flow and glomerular filtration rate and decrease in renal tubular reabsorption of sodium and water. Increases contractile force of heart and cardiac output by direct stimulation of myocardium. Also stimulates secretion of gastric acid and digestive enzymes.

THERAPEUTIC EFFECTS Effective in managing neonatal apnea, and as an adjuvant for pain control in headaches and following dural puncture. Relief of headache is perhaps due to mild cerebral vasoconstriction action and increased vascular tone. It acts as a bronchodilator in asthma and may improve psychomotor performance through CNS stimulation.

USES Orally as a mild CNS stimulant to aid in staying awake and restoring mental alertness, and as an adjunct in narcotic and nonnarcotic analgesia. Used parenterally as an emergency stimulant in acute circulatory failure, as a diuretic, and to relieve spinal puncture headache.

UNLABELED USES Topical treatment of atopic dermatitis; neonatal apnea.

CONTRAINDICATIONS Acute MI, symptomatic cardiac arrhythmias, palpitations; peptic ulcer; insomnia, panic attacks. Safe use during pregnancy (category C), in lactation, and in children not established.

CAUTIOUS USE Diabetes mellitus; hiatal hernia; hypertension with heart disease.

ROUTE & DOSAGE

Mental Stimulant

Adult: **PO** 100–200 mg q3–4h prn

Circulatory Stimulant

Adult: **IM** 200–500 mg prn

Spinal Puncture Headaches

Adult: **IV** 500 mg over 1 h; may repeat times 1 dose

Neonatal Apnea

Neonate: **PO/IV** 20–30 mg/kg caffeine citrate as a loading dose, followed by a maintenance dose 5 mg/kg citrate 24 h later of once daily up to max 10–12 d

ADMINISTRATION

Oral

- Give sustained-release oral preparations not less than 6 h before bedtime.
- Ensure that timed-release form of drug is not cut, chewed, or crushed. It must be swallowed whole.

Intramuscular

- Give deep IM into a large muscle.

Intravenous

- Note: IV route reserved for emergency situations only.

PREPARE **Direct:** Give undiluted.

ADMINISTER **Direct:** Emergency situations: IV push at a rate of 250 mg or fraction thereof over 1 min. With neonates use caffeine without sodium benzoate and check with prescriber regarding preferred rate.

ADVERSE EFFECTS (≥1%) **CV:** Tingling of face, flushing, palpitation, tachycardia or bradycardia, ventricular ectopic beats. **GI:** Nausea, vomiting; epigastric discomfort, gastric irritation (oral form), diarrhea, hematemesis, kernicterus (neonates). **CNS:** *Nervousness, insomnia,* restlessness, irritability, confusion, agitation, fasciculations, delirium, twitching, tremors, clonic convulsions. **Respiratory:** Tachypnea. **Special Senses:** Scintillating scotomas, tinnitus. **Urogenital:** Increased urination, diuresis.

DIAGNOSTIC TEST INTERFERENCE Caffeine reportedly may interfere with diagnosis of pheochromocytoma or neuroblastoma by increasing urinary excretion of ***catecholamines, VMA,*** and ***5-HIAA*** and may cause false-positive increases in ***serum urate*** (by ***Bittner method***).

INTERACTIONS Drug: Increases effects of **cimetidine;** increases cardiovascular stimulating effects of BETA-ADRENERGIC AGONISTS; possibly increases **theophylline** toxicity.

PHARMACOKINETICS Absorption: Rapidly absorbed. **Peak:** 15–45 min. **Distribution:** Widely distributed throughout body; crosses blood–brain barrier and placenta. **Metabolism:** Metabolized in liver. **Elimination:** Excreted in urine as metabolites; excreted in breast milk in small amounts. **Half-Life:** 3–5 h in adults, 36–144 h in neonates.

NURSING IMPLICATIONS

Assessment & Drug Effects

- Monitor vital signs closely because large doses may cause intensification rather than reversal of severe drug-induced depressions.
- Observe children closely following administration because they are more susceptible than adults to the CNS effects of caffeine.
- Lab tests: Monitor blood glucose and HbA_{1c} levels in diabetics.

Client & Family Education

- Caffeine in large amounts may impair glucose tolerance in diabetics.
- Do not consume large amounts of caffeine as headache, dizziness, anxiety, irritability, nervousness, and muscle tension may result from excessive use, as well as from abrupt withdrawal of coffee (or oral caffeine). Withdrawal symptoms usually occur 12–18 h following last coffee intake.

DEXTROAMPHETAMINE SULFATE

(dex-troe-am-fet'a-meen)

Dexampex, Dexedrine, Oxydess II ♣, Spancap No. 1

Classifications: CENTRAL NERVOUS SYSTEM AGENT; RESPIRATORY AND CEREBRAL STIMULANT; AMPHETAMINE; ANOREXIANT

Pregnancy Category: C

Controlled Substance: Schedule II

AVAILABILITY 5 mg, 10 mg tablets; 5 mg, 10 mg, 15 mg sustained-release capsules

ACTIONS Dextrorotatory isomer of amphetamine. Anorexigenic action is thought to result from CNS stimulation and possibly from loss of acuity of smell and taste.

THERAPEUTIC EFFECTS On a weight basis, has less pronounced effect on cardiovascular and peripheral nervous systems and is a more potent appetite suppressant than amphetamine. CNS stimulating effect approximately twice that of racemic amphetamine. In hyperkinetic children, amphetamines reduce motor restlessness by an unknown mechanism.

USES Adjunct in short-term treatment of exogenous obesity, narcolepsy, and attention deficit disorder with hyperactivity in children (also called minimal brain dysfunction or hyperkinetic syndrome).

UNLABELED USES Adjunct in epilepsy to control ataxia and drowsiness induced by barbiturates; to combat sedative effects of trimethadione in absence seizures.

CONTRAINDICATIONS Hypersensitivity to sympathomimetic amines, glaucoma, agitated states, psychoses (especially in children), advanced arteriosclerosis, symptomatic heart disease, moderate to severe hypertension, hyperthyroidism, history of drug abuse, during or within 14 d of MAOI therapy, as anorexiant in children <12 y, for attention deficit disorder in children <3 y, lactation.

CAUTIOUS USE Pregnancy (category C). Safety and efficacy in children <3 y have not been established.

ROUTE & DOSAGE

Narcolepsy

Adult: **PO** 5–20 mg 1–3 times/d at 4–6 h intervals

Child: **PO** *6–12 y,* 5 mg/d; may increase by 5 mg at weekly intervals; *>12 y,* 10 mg/d; may increase by 10 mg at weekly intervals

Attention Deficit Disorder

Child: **PO** *3–5y,* 2.5 mg 1–2 times/d; may increase by 2.5 mg at weekly intervals; *≥6 y,* 5 mg 1–2 times/d; may increase by 5 mg at weekly intervals (max 40 mg/d)

Obesity

Adult: **PO** 5–10 mg 1–3 times/d or 10–15 mg of sustained release once/d 30–60 min a.c.

ADMINISTRATION

Oral

- Ensure that sustained-release capsule is not cut, chewed, or crushed. It MUST be swallowed whole.
- Give 30–60 min before meals for treatment of obesity. Give long-acting form in the morning.
- Give last dose no later than 6 h before patient retires (10–14 h before bedtime for sustained-release form) to avoid insomnia.
- Store in tightly closed containers at 15°–30° C (59°–86° F) unless otherwise directed.

ADVERSE EFFECTS (≥1%) **CNS:** Nervousness, *restlessness,* hyperactivity, *insomnia,* euphoria, dizziness, headache; ***with prolonged use***—severe depression, psychotic reactions. **CV:** Palpitation, tachycardia, elevated BP. **GI:** Dry mouth, unpleasant taste, anorexia, weight loss, diarrhea, constipation, abdominal pain. **Other:** Impotence, changes in libido; unusual fatigue; increased intraocular pressure; marked dystonia of head, neck, and extremities; sweating.

DIAGNOSTIC TEST INTERFERENCE Dextroamphetamine may cause significant elevations in ***plasma corticosteroids*** (evening levels are highest) and increases in ***urinary epinephrine*** excretion (during first 3 h after drug administration).

INTERACTIONS Drug: Acetazolamide, sodium bicarbonate decrease dextroamphetamine elimination; **ammonium chloride, ascorbic acid** increase dextroamphetamine elimination; effects of both BARBITURATES and dextroamphetamine may be antagonized; **furazolidone** may increase BP effects of AMPHETAMINES—interaction may persist for several weeks after discontinuing **furazolidone;** antagonizes antihypertensive effects of **guanethidine, guanadrel;** MAOIS, **selegiline** can cause hypertensive crisis (fatalities reported)—do not administer AMPHETAMINES during or within 14 d of these drugs; PHENOTHIAZINES may inhibit mood-elevating effects of AMPHETAMINES; TRICYCLIC ANTIDEPRESSANTS enhance dextroamphetamine effects because of increased **norepinephrine** release; BETA-ADRENERGIC AGONISTS increase cardiovascular adverse effects.

PHARMACOKINETICS Absorption: Rapid. **Peak:** 1–5 h. **Duration:** Up to 10 h. **Distribution:** All tissues especially the CNS. **Metabolism:** Metabolized in liver. **Elimination:** Renal elimination; excreted in breast milk. **Half-Life:** 10–30 h.

NURSING IMPLICATIONS

Assessment & Drug Effects

- Monitor growth rate closely in children.
- Interrupt therapy or reduce dosage periodically to assess effectiveness in behavior disorders.
- Note: Tolerance to anorexiant effects may develop after a few weeks, however, tolerance does not appear to develop when dextroamphetamine is used to treat narcolepsy.

Client & Family Education

- Swallow sustained-release capsule whole with a liquid; do not cut, chew, or crush.
- Do not drive or engage in other potentially hazardous activities until response to drug is known.
- Taper drug gradually following long-term use to avoid extreme fatigue, mental depression, and prolonged sleep pattern.
- Do not breast feed while taking this drug.

METHAMPHETAMINE HYDROCHLORIDE

(meth-am-fet′a-meen)

Desoxyephedrine, Desoxyn

Classifications: CENTRAL NERVOUS SYSTEM AGENT; CEREBRAL STIMULANT; ANOREXIANT; AMPHETAMINE

Pregnancy Category: C

Controlled Substance: Schedule II

AVAILABILITY 5 mg tablets; 5 mg, 10 mg, 15 mg long-acting tablets

ACTIONS Sympathomimetic amine chemically related to amphetamine. CNS stimulant actions approximately equal to those of amphetamine, but accompanied by less peripheral activity. However, larger doses produce increased cardiac output, possibly reflex slowing of heart rate, and sustained increase in BP, chiefly by cardiac stimulation.

THERAPEUTIC EFFECTS CNS stimulant actions approximately equal to those of amphetamine, but accompanied by less peripheral activity.

USES Short-term adjunct in management of exogenous obesity, as adjunctive therapy in attention deficit disorder (ADD), narcolepsy, epilepsy, and postencephalitic parkinsonism, and in treatment of certain depressive reactions, especially when characterized by apathy and psychomotor retardation.

CONTRAINDICATIONS During pregnancy, especially first trimester (category C), lactation; as anorexiant in children <12 y; patients receiving MAOIS; arteriosclerotic parkinsonism.

CAUTIOUS USE Mild hypertension; psychopathic personalities; hyperexcitability states; history of suicide attempts; older adult or debilitated patients.

ROUTE & DOSAGE

Attention Deficit Hyperactivity Disorder

Child: **PO** $\geq$*6y,* 2.5–5 mg 1–2 times/d; may increase by 5 mg at weekly intervals up to 20–25 mg/d

Obesity

Adult: **PO** 2.5–5 mg 1–3 times/d 30 min before meals or 5–15 mg of long-acting form once/d

ADMINISTRATION

Oral

- Give early in the day to avoid insomnia, if possible.
- Ensure that long-acting tablets are not cut, chewed, or crushed; these need to be swallowed whole.
- Give 30 min before each meal when used for treatment of obesity. If insomnia results, advise patient to inform prescriber.
- Preserve in tight, light-resistant containers.

ADVERSE EFFECTS ($\geq$1%) **CNS:** Restlessness, tremor, hyperreflexia, insomnia, headache, nervousness, anxiety, dizziness, euphoria or dysphoria. **CV:** Palpitation, arrhythmias, hypertension, hypotension, circulatory collapse. **GI:** Dry mouth, unpleasant taste, nausea, vomiting, diarrhea, constipation. **Special Senses:** Increased intraocular pressure.

INTERACTIONS Drug: Acetazolamide, sodium bicarbonate decrease methamphetamine elimination; **ammonium chloride, ascorbic acid** increase methamphetamine elimination; effects of both methamphetamine and BARBITURATES may be antagonized; **furazolidone** may increase BP effects of AMPHETAMINES—interaction may persist for several weeks after discontinuing furazolidone; antagonizes antihypertensive effects of **guanethidine, guanadrel;** MAOIS, **selegiline** can cause hypertensive crisis (fatalities reported)—do not administer AMPHETAMINES during or within 14 d of administration of these drugs; PHENOTHIAZINES may inhibit mood-elevating effects of AMPHETAMINES; TRICYCLIC ANTIDEPRESSANTS enhance methamphetamine effects because they increase norepinephrine release; BETA-ADRENERGIC AGONISTS increase adverse cardiovascular effects of AMPHETAMINES.

PHARMACOKINETICS Absorption: Readily absorbed from the GI tract. **Duration:** 6–12 h. **Distribution:** All tissues, especially the CNS; excreted in breast milk. **Metabolism:** Metabolized in liver. **Elimination:** Renal elimination.

NURSING IMPLICATIONS

Assessment & Drug Effects

- Monitor weight throughout period of therapy.
- Be alert for paradoxic increase in depression or agitation in depressed patients. Report immediately; drug should be withdrawn.
- Do not exceed duration of a few weeks for treatment of obesity.

Client & Family Education

- Be alert for development of tolerance; it happens readily, and prolonged use may lead to drug dependence. Abuse potential is high. Methamphetamine is commonly known as "speed" or "crystal" among drug abusers.
- Withdrawal after prolonged use is frequently followed by lethargy that may persist for several weeks.
- Weigh every other day under standard conditions and maintain a record of weight loss.
- Do not breast feed while using this drug.

METHYLPHENIDATE HYDROCHLORIDE

(meth-ill-fen'i-date)

Concerta, Metadate CD, Metadate ER, Ritalin, Ritalin LA, Ritalin-SR

Classifications: CENTRAL NERVOUS SYSTEM AGENT; CEREBRAL STIMULANT

Pregnancy Category: C

Controlled Substance: Schedule II

AVAILABILITY 5 mg, 10 mg, 20 mg tablets; 20 mg, 30 mg, 40 mg sustained-release capsules; 27 mg sustained-release tablet

ACTIONS Piperidine derivative with actions and abuse potential qualitatively similar to those of amphetamine. Acts mainly on cerebral cortex to exert a stimulant effect.

THERAPEUTIC EFFECTS Results in mild CNS and respiratory stimulation with potency intermediate between amphetamine and caffeine. More prominent on mental than on motor activities. Also believed to have an anorexiant effect.

USES Adjunctive therapy in hyperkinetic syndromes characterized by attention deficit disorder, narcolepsy, mild depression, and apathetic or withdrawn senile behavior.

CONTRAINDICATIONS Hypersensitivity to drug; history of marked anxiety, agitation; motor tics, or Tourette's disease. Safety in pregnancy (category C), lactation, or in children <6 y of age is not established.

CAUTIOUS USE Alcoholic; emotionally unstable patient; history of drug dependence; hypertension; history of seizures.

ROUTE & DOSAGE

Narcolepsy

Adult: **PO** 10 mg b.i.d. or t.i.d. 30–45 min p.c. (range: 20–40 mg/d)

Attention Deficit Disorder

Child: **PO** 5–10 mg before breakfast and lunch, with a gradual increase of 5–10 mg/wk as needed (max 60 mg/d) or 20–40 mg sustained release q.d. before breakfast

Depression

Geriatric: **PO** 2.5 mg in morning before 9 a.m., may increase by 2.5–5 mg q2–3d (max 20 mg/d) divided 7 a.m. and noon

ADMINISTRATION

Oral

- Give 30–45 min before meals. To avoid insomnia, give last dose before 6 p.m.
- Ensure that sustained-release form is not cut, chewed, or crushed. It must be swallowed whole.
- Can open Metadate CD capsules and sprinkle on food.
- Store at 15°–30° C (59°–86° F).

ADVERSE EFFECTS (≥1%) **CNS:** Dizziness, drowsiness, *nervousness, insomnia*. **CV:** Palpitations, changes in BP and pulse rate, angina, cardiac arrhythmias. **Special Senses:** Difficulty with accommodation, blurred vision. **GI:** Dry throat, anorexia, nausea, <u>hepatotoxicity</u>, abdominal pain. **Body as a Whole:** Hypersensitivity reactions (rash, fever, arthralgia, urticaria, <u>exfoliative dermatitis</u>, erythema multiforme); growth suppression.

INTERACTIONS Drug: MAOIS may cause hypertensive crisis; antagonizes hypotensive effects of **guanethidine, bretylium;** potentiates action of CNS STIMULANTS (e.g., **amphetamine, caffeine**); may inhibit metabolism and increase serum levels of **fosphenytoin, phenytoin, phenobarbital,** and **primidone, warfarin,** TRICYCLIC ANTIDEPRESSANTS.

PHARMACOKINETICS Absorption: Readily absorbed from GI tract. **Peak:** 1.9 h; 4–7 h sustained release. **Duration:** 3–6 h; 8 h sustained release. **Elimination:** Excreted in urine.

NURSING IMPLICATIONS

Assessment & Drug Effects

- Monitor BP and pulse at appropriate intervals.
- Lab tests: Obtain periodic CBC with differential and platelet counts during prolonged therapy.
- Chronic abusive use can lead to tolerance, psychic dependence, and psychoses.
- Assess patient's condition with periodic drug-free periods during prolonged therapy.
- Supervise drug withdrawal carefully following prolonged use. Abrupt withdrawal may result in severe depression and psychotic behavior.

Client & Family Education

- Report adverse effects to prescriber, particularly nervousness and insomnia. These effects may diminish with time or require reduction of dosage or omission of afternoon or evening dose.
- Check weight at least 2 or 3 times weekly and report weight loss.
- Check height and weight in children; failure to gain in either should be reported to prescriber.
- Do not breast feed while taking this drug without consulting prescriber.

PEMOLINE

(pem′oh-leen)
Cylert
Classifications: CENTRAL NERVOUS SYSTEM AGENT; CEREBRAL STIMULANT
Pregnancy Category: B
Controlled Substance: Schedule IV

AVAILABILITY 18.75 mg, 37.5 mg, 75 mg tablets; 37.5 mg chewable tablets

ACTIONS Action qualitatively similar to those of amphetamine but with weak sympathomimetic activity.
THERAPEUTIC EFFECTS Capable of producing increased motor activity, mental alertness, diminished sense of fatigue, and mild euphoria. Also thought to have anorexigenic effect.

USES Adjunctive therapy to other remedial measures (psychologic, educational, social) in minimal brain dysfunction [attention deficit hyperactivity disorder (ADHD)] in carefully selected children.
UNLABELED USES Mild stimulant for geriatric patients.

CONTRAINDICATIONS Known hypersensitivity to pemoline; children <6 y. Safety during pregnancy (category B) or lactation is not established.
CAUTIOUS USE Impaired hepatic and kidney function; history of drug abuse; psychosis; emotional instability.

ROUTE & DOSAGE

Attention Deficit Disorder

Child: **PO** >6 y, 37.5 mg/d; may be increased by 18.75 mg at weekly intervals (max 112.5 mg/d)

ADMINISTRATION

Oral

- Give in morning to provide maximum effectiveness and to avoid insomnia.

ADVERSE EFFECTS (≥1%) **Body as a Whole:** Malaise, irritability, fatigue, dyskinetic movements, hallucinations, excitement, agitation, restlessness. **CNS:** *Insomnia,* mild depression, dizziness, headache, drowsiness, convulsions, nervousness. **CV:** Tachycardia. **GI:** *Anorexia,* abdominal discomfort, liver failure, nausea, diarrhea, elevated AST, ALT, and alkaline phosphatase (after several months of therapy); jaundice. **Skin:** Skin rash. **Special Senses:** Dyskinetic movements of eyes.

INTERACTIONS Drug: MAOIS (e.g., **selegiline, Parnate**) should be stopped 14 d before **sertraline** is started because of serious problems with other SEROTONIN-REUPTAKE INHIBITORS (shivering, nausea, diplopia, confusion, anxiety). **Tolbutamide** and **diazepam** clearance may be reduced. Use cautiously with other centrally acting CNS drugs. **Herbal: St. John's wort** may cause serotonin syndrome.

PHARMACOKINETICS Absorption: Readily absorbed from GI tract. **Onset:** 2–3 wk. **Peak:** 2–4 h. **Duration:** 8 h. **Metabolism:** Metabolized in liver. **Elimination:** Excreted in urine. **Half-Life:** 9–14 h.

NURSING IMPLICATIONS

Assessment & Drug Effects

- Monitor therapeutic effectiveness. Drug should be withdrawn if substantial clinical benefit is not seen following 3 wk of therapy.
- Note: Insomnia and anorexia (most frequent adverse effects) appear to be dose related.
- Monitor weight and height (growth rate) throughout therapy. Anorexia is often accompanied by weight loss.
- Be aware that careful clinical evaluation and supervision of patient are essential.
- Lab tests: Obtain baseline and biweekly liver function studies for patients receiving long-term therapy. Discontinue pemoline if significantly abnormal liver functions are noted.

Client & Family Education

- Report to prescriber immediately any sign of liver malfunction such as dark urine, jaundice, loss of appetite.

- Avoid potentially hazardous activities until the response to drug is known.
- Significant benefits of drug therapy may not be evident until third week of drug administration.
- Be aware that pemoline can produce tolerance and physical and psychologic dependence.

PHENTERMINE HYDROCHLORIDE

(phen-ter′meen)

Adipex-P, Fastin, Ionamin, Obe-Nix-30, Zantryl

Classifications: GASTROINTESTINAL AGENT; ANOREXIANT

Pregnancy Category: C

Controlled Substance: Schedule IV

AVAILABILITY 8 mg, 30 mg, 37.5 mg tablets; 15 mg, 18.75 mg, 30 mg, 37.5 mg capsules

ACTIONS Sympathetic amine with pharmacological similarity to amphetamine. Actions include CNS stimulation and blood pressure elevation.

THERAPEUTIC EFFECTS Appetite suppression or metabolic effects along with diet adjustment result in weight loss in obese individuals.

USES Short-term (8–12 wk) adjunct for weight loss.

CONTRAINDICATIONS History of hypertension, moderate to severe hypertension, advanced arteriosclerosis, cardiovascular disease; hyperthyroidism; known hypersensitivity to sympathetic amines; agitated states; history of drug abuse; during or within 14 d of administration of MAOI; concurrent administration of selective serotonin-reuptake inhibitors (SSRIs); valvular heart disease; glaucoma; pregnancy (category C), lactation, or children <16 y.

CAUTIOUS USE Mild hypertension, diabetes mellitus.

ROUTE & DOSAGE

Obesity

Adult: **PO** 8 mg t.i.d. 30 min before meals or 15–37.5 mg q.d. before breakfast or 10–14 h before retiring

ADMINISTRATION

Oral

- Ensure that at least 14 days have elapsed between the first dose of phentermine and the last dose of a MAOI.
- Give 30 min before meals.
- Do not administer if an SSRI is currently prescribed.
- Store in a tight container.

ADVERSE EFFECTS (≥1%) **Body as a Whole:** Hypersensitivity (urticaria, rash, erythema, burning sensation), chest pain, excessive sweating, clamminess, chills, flushing, fever, myalgia. **CV:** Palpitations, tachycardia, arrhythmias, hypertension or hypotension, syncope, precordial pain, pulmonary hypertension. **GI:** Dry mouth, altered taste, nausea, vomiting, abdominal pain, diarrhea, constipation, stomach pain. **Endocrine:** Gynecomastia. **Hematologic:** <u>Bone marrow suppression</u>, <u>agranulocytosis</u>, leukopenia. **Musculoskeletal:** Muscle pain. **CNS:** Overstimulation, nervousness, restlessness, dizziness, insomnia, weakness, fatigue, malaise, anxiety, euphoria, drowsiness, depression, agitation, dysphoria, tremor, dyskinesia, dysarthria, confusion, incoordination, headache, change in libido. **Skin:** Hair loss, ecchymosis. **Special Senses:** Mydriasis, blurred vision. **Urogenital:** Dysuria, polyuria, urinary frequency, impotence, menstrual upset.

INTERACTIONS Drug: MAOIS, **furazolidone** may increase pressor response resulting in hypertensive crisis. TRICYCLIC ANTIDEPRESSANTS may decrease anorectic response. May decrease hypotensive effects of **guanethidine.**

PHARMACOKINETICS Absorption: Absorbed from the small intestine. **Duration:** 4–14 h. **Elimination:** Excreted primarily in urine. **Half-Life:** 19–24 h.

NURSING IMPLICATIONS

Assessment & Drug Effects

- Assess for tolerance to the anorectic effect of the drug. Withhold drug and report to prescriber when this occurs.
- Lab tests: Periodic CBC with differential and blood glucose.
- Monitor periodic cardiovascular status, including BP, exercise tolerance, peripheral edema.
- Monitor weight at least 3 times/wk.

Client & Family Education

- Do not take this drug late in the evening because it could cause insomnia.
- Report immediately any of the following: Shortness of breath, chest pains, dizziness or fainting, swelling of the extremities.
- Tolerance to the appetite suppression effects of the drug usually develops in a few weeks. Notify prescriber, but do not increase the drug dose.
- Weigh yourself at least 3 times/wk at the same time of day with the same amount of clothing.
- Do not breast feed while taking this drug.

APPENDIXES

Schedule I

High potential for abuse and of no currently accepted medical use. Examples: heroin, LSD, marijuana, mescaline, peyote. Not obtainable by prescription but may be legally procured for research, study, or instructional use.

Schedule II

High abuse potential and high liability for severe psychlogical or physical dependence. Prescription required and cannot be renewed.[a] Includes opium derivatives, other opioids, and short-acting barbiturates. Examples: amphetamine, cocaine, meperidine, morphine, secobarbital.

Schedule III

Potential for abuse is less than that for drugs in Schedules I and II. Moderate to low physical dependence and high psychological dependence. Includes certain stimulants and depressants not included in the above schedules and preparations containing limited quantities of certain opioids. Examples: chlorphentermine, glutethimide, mazindol, paregoric, phendimetrazine. Prescription required.[b]

Schedule IV

Lower potential for abuse than Schedule III drugs. Examples: certain psychotropics (tranquilizers), chloral hydrate, chlordiazepoxide, diazepam, meprobamate, phenobarbital. Prescription required.[a]

Schedule V

Abuse potential less than that for Schedule IV drugs. Preparations contain limited quantities of certain narcotic drugs; generally intended for antitussive and antidiarrheal purposes and may be distributed without a prescription provided that:

1. Such distribution is made only by a pharmacist.
2. Not more than 240 ml or not more than 48 solid dosage units of any substance containing opium, nor more than 120 ml or not more than 24 solid dosage units of any other controlled substance may be distributed at retail to the same purchaser in any given 48-hour period without a valid prescription order.
3. The purchaser is at least 18 years old.
4. The pharmacist knows the purchaser or requests suitable identification.
5. The pharmacist keeps an official written record of: name and address of purchaser, name and quantity of controlled substance purchased, date of sale, initials of dispensing pharmacist. This record is to be

made available for inspection and copying by U.S. officers authorized by the Attorney General.
6. Other federal, state, or local law does not require a prescription order.

Under jurisdiction of the Federal Controlled Substances Act.
[a]Except when dispensed directly by a practitioner, other than a pharmacist, to an ultimate user, no controlled substance in Schedule II may be dispensed without a written prescription, except that in emergency situations such drug may be dispensed upon oral prescription and a written prescription must be obtained within the time frame prescribed by law. No prescription for a controlled substance in Schedule II may be refilled.
[b]Refillable up to 5 times within 6 mo, but only if so indicated by physician.

The FDA requires that all prescription drugs absorbed systemically or known to be potentially harmful to the fetus be classified according to one of five pregnancy categories (A, B, C, D, X). The identifying letter signifies the level of risk to the fetus and is to appear in the precautions section of the package insert. The categories described by the FDA are as follows:

Category A

Controlled studies in women fail to demonstrate a risk to the fetus in the first trimester (and there is no evidence of risk in later trimesters), and the possibility of fetal harm appears remote.

Category B

Either animal-reproduction studies have not demonstrated a fetal risk but there are no controlled studies in pregnant women, or animal-reproduction studies have shown an adverse effect (other than a decrease in fertility) that was not confirmed in controlled studies in women in the first trimester (and there is no evidence of a risk in later trimesters).

Category C

Either studies in animals have revealed adverse effects on the fetus (teratogenic or embryocidal effects or other) and there are no controlled studies in women, or studies in women and animals are not available. Drugs should be given only if the potential benefit justifies the potential risk to the fetus.

Category D

There is positive evidence of human fetal risk, but the benefits from use in pregnant women may be acceptable despite the risk (e.g., if the drug is needed in a life-threatening situation or for a serious disease for which safer drugs cannot be used or are ineffective). There will be an appropriate statement in the "warnings" section of the labeling.

Category X

Studies in animals or human beings have demonstrated fetal abnormalities or there is evidence of fetal risk based on human experience, or both, and the risk of the use of the drug in pregnant women clearly outweighs any possible benefit. The drug is contraindicated in women who are or may become pregnant. There will be an appropriate statement in the "contraindications" section of the labeling.

◆ APPENDIX C ORAL DOSAGE FORMS THAT SHOULD NOT BE CRUSHED

Some oral dosage forms should not be crushed or chewed. These dosage forms have been specially designed to release the drug slowly over several hours, to protect the drug from the low pH of the stomach, and/or to protect the stomach from the irritating effects of the drug.

Drugs may have an **enteric coating** which is designed to allow the drug to pass through the stomach intact with the drug being released in the intestines. This protects the stomach from the irritating effects of the drug, protects the drug from being destroyed by the acid pH of the stomach, and can delay the onset of action.

Extended-release (slow release, SR) formulations are designed to release the drug over an extended period of time. These formulations can include multiple-layer compressed tablets where drug is released as each layer dissolves, mixed-release pellets that dissolve at different time intervals, and special tablets that are themselves inert but are designed to release drug slowly from the formulation. Some extended-release dosage forms are scored and may be broken in half without affecting the release mechanism but still should not be crushed or chewed. Some mixed-release capsule formulations can be opened and the contents sprinkled on food. However, the pellets should not be crushed or chewed. Some extended-release formulations can be identified by common abbreviations used in their brand names. These abbreviations include: CR (controlled release), CRT (controlled-release tablet), LA (long acting), SR (sustained release), TR (time release), SA (sustained action), and XL or XR (extended release).

Occasionally, drugs should not be crushed because they are oral mucosa irritants, are extremely bitter, or contain dyes that may stain teeth or mucosal tissue.

The table contains a list of drugs found in the Guide that should not be crushed or chewed. A liquid dosage form may be available for many of these drugs. However, the dose or frequency of administration may be different from the slow-release product. Check with your pharmacist for liquid availability and dosing conversions.

	Generic Name	Comments
Accutane	isotretinoin	mucous membrane irritant
Acutrim	phenylpropanolamine	slow release
Adalat CC	nifedipine	slow release
Allerest 12 Hour	chlorpheniramine, phenylpropanolamine	slow release
Artane Sequels	trihexyphenydil	slow release; capsules may be opened and contents taken without chewing or crushing
Azulfidine Entabs	sulfasalazine	enteric coated

	Generic Name	Comments
Bayer Extra Strength Enteric 500	aspirin, enteric coated	enteric coated; slow release
Bayer Low Adult 81 mg	aspirin, enteric coated	enteric coated
Bayer Caplet	aspirin, enteric coated	enteric coated
Biphetamine	amphetamine, dextro-amphetamine	slow release
Bisacodyl	bisacodyl	enteric coated
Bisco-Lax	bisacodyl	enteric coated
Bromfed, Bromfed-PD	brompheniramine, pseudoephedrine	slow release
Calan SR	verapamil	slow release
Cama Arthritis Strength	aspirin, magnesium oxide, aluminum hydroxide	special table formulation
Cardizem, Cardizem CD, Cardizem SR	diltiazem	slow release; capsules may be opened and contents taken without chewing or crushing
Chloral Hydrate	chloral hydrate	liquid-filled capsule
Chlor-Trimeton Repetab	chlorpheniramine	slow release
Choledyl SA	oxytriphylline	slow release
Compazine Spansule	prochlorperazine	slow release; capsules may be opened and contents taken without chewing or crushing
Constant T	theophylline	slow release; capsules may be opened and contents taken without chewing or crushing
Contac	chlorpheniramine, phenylpropanolamine	slow release; capsules may be opened and contents taken without chewing or crushing
Cotazym S	pancrelipase	enteric coated; capsules may be opened and contents taken without chewing or crushing
Covera-HS	verapamil	slow release
Deconamine SR	chlorpheniramine, pseudoephedrine	slow release

	Generic Name	Comments
Depakene	valproic acid	slow release; mucous membrane irritant
Depakote	valproate disodium	enteric coated
Desoxyn Gradumets	methamphetamine	slow release
Dexatrim Max Strength	phenylpropanolamine	slow release
Dexedrine Spansule	dextroamphetamine	slow release
Diamox Sequels	acetazolamide	slow release
Dilacor XR	diltiazem	slow release
Dilatrate-SR	isosorbide dinitrate	slow release
Dimetane Extentab	brompheniramine, phenylephrine	slow release
Disophrol Chronotab	dexbrompheniramine, pseudoephedrine	slow release
Donnatol Extentab	atropine, scopolamine, hyoscyamine, phenobarbital	slow release
Donnazyme	pancreatin, pepsin, bile salts, atropine, scopolamine, hyoscyamine, phenobarbital	slow release
Drixoral	dexbrompheniramine, pseudoephedrine	slow release
Dulcolax	bisacodyl	enteric coated
Easprin	aspirin	enteric coated
Ecotrin	aspirin	enteric coated
E.E.S 400	erythromycin ethylsuccinate	enteric coated
Elixophyllin SR	theophylline	slow release; capsules may be opened and contents taken without chewing or crushing
E-Mycin	erythromycin	enteric coated
Ergostat	ergotamine	sublingual tablet
Eryc	erythromycin	enteric coated; capsules may be opened and contents taken without chewing or crushing
Ery-tab	erythromycin	enteric coated

	Generic Name	Comments
Erythrocin Stearate	erythromycin	enteric coated
Erythromycin Base	erythromycin	enteric coated
Eskalith CR	lithium	slow release
Fedahist Timecaps	chlorpheniramine, pseudoephedrine	slow release
Feldene	piroxicam	mucous membrane irritant
Feosol	ferrous sulfate	enteric coated
Feosol Spansule	ferrous sulfate	slow release; capsules may be opened and contents taken without chewing or crushing
Fergon	ferrous gluconate	slow release; capsules may be opened and contents taken without chewing or crushing
Ferro-Sequels	ferrous fumarate, docusate	slow release
Fero-Gradumet	ferrous sulfate	slow release
Festal II	pancrelipase	enteric coated
Glucotrol XL	glipizide	slow release
Gris-Peg	griseofulvin ultramicrosize	crushing may result in precipitation of drug as larger particles
Ilotycin	erythromycin	enteric coated
Inderal LA	propranolol	slow release
Inderide LA	propranolol, hydro-chlorothiazide	slow release
Indocin SR	indomethacin	slow release; capsules may be opened and contents taken without chewing or crushing
Isoptin SR	verapamil	slow release
Isordil Tembid	isosorbide dinitrate	slow release
Iso-Bid	isosorbide dinitrate	slow release
Isosorbide dinitrate SR	isosorbide dinitrate	slow release
Isuprel Glossets	isoproterenol	sublingual
Kaon CL 10	postassium chloride	slow release
Klor-Con	postassium chloride	slow release

	Generic Name	Comments
Klotrix	postassium chloride	slow release
K-Tab	postassium chloride	slow release
Levsinex Timecaps	hyoscyamine	slow release
Lithobid	lithium	slow release
Meprospan	meprobamate	slow release; capsules may be opened and contents taken without chewing or crushing
Mestinon Timespan	pyridostigmine	slow release
Micro K	postassium chloride	slow release
MS Contin	morphine	slow release
Naldecon	phenylepherine, phenylpropanolamine, chlorpheniramine, phenyltoloxamine	slow release
Nico-400	niacin	slow release
Nicobid	niacin	slow release
Nitro Bid	nitroglycerin	slow release; capsules may be opened and contents taken without chewing or crushing
Nitroglyn	nitroglycerin	slow release; capsules may be opened and contents taken without chewing or crushing
Nitrong SR	nitroglycerin	slow release
Nolamine	phenylpropanolamine, chlorpheniramine, phenindamine	slow release
Norflex	orphenadrine	slow release
Norpace CR	disopyramide	slow release
Novafed A	pseudoephedrine, chlorpheniramine	slow release
Oramorph SR	morphine	slow release
Ornade Spansule	phenylpropanolamine, chlorpheniramine	slow release
Pancrease	pancrelipase	enteric coated
Papaverine Sustained Action	papaverine	slow release

	Generic Name	Comments
Pavabid	papaverine	slow release
Pavabid Plateau	papaverine	slow release; capsules may be opened and contents taken without chewing or crushing
PBZ-SR	tripelennamine hydrochloride	slow release
Perdiem	psyllium hydrophilic mucioid	wax coated
Peritrate SA	pentaerythritol tetranitrate	slow release
Permitil Chronotab	fluphenazine	slow release
Phazyme, Phazyme 95	simethicone	slow release
Phyllocontin	aminophylline	slow release
Plendil	felodipine	slow release
Polaramine Repetabs	dexchlorpheniramine	slow release
Prevacid	lansoprazole	slow release; capsules may be opened and contents taken without chewing or crushing
Prilosec	omeprazole	slow release
Procainamide HCl SR	procainamide	slow release
Procan SR	procainamide	slow release
Procardia XL	nifedipine	slow release
Pronestyl SR	procainamide	slow release
Proventil Repetabs	albuterol	slow release
Prozac	fluoxetine	slow release; capsules may be opened and contents taken without chewing or crushing
Quibron-T SR	theophylline	slow release
Quinaglute Dura Tabs	quinidine gluconate	slow release
Quinidex Extentabs	quinidine sulfate	slow release
Respid	theophylline	slow release
Ritalin SR	methylphenidate	slow release

	Generic Name	Comments
Robimycin Robitab	erythromycin	enteric coated
Rondec TR	pseudoephedrine, carbinoxamine	slow release
Roxanol SR	morphine	slow release
Sinemet CR	levodopa, carbidopa	slow release; tablet is scored and may be broken in half
Slo-Bid Gyrocaps	theophylline	slow release; capsules may be opened and contents taken without chewing or crushing
Slo-Phyllin Gyrocaps	theophylline	slow release; capsules may be opened and contents taken without chewing or crushing
Slow-Fe	ferrous sulfate	slow release
Slow-K	potassium chloride	slow release
Sorbitrate SA	isosorbide dinitrate	slow release
Sudafed 12 hour	pseudoephedrine	slow release
Tavist-D	phenylpropanolamine, clemastine	multiple compressed tablet
Teldrin	chlorpheniramine	slow release; capsules may be opened and contents taken without chewing or crushing
Tepanil Ten-Tab	diethylpropion	slow release
Tessalon Perles	benzonatate	slow release
Theo-24	theophylline	slow release
Theobid, Theobid Jr.	theophylline	slow release
Theo-Dur	theophylline	slow release
Theo-Dur Sprinkle	theophylline	slow release; capsules may be opened and contents taken without chewing or crushing
Theolair SR	theophylline	slow release
Thorazine Spansule	chlorpromazine	slow release
Toprol XL	metoprolol	slow release
Trental	pentoxifylline	slow release

	Generic Name	Comments
Triaminic	phenylpropanolamine, chlorpheniramine	enteric coated
Triaminic 12	phenylpropanolamine, chlorpheniramine	slow release
Triaminic TR	phenylpropanolamine, pyrilamine, pheniramine	multiple compressed tablet
Trilafon Repetabs	perphenazine	slow release
Triptone Caplets	scopolamine	slow release
Uniphyl	theophylline	slow release
Valrelease	diazepam	slow release
Verelan	verapamil	slow release; capsules may be opened and contents taken without chewing or crushing
Volmax	albuterol	slow release
Welbutrin SR	bupropion	slow release
Wyamycin S	erythromycin stearate	slow release
ZORprin	aspirin	slow release

acute dystonia extrapyramidal symptom manifested by abnormal posturing, grimacing, spastic torticollis (neck torsion), and oculogyric (eyeball movement) crisis.

adverse effect unintended, unpredictable, and nontherapeutic response to drug action. Adverse effects occur at doses used therapeutically or for prophylaxis or diagnosis. They generally result from drug toxicity, idiosyncrasies, or hypersensitivity reactions caused by the drug itself or by ingredients added during manufacture, e.g., preservatives, dyes, or vehicles.

afterload resistance that ventricles must work against to eject blood into the aorta during systole.

agranulocytosis sudden drop in leukocyte count; often followed by a severe infection manifested by high fever, chills, prostration, and ulcerations of mucous membrane such as in the mouth, rectum, or vagina.

akathisia extrapyramidal symptom manifested by a compelling need to move or pace, without specific pattern, and an inability to be still.

analeptic restorative medication that enhances excitation of the CNS without affecting inhibitory impulses.

anaphylactoid reaction excessive allergic response manifested by wheezing, chills, generalized pruritic urticaria, diaphoresis, sense of uneasiness, agitation, flushing, palpitations, coughing, difficulty breathing, and cardiovascular collapse.

anticholinergic actions inhibition of parasympathetic response manifested by dry mouth, decreased peristalsis, constipation, blurred vision, and urinary retention.

bioavailability fraction of active drug that reaches its action sites after administration by any route. Following an IV dose, bioavailability is 100%; however, such factors as first-pass effect, enterohepatic cycling, and biotransformation reduce bioavailability of an orally administered drug.

blood dyscrasia pathological condition manifested by fever, sore mouth or throat, unexplained fatigue, easy bruising or bleeding.

cardiotoxicity impairment of cardiac function manifested by one or more of the following: hypotension, arrhythmias, precordial pain, dyspnea, electrocardiogram (ECG) abnormalities, cardiac dilation, congestive failure.

cholinergic response stimulation of the parasympathetic response manifested by lacrimation, diaphoresis, salivation, abdominal cramps, diarrhea, nausea, and vomiting.

circulatory overload excessive vascular volume manifested by increased central venous pressure (CVP), elevated blood pressure, tachycardia, distended neck veins, peripheral edema, dyspnea, cough, and pulmonary rales.

CNS stimulation excitement of the CNS manifested by hyperactivity, excitement, nervousness, insomnia, and tachycardia.

CNS toxicity impairment of CNS function manifested by ataxia, tremor, incoordination, paresthesias, numbness, impairment of pain or touch sensation, drowsiness, confusion, headache, anxiety, tremors, and behavior changes.

congestive heart failure (CHF) impaired pumping ability of the heart manifested by paroxysmal nocturnal dyspnea, cough, fatigue or dyspnea on exertion, tachycardia, peripheral or pulmonary edema, and weight gain.

Cushing's syndrome fatty swellings in the interscapular area (buffalo hump) and in the facial area (moon face), distension of the abdomen, ecchymoses following even minor trauma, impotence, amenorrhea, high blood pressure, general weakness, loss of muscle mass, osteoporosis, and psychosis.

dehydration decreased intracellular or extracellular fluid manifested by elevated temperature, dry skin and mucous membranes, decrease tissue turgor, sunken eyes, furrowed tongue, low blood pressure, diminished or irregular pulse, muscle or abdominal cramps, thick secretions, hard feces and impaction, scant urinary output, urine specific gravity above 1.030, an elevated hemoglobin.

disulfiram-type reaction Antabuse-type reaction manifested by facial flushing, pounding headache, sweating, slurred speech, abdominal cramps, nausea, vomiting, tachycardia, fever, palpitations, drop in blood pressure, dyspnea, and sense of chest con-striction. Symptoms may last up to 24 hours.

enzyme induction stimulation of microsomal enzymes by a drug resulting in its accelerated metabolism and decreased activity. If reactive intermediates are formed, drug-mediated toxicity may be exacerbated.

first-pass effect reduced bioavailability of an orally administered drug due to metabolism in GI epithelial cells and liver or to biliary excretion. Effect may be avoided by use of sublingual tablets or rectal suppositories.

fixed drug eruption drug-induced circumscribed skin lesion that persists or recurs in the same site. Residual pigmentation may remain following drug withdrawal.

half-life ($t_{1/2}$) time required for concentration of a drug in the body to decrease by 50%. Half-life also represents the time necessary to reach steady state or to decline from steady state after a change (i.e., starting or stopping) in the dosing regimen. Half-life may be affected by a disease state and age of the drug user.

heat stroke a life-threatening condition manifested by absence of sweating; red, dry, hot skin; dilated pupils; dyspnea; full bounding pulse; temperature above 40C (105F); and mental confusion.

hepatic toxicity impairment of liver function manifested by jaundice, dark urine, pruritus, light-colored stools, eosinophilia, itchy skin or rash, and persistently high elevations of alanine amino-transferase (ALT) and aspartate aminotransferase (AST).

hyperammonemia elevated level of ammonia or ammonium in the blood manifested by lethargy, decreased appetite, vomiting, asterixis (flapping tremor), weak pulse, irritability, decreased responsiveness, and seizures.

hypercalcemia elevated serum calcium manifested by deep bone and flank pain, renal calculi, anorexia, nausea, vomiting, thirst, constipation, muscle hypotonicity, pathologic fracture, bradycardia, lethargy, and psychosis.

hyperglycemia elevated blood glucose manifested by flushed, dry skin, low blood pressure and elevated pulse, tachypnea, Kussmaul's respirations, polyuria, polydipsia; polyphagia, lethargy, and drowsiness.

hyperkalemia excessive potassium in blood, which may produce life-threatening cardiac arrhythmias, including bradycardia and heart block, unusual fatigue, weakness or heaviness of limbs, general muscle weakness, muscle cramps, paresthesias, flaccid paralysis of extremities, shortness of breath, nervousness, confusion, diarrhea, and GI distress.

hypermagnesemia excessive magnesium in blood, which may produce cathartic effect, profound thirst, flushing, sedation, confusion, depressed deep tendon reflexes (DTRs), muscle weakness, hypotension, and depressed respirations.

hypernatremia excessive sodium in blood, which may produce confusion, neuromuscular excitability, muscle weakness, seizures, thirst, dry and flushed skin, dry mucous membranes, pyrexia, agitation, and oliguria or anuria.

hypersensitivity reactions excessive and abnormal sensitivity to given agent manifested by urticaria, pruritus, wheezing, edema, redness, and anaphylaxis.

hyperthyroidism excessive secretion by the thyroid glands, which increases basal metabolic rate, resulting in warm, flushed, moist skin; tachycardia, exophthalmos; infrequent lid blinking; lid edema; weight loss despite increased appetite; frequent urination; menstrual irregularity; breathlessness; hypoventilation; congestive heart failure; excessive sweating.

hyperuricemia excessive uric acid in blood, resulting in pain in flank; stomach, or joints, and changes in intake and output ratio and pattern.

hypocalcemia abnormally low calcium level in blood, which may result in depression; psychosis; hyperreflexia; diarrhea; cardiac arrhythmias; hypotension; muscle spasms; paresthesias of feet, fingers, tongue; positive Chvostek's sign. Severe deficiency (tetany) may result in carpopedal spasms, spasms of face muscle, laryngospasm, and generalized convulsions.

hypoglycemia abnormally low glucose level in the blood, which may result in acute fatigue, restlessness, malaise, marked irritability and weakness, cold sweats, excessive hunger, headache, dizziness, confusion, slurred speech, loss of consciousness, and death.

hypokalemia abnormally low level of potassium in blood, which may result in malaise, fatigue, paresthesias, depressed reflexes, muscle weakness and cramps, rapid, irregular pulse, arrhythmias, hypotension, vomiting, paralytic ileus, mental confusion, depression, delayed thought process, abdominal distension, polyuria, shallow breathing, and shortness of breath.

hypomagnesemia abnormally low level of magnesium in blood, resulting in nausea, vomiting, cardiac arrhythmias, and neuromuscular symptoms (tetany, positive Chvostek's and Trousseau's signs, seizures, tremors, ataxia, vertigo, nystagmus, muscular fasciculations).

hypophosphatemia abnormally low level of phosphates in blood, resulting in muscle weakness, anorexia, malaise, absent deep tendon reflexes, bone pain, paresthesias, tremors, negative calcium balance, osteomalacia, osteoporosis.

hypothyroidism condition caused by thyroid hormone deficiency that lowers basal metabolic rate and may result in periorbital edema, lethargy, puffy hands and feet, cool, pale skin, vertigo, nocturnal cramps, decreased GI motility, constipation, hypotension, slow pulse, depressed muscular activity, and enlarged thyroid gland.

hypoxia insufficient oxygenation in the blood manifested by dyspnea, tachypnea, headache, restlessness, cyanosis, tachycardia, dysrhythmias, confusion, decreased level of consciousness, and euphoria or delirium.

international normalizing ratio measurement that normalizes for the differences obtained from various laboratory readings in the value for thromboplastin blood level.

leukopenia abnormal decrease in number of white blood cells, usually below 5000 per cubic millimeter, resulting in fever, chills, sore mouth or throat, and unexplained fatigue.

liver toxicity manifested by anorexia, nausea, fatigue, lethargy, itching, jaundice, abdominal pain, dark-colored urine, and flu-like symptoms.

metabolic acidosis decrease in pH value of the extracellular fluid caused by either an increase in hydrogen ions or a decrease in bicarbonate ions. It may result in one or more of the following: lethargy, headache, weakness, abdominal pain, nausea, vomiting, dyspnea, hyperpnea progressing to Kussmaul breathing, dehydration, thirst, weakness, flushed face, full bounding pulse, progressive drowsiness, mental confusion, combativeness.

metabolic alkalosis increase in pH value of the extracellular fluid caused by either a loss of acid from the body (e.g., through vomiting) or an increased level of bicarbonate ions (e.g., through ingestion of sodium bicarbonate). It may result in muscle weakness, irritability, confusion, muscle twitching, slow and shallow respirations, and convulsive seizures.

microsomal enzymes drug-metabolizing enzymes located in the endoplasmic reticulum of the liver and other tissues chiefly responsible for oxidative drug metabolism, e.g., cytochrome P450.

myopathy any disease or abnormal condition of striated muscles manifested by muscle weakness, myalgia, diaphoresis, fever, and reddish-brown urine (myoglobinuria) or oliguria.

nephrotoxicity impairment of the nephrons of the kidney manifested by one or more of the following: oliguria, urinary frequency, hematuria, cloudy urine, rising BUN and serum creatinine, fever, graft tenderness or enlargement.

neuroleptic malignant syndrome (NMS) potentially fatal complication associated with antipsychotic drugs manifested by hyperpyrexia, altered mental status, muscle rigidity, irregular pulse, fluctuating BP, diaphoresis, and tachycardia.

orphan drug (as defined by the Orphan Drug Act, an amendment of the Federal Food, Drug, and Cosmetic Act which took effect in January 1983): drug or biological product used in the treatment, diagnosis, or prevention of a rare disease. A rare disease or condition is one that affects fewer than 200,000 persons in the United States, or affects more than 200,000 persons but for which there is no reasonable expectation that drug research and development costs can be recovered from sales within the United States.

ototoxicity impairment of the ear manifested by one or more of the following: headache, dizziness or vertigo, nausea and vomiting with motion, ataxia, nystagmus.

prodrug inactive drug form that becomes pharmacologically active through biotransformation.

protein binding reversible interaction between protein and drug resulting in a drug-protein complex (bound drug) which is in equilibrium with free (active) drug in plasma and tissues. Since only free drug can diffuse to action sites, factors that influence drug-binding (e.g., displacement of bound drug by another drug, or decreased albumin concentration) may potentiate pharmacological effect.

pseudomembranous enterocolitis life-threatening superinfection characterized by severe diarrhea and fever.

pseudoparkinsonism extrapyramidal symptom manifested by slowing of volitional movement (akinesia), mask facies, rigidity and tremor at rest (especially of upper extremities); and pill rolling motion.

pulmonary edema excessive fluid in the lung tissue manifestied by one or more of the following: shortness of breath, cyanosis, persistent productive cough (frothy sputum may be blood tinged), expiratory rales, restlessness, anxiety, increased heart rate, sense of chest pressure.

renal insufficiency reduced capacity of the kidney to perform its functions as manifested by one or more of the following: dysuria, oliguria, hematuria, swelling of lower legs and feet.

serotonin syndrome manifested by restlessness, myoclonus, mental status changes, hyperreflexia, diaphoresis, shivering, and tremor.

Somogyi effect rebound phenomenon clinically manifested by fasting hyperglycemia and worsening of diabetic control due to unnecessarily large p.m. insulin doses. Hormonal response to unrecognized hypoglycemia (i.e., release of epinephrine, glucagon, growth hormone, cortisol) causes insensitivity to insulin. Increasing the amount of insulin required to treat the hyperglycemia intensifies the hypoglycemia.

superinfection new infection by an organism different from the initial infection being treated by antimicrobial therapy manifested by one or more of the following: black, hairy tongue; glossitis, stomatitis; anal itching; loose, foul-smelling stools; vaginal itching or discharge; sudden fever; cough.

tachyphylaxis rapid decrease in response to a drug after administration of a few doses. Initial drug response cannot be restored by an increase in dose.

tardive dyskinesia extrapyramidal symptom manifested by involuntary rhythmic, bizarre movements of face, jaw, mouth, tongue, and sometimes extremities.

vasovagal symptoms transient vascular and neurogenic reaction marked by pallor, nausea, vomiting, bradycardia, and rapid fall in arterial blood pressure.

water intoxication (dilutional hyponatremia) less than normal concentration of sodium in the blood resulting from excess extracellular and intracellular fluid and producing one or more of the following: lethargy, confusion, headache, decreased skin turgor, tremors, convulsions, coma, anorexia, nausea, vomiting, diarrhea, sternal fingerprinting, weight gain, edema, full bounding pulse, jugular vein distension, rales, signs and symptoms of pulmonary edema.

ABGs	arterial blood gases
a.c.	before meals (*ante cibum*)
ACD	acid–citrate–dextrose
ACE	angiotensin-converting enzyme
ACh	acetylcholine
ACIP	Advisory Committee on Immunization Practices
ACLS	advanced cardiac life support
ACS	acute coronary syndrome
ACT	activated clotting time
ACTH	adrenocorticotropic hormone
ADD	attention deficit disorder
ADH	antidiuretic hormone
ADLs	activities of daily living
ad lib	as desired (*ad libitum*)
ADP	adenosine diphosphate
ADT	alternate-day drug (administration)
AIDS	acquired immunodeficiency syndrome
ALT	alanine aminotransferase (formerly SGPT)
AML	acute myelogenous leukemia
AMP	adenosine monophosphate
ANA	antinuclear antibody(ies)
ANC	acid neutralizing capacity
aPTT	activated partial thromboplastin time
ARC	AIDS related complex
ARDS	adult respiratory distress syndrome
ASHD	arteriosclerotic heart disease
AST	aspartate aminotransferase (formerly SGOT)
AT_1	angiotensin II receptor subtype I
AT_2	angiotensin II receptor subtype II
ATP	adenosine triphosphate
AV	atrioventricular
b.i.d.	two times a day (*bis in die*)
BM	bowel movement
BMD	bone mineral density
BMR	basal metabolic rate
BP	blood pressure
bpm	beats per minute
BSA	body surface area
BSE	breast self-exam
BSP	bromsulphalein
BT	bleeding time
BUN	blood urea nitrogen
C	centigrade, Celsius
CAD	coronary artery disease
cAMP	cyclic adenosine monophosphate
CBC	complete blood count
cc	cubic centimeter
CDC	Centers for Disease Control
CF	cystic fibrosis
CHF	congestive heart failure

Cl_{cr}	creatinine clearance
cm	centimeter
CMV	cytomegalovirus-I
CMVIG	cytomegalovirus immune globulin
CNS	central nervous system
Coll	collyrium (eye wash)
COMT	catecholamine-*o*-methyl transferase
COPD	chronic obstructive pulmonary disease
COX-2	cyclooxygenase-2
CPK	creatinine phosphokinase
CPR	cardiopulmonary resuscitation
CRF	chronic renal failure
C&S	culture and sensitivity
CSF	cerebrospinal fluid
CSP	cellulose sodium phosphate
CT	clotting time
CTZ	chemoreceptor trigger zone
CV	cardiovascular
CVA	cerebrovascular accident
CVP	central venous pressure
d	day
D5W	5% dextrose in water
D&C	dilation and curettage
DIC	disseminated intravascular coagulation
DKA	diabetic keto-acidosis
dl	deciliter (100 ml or 0.1 liter)
DM	diabetes mellitus
DNA	deoxyribonucleic acid
DTRs	deep tendon reflexes
DVT	deep venous thrombosis
ECG , EKG	electrocardiogram
ECT	electroconvulsive therapy
EEG	electroencephalogram
EENT	eye, ear, nose, throat
e.g.	for example (*exempli gratia*)
ENT	ear, nose, throat
EPS	extrapyramidal symptoms (or syndrome)
ER	estrogen receptor
ESR	erythrocyte sedimentation rate
F	Fahrenheit
FBS	fasting blood sugar
FDA	Food and Drug Administration
FSH	follicle-stimulating hormone
FTI	free thyroxine index
5-FU	5-fluorouracil
FUO	fever of unknown origin
g	gram
G6PD	glucose-6-phosphate dehydrogenase
GABA	gamma-aminobutyric acid
G-CSF	granulocyte colony-stimulating factor
GFR	glomerular filtration rate
GH	growth hormone

GI	gastrointestinal
GPIIb/IIIa	glycoprotein IIb/IIIa
GU	genitourinary
h	hour
HbA_{1c}	glycosylated hemoglobin
HCG	human chorionic gonadotropin
Hct	hematocrit
HDL	high density lipoprotein
HDL-C	high-density-lipoprotein cholesterol
HER	human epidermal growth factor
Hgb	hemoglobin
5-HIAA	5-hydroxyindoleacetic acid
HIT	heparin-induced thrombocytopenia
HIV	human immunodeficiency virus
HMG-CoA	3-hydroxy-3-methyl-glutaryl coenzyme A
HPA	hypothalamic-pituitary-adrenocortical (axis)
HPV	human papillomavirus
HR	heart rate
h.s.	nightly or at bedtime (*hora somni*)
HSV-1	herpes simplex virus type 1
HSV-2	herpes simplex virus type 2
5-HT	5-hydroxytryptamine (serotonin receptor)
I&O	intake and output
IBW	ideal body weight
IC	intracoronary
ICP	intracranial pressure
ICU	intensive care unit
ID	intradermal
IDDM	insulin-dependent diabetes mellitus (Type I diabetes)
IFN	interferon
Ig	immunoglobulin
IL	interleukin
IM	intramuscular
INR	international normalizing ratio
IOP	intraocular pressure
IPPB	intermittent positive pressure breathing
IU	international unit
IV	intravenous
kg	kilogram
17-KGS	17-ketogenic steroids
17-KS	17-ketosteroids
KVO	keep vein open
L	liter
LDH	lactic dehydrogenase
LDL	low density lipoprotein
LDL-C	low-density-lipoprotein cholesterol
LE	lupus erythematosus
LFT	liver function test
LH	luteinizing hormone
LSD	lysergic acid diethylamide
LTRA	leukotriene receptor antagonist

M	molar (strength of a solution)
m^2	square meter (of body surface area)
MAO	monoamine oxidase
MAOI	monoamine oxidase inhibitor
MBD	minimal brain dysfunction
MCH	mean corpuscular hemoglobin
MCHC	mean corpuscular hemoglobin concentration
mCi	millicurie
μg, mcg	microgram (1/1000 of a milligram)
μm	micrometer
MDI	metered dose inhaler
MDR	minimum daily requirements
mEq	milliequivalent
mg	milligram
min	minute
MI	myocardial infarction
MIC	minimum inhibitory concentration
ml	milliliter (0.001 liter)
mm	millimeter
mo	month
MRSA	methicillin-resistant *Staphylococcus aureus*
MS	multiple sclerosis
N	normal (strength of a solution)
NADH	reduced form of nicotine adenine dinucleotide
NAPA	*N*-acetyl procainamide
nb	note well (*nota bene*)
ng	nanogram (1/1000 of a microgram)
NIDDM	non-insulin-dependent diabetes mellitus (Type II diabetes)
NMS	neuroleptic malignant syndrome
NNRTI	nonnucleoside reverse transcriptase inhibitor
NPN	nonprotein nitrogen
NPO	nothing by mouth
NS	normal saline
NSAID	nonsteroidal antiinflammatory drug
NSR	normal sinus rhythm
OC	oral contraceptive
17-OHCS	17-hydroxycorticosteroids
OTC	over the counter (nonprescription)
PABA	*para*-aminobenzoic acid
PAS	*para*-aminosalicylic acid
PAWP	pulmonary artery wedge pressure
PBI	protein-bound iodine
PBP	penicillin-binding protein
p.c.	after meals (*post cibum*)
PCI	percutaneous coronary intervention
PERLA	pupils equal, react to light and accommodation
PG	prostaglandin
pH	hydrogen ion concentration
PID	pelvic inflammatory disease
PKU	phenylketonuria
PND	paroxysmal nocturnal dyspnea

PO	by mouth or orally (*per os*)
PPM	parts per million
PR	rectally (*per rectum*)
prn	when required (*pro re nata*)
PSA	prostate-specific antigen
PSP	phenolsulfonphthalein
PSVT	paroxysmal supraventricular tachycardia
PT	prothrombin time
PTH	parathyroid hormone
PTT	partial thromboplastin time
PUD	peptic ulcer disease
PVC	premature ventricular contraction
PVD	peripheral vascular disease
PZI	protamine zinc insulin
q	every
q.d.	every day
q.i.d.	four times daily
q.o.d.	every other day
RA	rheumatoid arthritis
RAI	radioactive iodine
RAST	radioallergosorbent test
RBC	red blood (cell) count
RDA	recommended (daily) dietary allowance
RDS	respiratory distress syndrome
REM	rapid eye movement
rem	radiation equivalent man
RIA	radioimmunoassay
RNA	ribonucleic acid
ROM	range of motion
RSV	respiratory syncytial virus
RT_3U	total serum thyroxine concentration
s	second
S&S	signs and symptoms
SA	sinoatrial
SBE	subacute bacterial endocarditis
SC	subcutaneous
Scr	serum creatinine
SGGT	serum gamma-glutamyl transferase
SGOT	serum glutamic-oxaloacetic transaminase (*see* AST)
SGPT	serum glutamic-pyruvic transaminase (*see* ALT)
SIADH	syndrome of inappropriate antidiuretic hormone
SI Units	International System of Units
SK	streptokinase
SL	sublingual
SLE	systemic lupus erythematosus
SMA	sequential multiple analysis
SOS	if necessary (*si opus cit*)
sp	species
SPF	sun protection factor
sq	square

SR	sedimentation rate
SRS-A	slow-reactive substance of anaphylaxis
SSRI	selective serotonin reuptake inhibitor
stat	immediately
STD	sexually transmitted disease
$t_{1/2}$	half-life
T_3	triiodothyronine
T_4	thyroxine
TCA	tricyclic antidepressant
TG	total triglycerides
TIA	transient ischemic attack
t.i.d.	three times a day (*ter in die*)
TNF	tumor necrosis factor
tPA	tissue plasminogen activator
TPN	total parenteral nutrition
TPR	temperature, pulse, respirations
TSH	thyroid-stimulating hormone
TT	thrombin time
URI	upper respiratory infection
USP	United States Pharmacopeia
USPHS	United States Public Health Service
UTI	urinary tract infection
UV-A, UVA	ultraviolet A wave
VDRL	venereal disease research laboratory
VLDL	very low density lipoprotein
VMA	vanillylmandelic acid
VS	vital signs
wk	week
WBC	white blood (cell) count
WBCT	whole blood clotting time
y	year

Bibliography

American Hospital Formulary Service (AHFS) Drug Information 04. Bethesda, MD: American Society of Health-System Pharmacists. 2004.

American Nurses Association. *Scope and standards of psychiatric–mental health nursing*. Washington, DC: Author. 2000.

American Nurses Association Task Force on Psychopharmacology. *Psychiatric–mental health nursing psychopharmacology project*. Washington, DC: American Nurses Association. 1994.

Bagnall A, Jones L, Ginnelly L, Lewis R, Glanville J, Gilbody S, Davies L, Torgerson D, Kleijnen J. A systematic review of atypical antipsychotic drugs in schizophrenia. *Health Technology Assessment*. 2003; 7(13):1–193.

Bain KT, Weschules DJ, Knowlton CH, Gallagher R. Pharmaceutical update. Toward evidence-based prescribing at end of life: a comparative review of temazepam and zolpidem for the treatment of insomnia. *American Journal of Hospice & Palliative Care*. 2003; 20(5):382–388, 400.

Bernstein JG. *Handbook of drug therapy in psychiatry*. (1995). 3rd ed. St. Louis, MO: Mosby.

Boyd M. Atypical antipsychotics: Impact on overall health and quality of life. *Journal of the American Psychiatric Nurses Association*. 2002; 8(4), Suppl:S9-17.

Caroff SN, Mann SC, Keck PE, Francis A. Residual catatonic state following neuroleptic malignant syndrome. *Journal of Clinical Psychopharmacology*. 2000; 20:257–259.

Carrese JA, Rhodes LA. Bridging cultural differences in medical practice: The case of discussing negative information with Navajo patients. *Journal of General Internal Medicine*. 2000; 15:92–96.

Denvir MA, Sood A, Dow R, Brady AJ, Rankin AC. Thioridazine, diarrhea, and torsades de pointe. *Journal of Social Medicine*. 1998; 91:145–147.

Dimsdale, JE. Stalked by the past: The influence of ethnicity on health. *Psychosomatic Medicine*. 2000; 62:161–170.

Drug Facts and Comparisons. St. Louis: Facts and Comparisons. 2004.

Erkinjuntti T, Skoog I, Lane R, Andrews C. Potential long-term effects of rivastigmine on disease progression may be linked to drug effects on vascular changes in Alzheimer brains. *International Journal of Clinical Practice.* 2003; 57(9):756–760.

Expert Consensus Guideline Series. Updated guidelines for pharmacologic treatment of bipolar disorder. *Postgraduate Medicine.* 2000.

Flores G. Culture and patient-physician relationship: Achieving cultural competency in health care. *The Journal of Pediatrics.* 2000; 136:14–23.

Gaskin CJ, O'Brien AP, Hardy DJ. The development of a professional practice audit questionnaire for mental health nursing in Aotearoa/New Zealand. *International Journal of Mental Health Nursing.* 2003; 12(4):259–270.

Gelman CR, Rumack BH. Eds. *DrugDex Information System.* Denver: Micromedex 2003.

Gerrish K. Individualized care: Its conceptualization and practice within a multiethnic society. *Journal of Advanced Nursing.* 2000; 32:91–99.

Gold Standard Media http://www.gms.com *Clinical Pharmacology 2004*

Gurrera RJ. Sympathoadrenal hyperactivity and the etiology of neuroleptic malignant syndrome. *The American Journal of Psychiatry.* 2000; 156:169–180.

Jeste DV, Okamoto A, Napolitano J, Kane JM, Martinez RA. Low incidence of persistent tardive dyskinesia in elderly patients with dementia treated with risperidone. *The American Journal of Psychiatry.* 2000; 157:1150–1155.

Kilian JG, Lawrence C. Myocarditis and cardiomyopathy associated with clozapine. *Lancet.* 1999; 354:1841–1845.

Koth C. Drug interactions with grapefruit juice. *Clinical Pharmacology and Therapeutics.* 2000; 1:1–2.

Kralik D, Koch T. "It's just the way I am": Life with schizophrenia. *Australian Journal of Holistic Nursing.* 2003; 10(2):11–18.

Lambert CE, Lambert VA, Davidson PM, Anders R, O'Brien L, Yunibhand J, Wong TKS, Lee S, Kim S, Kawano M. Nurse faculty perceptions regarding psychiatric-mental health nursing behavioral interventions: a cross-cultural comparison. *Contemporary Nurse.* 2003; 15(3):333–346.

Laraia MT, et al. *Psychiatric Mental Health Nursing Psychopharmacology Project.* Washington, DC: American Nurses Association. 1994.

Leighton K. A social conflict analysis of collective mental health care: Past, present, and future. *Journal of Mental Health.* 2003; 12(5):475–488.

Lin KM, Smith MW, Ortiz V. Culture and psychopharmacology. *Psychiatric Clinics of North America*. 2001; 24(3):523–538.

List T, Axelsson S, Leijon G. Pharmacologic interventions in the treatment of temporomandibular disorders, atypical facial pain, and burning mouth syndrome. A qualitative systematic review. *Journal of Orofacial Pain*. 2003; 17(4):301–310.

Littrell KH, Petty RG, Hilligoss NM, Peabody CD, Johnson CG. Weight loss associated with olanzapine treatment. *Journal of Clinical Psychopharmacology*. 2002; 22:436–437.

Lopez SR, Guarnaccia P. Cultural psychopathology: Uncovering the social world of mental illness. *Annual Review of Psychology*. 2000; 51:571–598.

McCabe S. Advances in the pharmacological treatment of bipolar affective disorders. *Perspectives in Psychiatric Care*. 2003; 39(3):95–103.

McGrath JJ, Soares-Weiser KVS. Neuroleptic reduction and/or cessation and neuroleptics as specific treatments for tardive dyskinesia. *The Cochrane Library (Oxford)*. 2004; 1 (ID #CD000459).

Morita S, Shimoda K, Someya T, Yoshimura Y, Kamijima K, Kato N. Steady-state plasma levels of nortriptyline and its hydroxylated metabolites in Japanese patients: Impact of CYP2D6 genotype on the hydroxylation of nortriptyline. *Journal of Clinical Psychopharmacology*. 2000; 20:141–149.

Opolka JL, Rascati KL, Brown CM, Barner JC, Johnsrud MT, Gibson PJ. Ethnic differences in use of antipsychotic medication among Texas medicaid clients with schizophrenia. *Journal of Clinical Psychiatry*. 2003; 64(6):635–639.

Perese EF, Perese K. Health problems of women with severe mental illness. *Journal of the American Academy of Nurse Practitioners*. 2003; 15(5):212–219.

Physicians' Desk Reference. 58th ed. Oradell, NJ: Medical Economics Co. 2004.

Quitkin FM, Rabkin JG, Gerald J, Davis JM, Klein DF. Validity of clinical trials of antidepressants. *American Journal of Psychiatry*. 2000; 157:327–337.

Qureshi NA, Al-Habeeb TA. Sympathoadrenal hyperactivity and neuroleptic malignant syndrome. *American Journal of Psychiatry*. 2000; 157:310–311.

Rosner F. *Julius Preuss's Biblical and Talmudic Medicine*. 1978; New York: Sanhedrin Press.

Rummel C, Hamann J, Kissling W, Leucht S. New generation antipsychotics for first episode schizophrenia. *The Cochrane Library, (Oxford)* 2004: 1 (ID #CD004410).

Schaafsma ES, Raynor TD, de Jong-van den Berg LT. Accessing medication information by ethnic minorities: barriers and possible solutions. *Pharmacy World & Science.* 2003; 25(5):185–190.

Schreiber R, Stern PN, Wilson C. Being strong: How black West-Indian Canadian women manage depression and its stigma. *Journal of Nursing Scholarship First Quarter.* 2000; 39–45.

Semla TP, Beizer JL, Higbee MD. *Geriatric Dosage Handbook.* 4th ed. Hudson, OH: Lexi-Comp. 1998.

Skaer TL. Insomnia pharmacotherapy: Selecting a hypnotic agent. *Pharmacy & Therapeutics.* 2000; 25:93–102.

Silva RR, Munoz DM, Alpert M, Perlmutter IR, Diaz J. Neuroleptic malignant syndrome in children and adolescents. *Journal of the American Academy of Child and Adolescent Psychiatry.* 2000; 38:184–194.

Sirota P, Mosheva T, Shabtay H, Giladi N, Korczyn A. Use of the selective serotonin 3 receptor antagonist ondansetron in the treatment of neuroleptic-induced tardive dyskinesia. *American Journal of Psychiatry.* 2000; 157:287–289.

Smock TK, *Physiological psychology: A neuroscience approach.* 1999; Upper Saddle River, NJ: Prentice Hall.

Taketomo CK, Hodding JH, Kraus DM. *Pediatric Dosage Handbook.* 5th ed. Hudson, OH: Lexi-Comp. 1998.

Terrill KR, Wheeler M, Rollins DE, Beckwith MC. Drug interactions reported with grapefruit juice. *Journal of Pharmaceutical Care in Pain & Symptom Control* 2000; 8:39–48.

Tramontina S, Schmitz M, Polanczyk G, Rohde LA. Juvenile bipolar disorder in Brazil: clinical and treatment findings. *Biological Psychiatry.* 2003; 53(11):1043–1049.

Trigoboff, E. Psychopharmacology. In Kneisl C, Wilson H, Trigoboff E Eds. *Contemporary Psychiatric-Mental Health Nursing.* 1st ed. Upper Saddle River, NJ: Prentice Hall. 2004.

Trissel LA. *Handbook of Injectable Drugs.* 12th ed. Bethesda, MD: American Society of Health-System Pharmacists. 2003.

Trissel, LA, Gilbert, DK, Williams, KY. Compatibility of screening of gatifloxacin during simulated Y-site administration with other drugs. *Hospital Pharmacy* 1999; 34(12):1409–1416.

Trissel LA, Zhang Y, Xu QA. Incompatibility of erythromycin lactiobionate and sulfamethoxazole/trimethoprim with linezolid injection. *Hospital Pharmacy.* 2000; 35:1192–1196.

USP DI: Advice to Patients. Rockville, MD: US Pharmacopeial Convention. 2004.

USP DI: Drug Information for the Health Care Professional. Rockville, MD: US Pharmacopeial Convention. 2004.

Wahlbeck K, Cheine M, Essali MA. Clozapine versus typical neuroleptic medication for schizophrenia. *The Cochrane Library, (Oxford)* 2004; 1 (ID #CD000059).

Wilson BA, Shannon MT, Stang CL. *Nurse's Drug Guide 2005*. Upper Saddle River, NJ: Pearson Education. 2005.

Xu QA, Trissel LA, Williams KY. Compatibility and stability of linezolid injection admixed with three cephalosporin antibiotics. *Journal of the American Pharmaceutical Association*. 2000; 40(40):509–514.

INDEX

Drug categories are in SMALL CAPS.
Generic drug names are given in parentheses.

Drug categories are in SMALL CAPS.
Generic drug names are given in parentheses.

Drug categories are in SMALL CAPS.
Generic drug names are given in parentheses.

	PHYLLINE	MINE	DOPAMINE	HEPARIN	MEPERIDINE	MORPHINE	GLYCERIN	SETRON	IN D5W OR NS
acyclovir		I	I	C	C	I/C		I	C
alteplase		I	I	I		I	I		
amikacin	C			I	C	C		C	
amino acids (TPN)	C	C	C	C	C	C			
aminophylline	C	I	I	C	I	C	C	I	C
amiodarone	I	C	C	I		C	C		C
ampicillin	C			C	C	C		I	C
ampicillin/sulbactam				C	C	C		I	
amrinone	C	C	C				C		C
aztreonam				C	C	C		C	
bretylium	C	C	C				C		C
bumetanide		I		C	C	C			
calcium chloride	I	C	C			C			
cefamandole					C	C			C
cefazolin	C			C	C	C		C	C
cefoperazone	C	I			I	C		I	
cefotaxime					C	C		C	
cefotetan	C		C	C	C	C			
cefoxitin					C	C		C	
ceftazidime	C			C	C	C		C	C
ceftizoxime					C	C		C	
ceftriaxone	C			C	C	C			
cefuroxime	C			C	C	C		C	C
cephalothin	I		C	C	C	C			
chloramphenicol			C	C	C	C			C
cimetidine	C	C		C	C	C		C	C
ciprofloxacin	I	C	C	I					C
clindamycin	I			C	C	C		C	
dexamethasone	C			C	C	C		C	C

	AMINO-PHYLLINE	DOBUTA-MINE	DOPAMINE	HEPARIN	MEPERIDINE	MORPHINE	NITRO-GLYCERIN	ONDAN-SETRON	POTASSIUM IN D5W OR NS
diazepam		I/C		I	I				I/C
digoxin	C			C	C	C			C
diltiazem	I	C	C	C	C	C	C		C
diphenydramine	C			I	C	C		C	C
dobutamine	I	C	C	I/C	C	C	C		C
dopamine	I	C	C	C	C	C	C		C
doxycycline			I	I	C	C		C	
enalapril/enalaprilat	C	C	C	C		C			C
epinephrine	I			C					C
eptifibatide									
erythromycin	I			I	C	C			
esmolol	C	C	C	C		C	C		C
famotidine	C	C	C	C	C	C	C	C	C
filgrastim	C			I	C	C		C	C
fluconazole	C	C	C	C	C	C	C	C	
foscarnet	C	I	C	C		C			
fosphenytoin									
furosemide	C	I/C		C	I/C	I	C	I	C
ganciclovir								I	
gentamicin	C		C	I	C	C		C	
heparin	C	I/C	C	C	C	C	I	C	C
hydrocortisone	C		C	C	C	C		C	C
hydromorphone								C	
imipenem/cilastatin				C	I			C	
insulin		C		C	C	C			C
isoproterenol				C					C
labetolol	C	C	C	C	C	C	C		C
lidocaine	C	C	C	C	C	C	C		C

metoclopramide	C			C	C	C		C	C
metoprolol					C	C			
metronidazole	C				C	C			
mezlocillin					I	C		I	
midazolam		I	C		C	C			
milrinone						C			
morphine	I/C	C	C	C				C	C
moxalactam					C	C			
nafcillin		I		C	I	C			C
nitroglycerin	C	C	C	I			C		
nitroprusside		C	C	C			C		
norepinephrine	I	C		C					C
ondansetron	I			C	C	C			C
penicillin G			C	C	C	C			C
phenylephrine		C							
phenytoin		I		I	I	I	I		I
piperacillin	C			C	C	C		I	C
piperacillin/tazobactam	C	I	C	C	C	C		C	C
potassium Cl in D5W or NS	C	C	C		C	C		C	C
procainamide		C		C					C
propofol						C			
ranitidine	C	C	C	C	C	C	C	C	C
sargramostim	C		C	C	C	I		I	C
sodium bicarbonate	C	I	I	C		C		I	C
ticarcillin				C	C	C		C	
tobramycin				I	C	C			
trimethoprim/sulfa-methoxazole					C	C			
vancomycin	I			I	C	C		C	

C = compatible; I = incompatible; I/C = conflicting data